Modern Trends in Pharmacopsychiatry

Vol. 29

Series Editor

B.E. Leonard Galway

Anxiety Disorders

Volume Editors

D.S. Baldwin Southampton/Cape Town
B.E. Leonard Galway

8 figures, 2 in color, and 5 tables, 2013

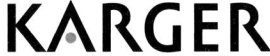

Basel · Freiburg · Paris · London · New York · New Delhi · Bangkok ·
Beijing · Tokyo · Kuala Lumpur · Singapore · Sydney

Modern Trends in Pharmacopsychiatry

(Formerly published as 'Modern Problems in Pharmacopsychiatry')

Prof. David S. Baldwin
University of Southampton
Faculty of Medicine
University Department of Psychiatry
Southampton (UK)

Prof. Brian E. Leonard
Department of Pharmacology
National University of Ireland
Galway (Ireland)

Library of Congress Cataloging-in-Publication Data

Anxiety disorders (Baldwin)
  Anxiety disorders / volume editors, D.S. Baldwin, B.E. Leonard.
     p. ; cm. -- (Modern trends in pharmacopsychiatry, ISSN 1662-2685 ;
vol. 29)
  Includes bibliographical references and index.
  ISBN 978-3-318-02463-0 (hard cover : alk. paper) -- ISBN 978-3-318-02464-7
(electronic version)
  I. Baldwin, David S., editor of compilation. II. Leonard, B. E., editor of
compilation. III. Title. IV. Series: Modern trends in pharmacopsychiatry ;
v. 29. 1662-2685
  [DNLM: 1. Anxiety Disorders--therapy. W1 MO168P v.29 2013 / WM 172]
  RC531
  616.85'22--dc23
                                                        2013029183

Bibliographic Indices. This publication is listed in bibliographic services, including Current Contents® and Index Medicus.

© Copyright 2013 by S. Karger AG, P.O. Box, CH–4009 Basel (Switzerland)
www.karger.com
Printed in Germany on acid-free and non-aging paper (ISO 9706) by Kraft Druck, Ettlingen
ISSN 1662–2685
e-ISSN 1662–4505
ISBN 978–3–318–02463–0
e-ISBN 978–3–318–02464–7

Contents

Preface

Concerted Efforts to Improve the Understanding and Treatment of Anxiety Disorders

Anxiety disorders are common, usually have an early onset, often take a prolonged course, cause much personal distress, impair everyday function, lower quality of life, and carry a considerable economic burden. They are often 'co-morbid' with other forms of mental disorder – including major depression, bipolar disorder, schizophrenia, substance misuse – and with physical illness, and many anxiety disorders are associated with an increased risk of self-harm. It is hard not to regard anxiety disorders as a significant public health problem which requires the attention of health professionals and health policy makers [1].

Knowledge of the underlying causes of anxiety disorders is incomplete, and this hinders reliable diagnosis and accurate prediction of prognosis, and the refinement of treatment approaches. Many individuals with recognisable anxiety disorders do not present to health professionals, or do present but are not diagnosed correctly. Even when recognised as having an anxiety disorder, the standard of care received by many patients is less than ideal. Unfortunately, the effectiveness and acceptability of current pharmacological and psychological treatments in real-world clinical practice is often disappointing. It is reasonable to contend that one way to address the current unmet public health, clinical and research needs in anxiety disorders is through the development of independent collaborative networks [2].

There are many world-leading centres of research excellence within Europe, some with clinical and research databases that are sufficiently large and detailed to have already led to step-changing insights into anxiety disorders. But methodologies vary across centres, and this reduces the ability to confirm or refute new findings. There seems much scope for developing multi-centre collaborative patient databases and for harmonising research methodologies, to bring new insights and other perspectives on current debates about the diagnosis and treatment of mental disorders. The European College of Neuropsychopharmacology (ECNP) has been concerned to support the development of such independent collaborative international research networks of basic scientists and practising clinicians, has established the ECNP Network Initiative (ECNP-NI) to help meet this goal, and has adopted and supported the Anxiety Disorders Research Network (ADRN) [1].

There is a parallel need for similar networks in low- and middle-income countries. South Africa offers many opportunities to gain additional insights into the mechanisms that underlie and maintain anxiety disorders. These include access to a range of clinical groups that allow important questions about anxiety to be explored in more detail: such as the influence of HIV/AIDS, the effect of traumatic experiences and societal deprivation, and role of common South African substances of abuse in precipitating and maintaining anxiety symptoms. Through its Marie Curie Actions International Research Staff Exchange Scheme funding stream, the European Union is supporting the Joint European South African Research Network in Anxiety Disorders (EUSARNAD) programme to strengthen existing links and foster new collaborative research configurations, and to enhance the relevance of translational research activity jointly conducted within Europe and South Africa to other developed and developing societies [3].

Contributors to this book are drawn from participating centres within the ADRN: many chapters include authors from a range of centres, including the University of Cape Town in South Africa, reflecting the collaborative and international nature of the ADRN. The early chapters provide updates on the nature and origin of anxiety and related symptoms and insights from genetic and neuroimaging research, and from investigations of cardiovascular and immunological factors; subsequent chapters consider the early phases of anxiety disorders, and the effects of prolonged illness before undergoing treatment; the later chapters provide succinct but comprehensive accounts of the evidence-based pharmacological treatment of generalised anxiety disorder, panic disorder, social anxiety disorder, post-traumatic stress disorder and obsessive-compulsive disorder.

The development of new treatments for patients with mental disorders is often described as being 'in crisis'. An ECNP Summit on the future of neuropsychopharmacological research in Europe recommended that research efforts and productivity could be enhanced by setting up and supporting specialist centres of excellence in clinical neuroscience, experimental medicine research, and brain imaging, in which early-phase trials could be conducted, with the accumulation of experience and training of new researchers [4]. We believe that research networks such as the ADRN can play a role in meeting these recommendations, whilst providing a framework for the training of the next generation of pre-clinical and clinical researchers.

Jules Angst, Zurich
David S. Baldwin, Southampton/Cape Town

Acknowledgements

The Anxiety Disorders Research Network is part of the European College of Neuropsychopharmacology Network Initiative (ECNP-NI) and receives financial support from the ECNP to support its development. Current (July 2013) centres within the ADRN are located in Amsterdam, Athens, Bristol, Florence, Göttingen, Gothenburg, Groningen, Leiden, London, Milan, Münster, Paris, Pisa, Santander, Southampton, Stockholm, Tartu, Tel Aviv, Uppsala, Welwyn Garden City, Würzburg, and Zurich. Administrative support to the ADRN is provided by Miss Magda Nowak, through a grant from the ECNP-NI; she provided invaluable assistance to the Editors in the development of this book.

References

1 Baldwin DS, Allgulander C, Altamura AC, Angst J, Bandelow B, den Boer J, Boyer P, Davies S, Dell'Osso B, Eriksson E, Fineberg N, Fredrikson M, Herran A, Maron E, Metspalu A, Nutt D, van der Wee N, Vázquez-Barquero JL, Zohar J: Manifesto for a European anxiety disorders research network. Eur Neuropsychopharmacol 2010;20:426–432.

2 Baldwin DS, Pallanti S, Zwanzger P: Developing a European research network to address unmet needs in anxiety disorders. Neurosci Biobehav Rev DOI: 10.1016/j.neubiorev.2013.01.009.

3 Baldwin DS, Stein DJ: A joint European and South African research network in anxiety disorders (editorial). Hum Psychopharmacol 2012;27:4–5.

4 Nutt D, Goodwin G: ECNP Summit on the future of CNS drug research in Europe 2011: report prepared for ECNP by David Nutt and Guy Goodwin. Eur Neuropsychopharmacol 2011;21:495–499.

Baldwin DS, Leonard BE (eds): Anxiety Disorders.
Mod Trends Pharmacopsychiatry. Basel, Karger, 2013, vol 29, pp 1–15 (DOI: 10.1159/000351929)

On the Nature of Obsessions and Compulsions

Sanneke de Haan[a] · Erik Rietveld[a, b] · Damiaan Denys[a, c]

[a]Department of Psychiatry, Academic Medical Center, and [b]Department of Philosophy,
University of Amsterdam, [c]The Netherlands Institute for Neuroscience,
The Royal Netherlands Academy of Arts and Sciences, Amsterdam, The Netherlands

Abstract

In this chapter, we give an overview of current and historical conceptions of the nature of obsessions and compulsions. We discuss some open questions pertaining to the primacy of the affective, volitional or affective nature of obsessive-compulsive disorder. Furthermore, we add some phenomenological suggestions of our own. In particular, we point to the patients' need for absolute certainty and the lack of trust underlying this need. Building on insights from Wittgenstein, we argue that the kind of certainty the patients strive for is unattainable in principle via the acquisition of factual knowledge. Moreover, we suggest that the patients' attempts to attain certainty are counterproductive as their excessive conscious control in fact undermines the trust they need.

Obsessions and compulsions are easily comprehensible and utterly elusive. They are comprehensible because we are all familiar with their mild variants. When we go on vacation, we double check whether we locked the door – just to be sure. Of course we know it is nonsense, but still, we knock on wood when we talk about our hopes. After all, it will not do any harm either. We may have superstitious rituals, lucky numbers, unlucky numbers and the like, and even be a little upset when we cannot indulge these preferences. In this sense, we can understand the urge to do something that we recognize as not being entirely reasonable. Likewise, we may also be familiar with annoying thoughts or images that keep on popping up. In fact, it is our everyday experience that thoughts and images pop up rather than that we deliberately develop them. This lack of control is usually no problem – until it is our explicit intention *not* to think of some-

thing. Wegner et al. [1] described the now classical experiment in which they instructed participants NOT to think of a white bear. Paradoxically, this and other experiments [2] show that the attempts to suppress a specific thought or image in fact lead
to its more persistent reappearance. So, the uncontrollability of our thoughts and
imagination and the concomitant adverse effects, which appear if one does try to keep
them under control, is not alien to us either.

However, when obsessions and compulsions get out of hand, when people devote
their whole day endlessly moving chairs so that they form a perfectly straight line
with the table, or cement them to avoid changes, this seems to be something completely different. Patients with obsessive-compulsive disorder (OCD) may wash
their hands until they bleed, may not leave their houses for fear of contamination,
or may check on the oven or windows for hours on end. It is not that they *want* to
do these things: they regard their compulsive behavior as pointless – or at least as
completely disproportional. They feel compelled to do so since *not* doing these
things brings forth an extreme experience of tension and anxiety. They agree that it
is nonsense and that their compulsive activities are not helping them, and this actually makes their condition all the more elusive. For instance, when we compare their
behavior to that of schizophrenic patients, the latter may act in strange ways, but at
least that is in line with their delusions: their behavior is coherent with their thoughts.
People suffering from OCD are rather 'split' in that they do things they do not want
to do. Understandably, this increases their suffering, their feeling of being unfree,
and the shame for their behavior, in particular since they are otherwise completely
healthy.

In this chapter, we will explore the nature of obsessions and compulsions. We start
by looking at the criteria for OCD as laid down in the fourth edition of the Diagnostic
and Statistical Manual of Mental Disorders (DSM-IV). We will then give a historical
overview over the general development of thinking about what we now call OCD. In
the last sections, we will point to some open questions, and add some of our own in-
terpretations.

DSM Criteria

According to the DSM-IV, *obsessions* are recurrent and persistent thoughts, impulses,
or images that are experienced as intrusive and inappropriate and that cause marked
anxiety or distress [3]. Moreover, the person attempts to ignore or suppress such
thoughts, impulses, or images, or tries to neutralize them with some other thought or
action. Also, the person recognizes that the obsessional thoughts, impulses, or images
are a product of his or her own mind (thus not imposed from without as in schizophrenic thought insertion) [3].

In an attempt to cope with the anxiety and distress that are caused by the obsessions, people start to develop repetitive acts or specific rituals. *Compulsions* are de-

fined as repetitive behaviors or mental acts (e.g. praying, counting, repeating words silently) that the person feels driven to perform. These mental acts and behaviors are aimed at preventing or reducing distress or at preventing some dreaded event or situation, but they are either not connected in a realistic way with what they are designed to prevent or they are clearly excessive [3].

Moreover, the diagnosis of OCD requires that, at some point during the course of the disorder, the person has recognized that the obsessions or compulsions are excessive or unreasonable.[1] The obsessions and compulsions must also induce some impairment: they cause marked distress, are time consuming (take more than 1 h a day), or significantly interfere with the person's normal routine, occupational functioning, or social activities or relationships [3].

The insight into the unreasonableness of their behavior is an important characteristic to set OCD apart from both delusions and obsessive-compulsive personality disorder (OCPD). The outward behavior may be very similar, and accordingly it may require careful phenomenological analysis of the person's experiences to arrive at an adequate diagnosis [4]. Bürgy [5] describes an exemplary case in which OCD and paranoid delusion could easily be confused. The patient concerned suffers from repetitive hand washing and endless dressing rituals: two common forms of compulsions for OCD patients. The patient moreover explains that he acts this way because 'he is not sure whether he had done it properly' [5, p. 294] – again a worry that many OCD patients also voice. However, further exploration revealed that this patient actually had the suspicion that it was someone else who was performing these actions. What had led him to these endless repetitions was the uncertainty whether they 'were still his own hands and movements' [5, p. 295].

The distinction between OCD and OCPD may be complicated as well. In OCD, patients experience their compulsions as not belonging to them, that is, as 'ego-dystonic'. In OCPD patients, there is no such split or estrangement: their compulsive behavior is rather part of how they see themselves, or 'ego-syntonic'. Typically, OCPD patients do not see their own behavior as problematic: being perfectionistic themselves, they rather have problems with the lack of orderliness of their loved ones. For most patients, it will be clear whether or not their compulsions seem alien to them. But there are also patients who have a more ambiguous relation to their need to clean, order, or control things. They would for instance admit that their behavior is excessive, but at the same time stress that it is also important to be tidy and meticulous. Accordingly, in these patients, the distinction between OCD and OCPD will be harder to make.

As Denys [6] points out, we can distinguish three main conceptualizations of OCD depending on which faculty is taken as central: affective (anxiety), volitional (compulsive), or cognitive (obsessional). Traditionally, OCD is classified as an anxiety disor-

[1] This does not apply to children.

der. This is reasonable, given the driving force of tension and anxiety that most patients experience. However, not all patients report anxious feelings [7, 8]. Some argue that OCD is more akin to disorders of impulse control such as addictions – which puts the volitional component at center stage [9]. Others point to the cognitive disturbances of OCD patients, in particular their lack of cognitive flexibility [10].

The classification of OCD was discussed in the run-up to the publication of the DSM-5. On the official website of the American Psychiatric Association, one can find the proposed revisions [11]. It is proposed that OCD is no longer subsumed under Anxiety disorders, but that a separate chapter of 'Obsessive-compulsive and related disorders' is formed which brings OCD and all OC spectrum disorders under one heading. With regard to the definition of OCD, the proposal acknowledges that obsessions usually, but not always cause marked anxiety or distress. The main difference is the proposed amendment of a differentiation in the level of insight – good, fair, poor, or absent. In the case of absent insight, the question is whether such delusional beliefs should not be categorized as a psychotic disorder rather than OCD, as the current definition implies. In 2010, the DSM-V workgroup 'Anxiety, Obsessive-Compulsive Spectrum, Post-traumatic, and Dissociative Disorders' [8] recommended the elimination of 'OCD's delusional variant' (p. 513) from the psychosis section, but this question is not yet resolved [11].

Historical Overview

In hindsight, we can distinguish obsessions and compulsions in various historical cases, most of which are of a religious nature (probably also because clerics were the writing class, and thus these cases are more likely to be reported, as Berrios [12] rightly remarks). However, even though the development of psychiatry as a medical discipline had been taking shape for some decades, it was not until 1838 that the first case description of what we would now call OCD was published by the French psychiatrist Esquirol [13]. Thirty years later, in 1868, the German psychiatrist Griesinger still speaks of 'a little known psychopathical condition' [14] when he describes 3 patients suffering from obsessions and compulsions. Their condition may be so unknown because these patients cannot be found in a mental asylum, but still move around freely, as Griesinger remarks.

A growing recognition of obsessions and compulsions lead to varying conceptualizations and definitions during the 19th century, mostly by French and German psychopathologists. Drawing on case studies, they tried to understand the nature of the problems of their patients and to carve out a common structure that would justify grouping these problems together as different instances of the same disorder. At the same time, they were concerned with classification: they wanted to find out not only whether these problems could be united as one disorder, but also how this disorder could be distinguished from other psychiatric conditions. As noted earlier, OCD may be conceptualized according to its affective, cognitive and volitional nature, and so can its historical development. We can distinguish those who regarded *emotions* (especially anxiety) as central, those who regarded the problems as stemming from a lack of *will power*, and those who considered the *intellect* to be at the root of the problems.

Early Developments

In 1838, Esquirol [13] wrote about one of his patients, 'Mademoiselle F', and therewith provided the first description of a classical case of what we now call OCD. He described her fear that she might steal what she touched and how she tried to keep her thoughts under control by washing her hands or standing on one leg for hours. Her behavior appears to be 'involuntary, irresistible and instinctive'. She consciously rejects these actions, but her will does not succeed in trying to resist. Esquirol points out that her rejection of these activities signals that she has some insight. He therefore characterized her condition as a *'délire partiel'*, a partial madness. According to Esquirol, these problems were neither due to reason nor emotion, but rather reflected a *weakness of the will*. He concluded that Mademoiselle F. suffered from a form of volitional *'monomanie'*.

In 1866, Jules Falret [15, 16] introduced the term *'maladie du doute'* (also called *'folie du doute'*), pointing to the pathological doubt involved. In that same year, Morel's analysis of 7 patients was published. Like Esquirol, Morel [17] also regarded the insight of the patients into the foolishness of their actions to be a major characteristic of their condition. He however disagreed with Esquirol's analysis of the problem: Morel thought their condition was rather a 'disease of the emotions' [12] – with anxious doubt being the central emotion. This *'délire émotif'* would stem from disturbances of the central nervous system. For Morel, the patients' insight implied that they do not suffer from a 'true' madness. He studied the disorder quite extensively and listed some predisposing factors for its development: (1) suffering or a great loss; (2) stopping with an active life; (3) long-lasting insomnia; (4) excessive intellectual efforts; (5) heredity [18].

A year later, Von Krafft-Ebing [19] introduces the word 'compulsion' *(Zwangsvorstellung)*. He generally agrees with Morel's perspective: he too thinks the central nervous system plays a crucial role. He also agrees with Morel that a traumatic experience can trigger the disorder – although some patients develop these symptoms 'out of the blue': in those cases it must be a genetic disposition that is at work.

It is important to realize that both Morel and Von Krafft-Ebing did not draw the boundaries of the disorder in the way that we do now. As Berrios [12] points out, Morel's category of *'délire émotif'* was very broad and included also 'vasomotor and digestive symptomatology, phobias, dysphoria, unmotivated fears, fixed ideas, and compulsions' (p. 285). Morel's main criterion was the lack of cognitive impairment. Von Krafft-Ebing too was not referring to our present-day definition of OCD when he introduced the word 'compulsion': he used it to describe a phenomenon concerning the structure of the course of thinking. In fact, he used *'Zwangsvorstellung'* as it occurred in a patient suffering from melancholic mood to describe the compelling force with which certain mental acts result in other mental acts, such as melancholic thoughts following melancholic mood.

Westphal

It is Westphal's [20] definition from 1878 which stands at the basis of our present definition of OCD. He writes:

'By obsessive images I understand those which, with intelligence being otherwise intact and without being conditioned by an emotional or affect-like state, step into the foreground of consciousness against the will of the person concerned and cannot be chased away and which hinder or interfere with the normal course of images, which the person affected continually acknowledges as abnormal and alien to him and which he faces with his sane consciousness' (p. 734).

Like his predecessors, he sees the patients' insight in their condition as a crucial and distinguishing feature. And like Griesinger, he relates this insight to the patients' experience of shame and their efforts to hide their problems from others. However, his analysis of what constitutes the core of the disorder differs. Contrary to Morel and Von Krafft-Ebing, Westphal regards the anxiety of the patients as a secondary effect of the obsessive thoughts. The disorder does not have an emotional basis: it is rather a disorder of the *course of thinking*. It is the occurrence of obsessive thoughts that subsequently frightens the patients. Accordingly, he does not think that emotional experiences can trigger the disorder.

Similarly, Westphal considers the weakness of the will a secondary phenomenon too. The obsessions can acquire such intensity that, for the time being, they force back all healthy thoughts and images, and thus direct the will accordingly: either by acting in a particular manner, or by avoiding specific actions. He acknowledges that patients themselves think it is their weakness of the will that is their problem, but when they say that, they mean the same thing, he says, namely that their healthy thoughts are too weak to fight the impulses that accompany the obsessive images [20, footnote 4]. In the battle between the will and the obsessions, the obsessions win. Because the obsessions are too strong, says Westphal. Because the will is too weak, says Esquirol.

Westphal has also been influential by introducing the sequence of the primacy of the obsessions, which subsequently may lead the patient to perform (or avoid) certain activities. He also distinguished a third, very severe stage of the illness, namely those patients for whom a 'direct connection' between obsession and impulses of the will (hence activities) takes place. However, he regards this third category as very rare and in his text does not further explain this condition. As we saw, the DSM-IV adopted only the two-stage view, but applied it less flexibly than Westphal did, largely influenced by the paradigmatic anxiety conditioning theory of behavior therapists. Besides, Westphal approached OCD in terms of the development of the disorder, which was a popular approach at that time, whereas the DSM-IV gives a more static definition, neglecting the evolution of symptoms.

Janet and Von Gebsattel

At the turn of the 20th century, with the rise of phenomenological psychiatry, some interesting phenomenological analyses of obsessions and compulsions have been put forward. We restrict ourselves here to the descriptions provided by Janet and Von Gebsattel. Like Westphal, Janet [21] also argues for three stages of illness: psychasthenic state, forced agitations, and obsessions and compulsions. And Janet too regards anxiety as a secondary phenomenon. In his opinion, the most basic factor in the illness is that patients feel that 'actions they perform are incompletely achieved, or that they do not produce the sought-for satisfaction' [22, p. 226]. They are 'continually tormented by an inner sense of imperfection' [22, p. 226]. This sense of incompleteness often pertains to their perceptions too, leading to doubts, and even derealization. In this way, Janet's account suggests that this feeling of incompleteness is at the root of the insatiable doubts.

Several decades later, the German psychiatrist and philosopher Von Gebsattel [23] took a more phenomenological approach to the disorder, which means that he tried to understand the disorder by investigating the way in which the patient relates to the world, to people, and to him-/herself. Von Gebsattel characterizes the relation between obsessive and compulsive patients to their world as one of 'fearful disgust' *(phobischer Ekel)*. This disgust not only pertains to things having to do with death and decay (all that is 'aversive to life' and that we cannot possibly sympathize with), but is also related to dirt in the metaphorical, moral sense of that which is sinful. The world of people suffering from obsessions and compulsions is one filled with dangerous or repulsive objects and possibilities for action. We may all know how the physiognomy of the world may suddenly change, Von Gebsattel writes, for instance when we are drawn to a friendly meadow to rest there and all of a sudden a poisonous snake crawls up. We are then confronted with the threatening side of the environment where we felt so at ease only a minute ago. This is what the world of obsessive-compulsive patients looks like all the time: they constantly perceive lurking dangers, reasons to worry, and potentially harmful events. Consequently, they feel unsafe in their world. As Von Gebsattel remarks: 'their world lacks the peaceful foundation' (p. 99) that we are used to rely upon. We take things for granted in normal life and unthinkingly assume harmless scenarios, in contrast to patients suffering from OCD.

Patients continuously try to dispel the chaos and potential destruction through their overly ordered, repetitive rituals. Their activities are not actions in the strict sense of the word because they are aimless, they serve no purpose. There is no progression, no future directedness, only a repetition of a series of instances of 'now'. Commenting on Von Gebsattel, Glas [24] points out that this obstruction of time leading anywhere can be seen as an ultimate attempt to stop the perpetual decay and destruction that comes with the passing of time. With these endless and sterile activities, patients try to control their worlds, to keep the destructive chaos at bay.

We can add here a distinction that Arendt [25] makes between labor, work, and action. Labor refers to activities that are aimed purely at staying alive and keeping our world liveable, like cooking and cleaning. These are the necessary everyday routines that we need to perform over and over again because otherwise decay (of food) or chaos (of our home) would follow. It forms the precondition for the other forms of activity. When we work, we aim to produce something longer lasting, like tools, or clothing. Here, the timescale is one of decades rather than days. Lastly, we humans are capable of actions. For Arendt, actions refer to our political and societal deeds: our participation in a community. It is through our public engagement that we can actualize our human freedom. Although labor is necessary for survival, and work is necessary for shaping our worlds, it is our capacity for acting that characterizes us as humans. Undertaking actions, engaging oneself in a community is however also the least controllable of all activities. We can never predict exactly how our actions will turn out, because this will depend on the other citizens in our community. To prevent that this unexpectedness leads to chaos, we have the possibility to make promises on the one hand, and to forgive on the other hand [25].

When we consider the activities that OCD patients perform, they are all in the realm of labor: cleaning the house, ordering, and washing oneself. For Arendt labor serves the continuous securing of our environment. Indeed, cleaning your house is reconquering your home, reestablishing your home as yours. The compulsions appear to be an attempt to reconquer the world. Von Gebsattel similarly speaks of a fight against the 'unworlding' (*Entweltlichung*) of the world. However, if one does not get past the stage of labor, and does not succeed to act in the sense of participating in a community, one thus cannot 'actualize one's freedom' as Arendt calls it. This is exactly what Von Gebsattel notices: being busy all day with their compulsive activities, patients do not partake in the 'real life'. Social participation is after all the least controllable of activities. In this way, patients obstruct their own self-realization. This fits with the fact that typically, in severe OCD patients, social isolation is one of the most characteristic traits, and the most difficult to treat.

Summary

Several defining and distinguishing characteristics emerge from this debate. First of all, patients suffer from recurrent thoughts or images that upset them and which they cannot control, and/or they perform certain activities that they acknowledge to be senseless. This acknowledgment or insight means that patients do not have delusions. Moreover, the insight into their condition goes hand in hand with their experience of shame. As a result, patients make every effort to conceal their problems to others, and

de Haan · Rietveld · Denys

will usually come for help only at a late stage. It is also apparent that the specific contents of thoughts and kinds of activities may vary widely. Still, the structure of their experiences is the same. The psychopathologists reported the anxiety that patients experience: some regarded it as the basic feature of this condition; others judged it to be a secondary phenomenon. There has also been debate about the role of the will and of the course of thoughts: is these patients' will too weak to control their thoughts, or are their thoughts of such an unusual kind that the will is no match for them? In any way, patients experience themselves as unfree.

Concerning the phenomenology of the disorder, Janet added the observation that patients suffer from a feeling of incompleteness. Von Gebsattel highlighted the role of disgust and fear of decay and chaos and the patients' experience of their worlds as unsafe. He also points to obstruction of self-actualization that is implicated in the patients' behavior.

Open Questions and Suggestions for Answers

Our historical overview has shown a quest for determining the primary or basic nature of OCD: is it a disorder of the will, of emotions, or rather of the course of thinking? All three conceptions have their limitations. It is obvious that anxiety and tension play an important role in the development and sustenance of the disorder – but is it primary? One could still ask where this anxiety comes from. Here, the proponents of a more 'cognitive' understanding of OCD do have a story to tell: the anxiety is secondary to the abnormal course of thinking. And compulsions in turn develop because of the anxiety aroused by the obsessions. Although this analysis of the reactive nature of compulsions indeed seems to be true for the majority of patients, one might again ask where the obsessions come from. Are they the result of a weakness of the will after all, as Esquirol thought? Indeed, patients attempt to keep their obsessions and compulsions under control and fail. But should we explain this as a lack of will power or rather as an erroneous attempt?

Little attention is paid to the fact that our normal course of thinking is characterized by a very limited amount of control. In other words, it is only natural that our stream of consciousness unfolds without conscious steering or control. Sometimes, we will direct our thoughts explicitly to a specific topic, but even then, it is more like a funneling of the thoughts than that we actually steer or control them [26]. Moreover, it is just as normal that our attempts to exert control over our thoughts in fact end up being counterproductive. As Dagonet pointed out in 1875: 'the more one tries to discard an idea, the more it becomes imposed upon the mind, the more one tries to get rid of an emotion of tendency, the more energetic it becomes' [12]. Or as we now would say: anything you pay attention to will grow. This is a common mechanism too, nothing unusual. Consequently, popular definitions such as the one by Kurt Schneider – 'Obsession is when someone can not repress contents of consciousness although he judges them as being nonsensical or dominating for no reason' [5, p. 292] – seem to miss an important point. Namely, the problem is not the inability to repress thoughts or images (we are all bad at that), but rather the wish or even need to try to do so.

Thoughts and images (even repulsive ones) pop up all the time – that is normal. So, how come these images and thoughts gain such force and cause such anxiety? It seems that patients attach much more value to these images and thoughts. In fact, having inappropriate thoughts or fantasies alone does not yet make for an obsession. It is only when one starts to worry excessively *about* having these thoughts that obsessions develop. Obsessions thus depend on the *attitude* of persons to their unwanted thoughts and images. Instead of discarding them as mere silly fantasies, patients assume that these images and thoughts reveal something about them: might they be a memory? Or do they reveal what I actually want to do if I would let myself go? How can I know for sure that I won't do all these terrible things? Or have not already done them? Otherwise, why would I have these ideas and images?

And yet again, we may ask why patients would attach too much value to their images and thoughts. Why would I shrug my shoulders over a sexual or aggressive fantasy and do away with it as merely a fantasy – as opposed to someone who believes these fantasies convey something about who they really are? It might be that patients are less able to compartmentalize: that is, to tolerate parts of themselves that are at odds with their general self-concept. In other words: we normally succeed to ignore the incoherencies between what we think and do and our image of who we are.[2] More in general, as Denys [6] points out, patients suffering from OCD seem to have difficulties in tolerating uncertainty. This was already apparent from one of the first characterizations of this condition as '*maladie de doute'*. What bothers them is that they cannot be *absolutely* certain whether or not their thoughts may be revealing something after all, or whether or not they might get infected, or whether or not they infected somebody else. They feel they cannot be entirely sure, and this feeling of uncertainty is tantamount to experiencing tension.[3] In OCD, there is a desire for *absolute* certainty.

Certainty and Trust

The experiences of patients with OCD reveal how much we usually take for granted. We do not consider every possible worst-case scenario before we take action, we are blissfully oblivious to all the germs and bacteria that surround us, we ignore things we

---

[2] This explanation was suggested to us by Prof. Martin Stokhof [pers. commun.].
[3] Of course, the question remains where this uncertainty then comes from, but this is a question at a different etiological (causal) level of analysis. Several hypotheses could be formulated, for instance that these patients' sense of agency is disturbed as a result of disordered feed-forward mechanisms [27]. But the quest for finding THE primary root or cause of the disorder could lead to a continuous shift of the etiological question. We would like to point out that the development of a complex psychiatric disorder like OCD may well consists of several, mutually influencing processes, rather than just one primary, common cause of everything. We therefore sympathize with recent network approaches to psychiatric disorders. See for instance Cramer et al. [28].

de Haan · Rietveld · Denys

do not fully understand and accept that we make mistakes. As one patient blurted out: ordinary folks are so superficial! They do not think about anything! Normal people are blissfully ignorant. They just go about doing things, without properly investigating all the risks involved! Although he was fairly invalidated by his compulsions and longed for a normal life, he was at the same time ambivalent whether he would want to be 'cured' if that would entail becoming just as superficial – which puts him at the border between OCD and OCPD.

Moreover, patients' experiences also make clear that the uncertainty at stake in OCD goes much deeper than a temporal lack of knowledge. In fact, knowledge will in general not help much. Suppose one worries whether one could get diseases from sitting on a toilet. Many people would not even consider this possibility, but suppose one does, one could look for information on the internet, or more reliably, ask an expert. Some patients indeed search for assurance in this way. But if it helps at all, it will not last. For who knows, the expert may be wrong. Experts may disagree: whom to trust? Even of so-called facts, commonly accepted pieces of knowledge, one cannot be entirely sure, for even these facts may need revision once in a while. Even scientific facts are only true within a particular paradigm. What patients suffering from OCD lack is not so much knowledge, but trust. Knowing the facts does not suffice: one still needs to surrender to them in daily life.

In his book *On Certainty*, Wittgenstein [29] points to the difference between knowledge claims (facts) and well-founded yet unexpressed basic assumptions. We can have knowledge about certain facts, but in the end, these facts are founded on basic assumptions which are grounded in sociocultural practices[4]. Without doubt we normally presume these basic assumptions, which are typically not articulated linguistically, and act upon them: 'The assumption (…) forms the basis of action, and therefore, naturally, of thought' [29, p. 411, see also p. 134]. Interestingly, Wittgenstein states that doubting is only meaningful with regard to facts or knowledge claims – but not with regard to basic assumptions. We suggest that doubting basic assumptions is indeed not doubt proper: it is rather a form of anxiety. Doubting facts is normal, doubting basic assumptions is either philosophy or pathology.

Wittgenstein gives the following example, highlighting the difference between doubting a fact and doubting a basic assumption:

'If the water over the gas freezes, of course I shall be as astonished as can be, but I shall assume some factor I don't know of, and perhaps leave the matter to physicists to judge. But what could make me doubt whether this person here is N.N., whom I have known for years? *Here doubt would seem to drag everything with it and plunge it into chaos*' [29, p. 613, our italics].

If I start to doubt something as basic and fundamental as the identity of my friend, then innumerable things normally taken for granted will become uncertain as well. If

---

[4] Wittgenstein [29] points out that there is no 'sharp division' (p. 97) between what counts as a 'fact' and what as an 'assumptions'. He uses the metaphor of the flowing river and the riverbed: the knowledge claims are changeable like the water of the river, but even the 'river-bed of thoughts' (p. 97) may shift at some point.

I doubt *that*, what can I still rely on? The ensuing world would indeed resemble the unsafe world that Von Gebsattel described. Wittgenstein emphasizes that normally we simply do not doubt these basic assumptions: we rather unreflectively trust that these are my two hands, that my friend is the same person as he was yesterday, and that the ground beneath us will not disappear. One needs a foundation of trust in order to even be able to doubt specific knowledge claims.[5] From this perspective, the experience of the unsafe world that Von Gabsattel described is the phenomenological counterpart of an individual who lacks the foundation of trustful reliance on the practices that we normally take for granted; on the 'basic assumptions' of our sociocultural practices.

Moreover, Wittgenstein points out that 'doubting' such a basic assumption would have spill-over effects and could undermine one's whole framework of everyday assumptions. We would lose the ground of our actions and thoughts. This is expressed in a different example:

'If I wanted to doubt the existence of the earth long before my birth, I should have to doubt all sorts of things that stand fast for me' [29, p. 234].

'Doubt' would not come to an end and chaos would result, Wittgenstein suggests. Could it be that the OCD undermines some basic assumption that has a spill-over effect on the person's whole fabric or 'nest' [29, p. 134] of assumptions, inducing anxiety?[6]

Wittgenstein's distinction between facts and basic assumptions clarifies why knowledge of the facts does not help to reduce the compulsions of OCD patients: the anxiety that motivates the compulsions concerns the *assumptions* rather than the *facts* of our existence. If our acceptance of the facts rests upon our trust in our basic assumptions, what can we say about where this trust comes from? Is this trust then completely unfounded? No, says Wittgenstein, there is a ground for our trust, namely the way in which we act: 'Why do I not satisfy myself that I have two feet when I want to get up from a chair? There is no why. I simply don't. This is how I act' [29, p. 148]. Our daily practices form both the foundation and the affirmation [29, p. 509] of our trust. We trust on the basis of our practical familiarity.

The problem for patients with OCD is that they want to attain absolute certainty whereas the experience of certainty can never be absolute, but will always depend on basic trust. They are right that we can never be sure; that some disaster could happen, or that we might cause an accident, or that someone might be offended by something we say. Indeed, one cannot be absolutely certain about these things: we need to trust in that which we can never be entirely certain of. As a consequence, the striving for

---

[5] Wittgenstein [29] distinguishes between a subjectively experienced or 'psychological' certainty and certainty in a logical sense (p. 447, 448). The former applies to specific knowledge claims, the latter to basic assumptions.

[6] Again, it is a different kind of question where the pathological doubt that undermines this basic trust comes from. How come that these patients' basic trust is eroded? Is there a very basic perceptual process that is disturbed? And how would that have come about? These are questions at another, etiological, causal, level of analysis. Amongst other things, it requires an investigation of (and comparison with) the nature of normal unreflective, trusting action.

certainty via the acquisition of factual knowledge is doomed to fail. Both certainty and meaningful doubt depend on the acceptance of the possibility of the truth, which requires trust rather than science.

The Role of Reflection

The patients' striving for certainty via the acquisition of facts is thus an unattainable goal, and unfortunately the attempts to reach it via conscious control even have opposite effects. Their experience of uncertainty prompts them to pay extra attention to their actions: to remain conscious of all their movements rather than thoughtlessly repeating an old habit. This is a normal reaction: for instance when you go on vacation, you will make sure that you very deliberately locked the door, so that you will not have to worry about it later. But normally, such deliberately controlled actions are the exceptions and unthinking performance of habits is the norm. For people suffering from OCD, it is the other way around: reflective deliberation becomes the norm. As the disorder worsens, fewer activities can be performed spontaneously: conscious control colonizes the bodily know-how.

In OCD, the balance between unreflective action and reflective deliberation is disturbed: patients think all the time (mostly of what might go wrong) and constantly try to pay attention to what they are doing. This is not some form of enlightened 'mindfulness', but rather an extremely tiresome and stressful attempt to attain maximal control over things. Such exaggerated reflection and deliberate attention to what you are doing is called 'hyperreflectivity'. Every act becomes a conscious, deliberate decision instead of just a spontaneous reaction. What is normally taken for granted, unthinkingly relied upon, is now brought to awareness. As Fuchs [30] points out, making such tacit processes explicit actually disturbs their functionality. In other words: too much reflection undermines trust. Fuchs [30] writes: 'Self-centeredness and hyper-reflection are thus, on the one hand, the result of the illness, but on the other hand, they often additionally contribute to it' (p. 239).

This process of hyperreflection can be recognized in many different forms of psychopathology – it was first described by Frankl [31] with regard to anxiety disorders, OCD, sexual disorders, and sleeping disorders, and by Laing [32] and later by Sass and Parnas [33] with regard to schizophrenia. In the case of OCD patients, we can also see such a negative spiral at work. As Denys [6] points out: 'Typically, someone suffering from OCD will attempt to gain absolute control by total conscious awareness that, ironically, only leads to more dyscontrol' [34]. We propose to call this mechanism the 'hyperreflectivity trap'. It proceeds through several stages:
1 First, there is the feeling of uncertainty, anxiety, or tension.
2 This feeling leads to attempts to regain control through deliberation (What might go wrong? How could I prevent that?), and reflective action (trying to perform all actions with maximal attention).

3   But too much reflection can be dangerous: analyzing and paying attention to your actions may lead to estrangement and typically *augments* insecurity.[7]
4   As a last step, the increase in insecurity brings us back to the first step.

Too much reflection thus disturbs the balance that is required to feel in control and it may even lead to a negative self-reinforcing spiral of feelings of anxiety and insecurity and subsequent attempts of reflective control. As we can see from the experiences of OCD patients, getting a grip on things requires letting go as well – and trust in one's unreflective actions.

Conclusion

In this chapter, we gave an overview of current and historical conceptions of the nature of obsessions and compulsions. We also discussed some open questions and added some phenomenological suggestions of our own. In particular, we pointed to the patients' need for absolute certainty and the lack of trust underlying this need. Building on insights from Wittgenstein, we argued that the kind of certainty the patients strive for is unattainable in principle via the acquisition of factual knowledge. Moreover, we suggested that the patients' attempts to attain certainty are counterproductive as their excessive conscious control in fact undermines the trust they need.

References

1   Wegner DM, Schneider DJ, Carter SR, White TL: Paradoxical effects of thought suppression. J Pers Soc Psychol 1987;53:5.
2   Abramowitz JS, Tolin DF, Street GP: Paradoxical effects of thought suppression: a meta-analysis of controlled studies. Clin Psychol Rev 2001;21:683–703.
3   American Psychiatric Association: Diagnostic and Statistical Manual of Mental Disorders, ed 4, DSM-IV-TR (text revision). Washington, American Psychiatric Association, 2000.
4   Denys D: Obsessionality & compulsivity: a phenomenology of obsessive-compulsive disorder. Philos Ethics Humanit Med 2011;6:3.
5   Bürgy M: Psychopathology of obsessive-compulsive disorder: a phenomenological approach. Psychopathology 2005;38:291–300.
6   Denys D: On Certainty: Studies in Obsessive-Compulsive Disorder. Utrecht, Universiteit Utrecht, 2004.
7   Stein DJ, Fineberg NA, Bienvenu OJ, Denys D, Lochner C, Nestadt G, Leckman JF, Rauch SL, Phillips KA: Should OCD be classified as an anxiety disorder in DSM-V? Depress Anxiety 2010;27:495–506.
8   Leckman JF, Denys D, Simpson HB, Mataix-Cols D, Hollander E, Saxena S, Miguel EC, Rauch SL, Goodman WK, Phillips KA, Stein DJ: Obsessive-compulsive disorder: a review of the diagnostic criteria and possible subtypes and dimensional specifiers for DSM-V. Depress Anxiety 2010;27:507–527.
9   Hollander E, Kim S, Khanna S, Pallanti S: Obsessive-compulsive disorder and obsessive-compulsive spectrum disorders: diagnostic and dimensional issues. CNS Spectrums 2007;12:5–13.
10 Chamberlain S, Fineberg N, Blackwell A, Robbins T, Sahakian B: Motor inhibition and cognitive flexibility in obsessive-compulsive disorder and trichotillomania. Am J Psychiatry 2006;163:1282–1284.

---

[7]   Research on memory shows that patients with OCD do not have memory impairments per se, but rather distrust their memory: it is thus the attitude towards their memory that is affected. Interestingly, the same happens to normal controls who are instructed to repeatedly check their tasks. The checking thus augments the feeling of insecurity. See Van den Hout and Kindt [35].

11 American Psychiatric Association: Proposed Revision of OCD in DSM-V. Washington, American Psychiatric Association, 2012.

12 Berrios GE: Obsessive-compulsive disorder: its conceptual history in France during the 19th century. Compr Psychiatry 1989;30:283–295.

13 Esquirol E: Des maladies mentales considérées sous les rapports médical, hygiénique et médico-légal. Paris, JB Baillière, 1838.

14 Griesinger W: Ueber einen wenig bekannten psychopathischen Zustand Vortrag. Eur Arch Psychiatry Clin Neurosci 1868;1:626–635.

15 Falret J: Folie raisonnante ou folie morale. Ann Med Psychol 1866;24:382.

16 Falret J: Études cliniques sur les maladies mentales et nerveuses. Paris, JB Baillière, 1980, pp 475–525.

17 Morel BA: Du délire émotif. Névrose du système nerveux ganglionnaire viscéral. Paris, P Asselin, 1866.

18 Hovens H: Geschiedenis van de diagnose obsessieve-compulsieve stoornis; in Denys D, de Geus F (eds): Handboek Obsessieve-Compulsieve Stoornissen. Utrecht, De Tijdstroom, 2007, pp 1–13.

19 Von Krafft-Ebing R: Beiträge zur Erkennung und richtigen forensischen Beurteilung krankhafter Gemützustände für Ärzte, Richter, und Verteidiger. Erlangen, Enke, 1867.

20 Westphal C: Über Zwangsvorstellungen. Arch Psychiatr Nervenkr 1878;7:734–750.

21 Janet P: Les Obsessions et la psychasthénie. Paris, Alcan, 1903.

22 Pitman RK: Pierre Janet on obsessive-compulsive disorder (1903). Review and commentary. Arch Gen Psychiatr 1987;44:226–232.

23 Von Gebsattel VE: Die Welt des Zwangskranken; Prolegomena einer medizinischen Anthropologie. Berlin, Springer, 1954.

24 Glas G: Angst. Beleving, Structuur, Macht. Amsterdam, Boom, 2002.

25 Arendt H: The Human Condition. University of Chicago Press, Chicago, 1958/1998.

26 De Haan S, De Bruin L: Reconstructing the minimal self, or how to make sense of agency and ownership. Phenomenol Cogn Sci 2010;9:373–396.

27 Gentsch A, Schütz-Bosbach S, Endrass T, Kathmann N: Dysfunctional forward model mechanisms and aberrant sense of agency in obsessive-compulsive disorder. Biol Psychiatry 2012;71:652–659.

28 Cramer AOJ, Waldorp LJ, van der Maas HLJ, Borsboom D: Comorbidity: a network perspective. Behav Brain Sci 2010;33:178–193.

29 Wittgenstein L: On Certainty. Oxford, Blackwell, 1975.

30 Fuchs T: The psychopathology of hyperreflexivity. J Speculative Philos 2011;24:239–255.

31 Frankl VE: Ärztliche Seelsorge. Grundlagen der Logotherapie und Existenzanalyse, mit den zehn Thesen über die Person. München, Deutscher Taschenbuch Verlag, 1946/2009.

32 Laing RD: The Divided Self, ed 1990 (incl 1965 preface). London, Penguin Books, 1959/1990.

33 Sass LA, Parnas J: Schizophrenia, consciousness, and the self. Schizophr Bull 2003;29:427–444.

34 Denys D, Prosée R, Stein D: Obsessive-compulsive disorder and certainty; in Mishara A, Corlett P, Fletcher P, Schwartz M (eds): Phenomenological Neuropsychiatry: How Patient Experience Bridges Clinic with Clinical Neuroscience. New York, Springer, in press.

35 Van den Hout M, Kindt M: Repeated checking causes memory distrust. Behav Res Ther 2003;41:301–316.

Sanneke de Haan
AMC Psychiatrie
Postbus 22660
NL–1100 DD Amsterdam (The Netherlands)
E-Mail Sanneke.deHaan@amc.uva.nl

Baldwin DS, Leonard BE (eds): Anxiety Disorders.
Mod Trends Pharmacopsychiatry. Basel, Karger, 2013, vol 29, pp 16–23 (DOI: 10.1159/000351919)

The Origin of Anxiety Disorders – An Evolutionary Approach

Lisette E.W.G. Willers[b] · Nienke C. Vulink[b] · Damiaan Denys[b] · Dan J. Stein[a]

[a]Department of Psychiatry, University of Cape Town, Cape Town, South Africa, and
[b]Department of Psychiatry, University of Amsterdam, Amsterdam, The Netherlands

Abstract

There is growing interest in the application of evolutionary theory to medicine. In this review, we outline an evolutionary approach to the anxiety disorders. We begin by considering the nature of fear and anxiety, and their evolutionary benefits. We emphasize that fear and anxiety exist in multiple organisms, and note the implications of brain complexity in *Homo sapiens* for the anxiety disorders. This account emphasizes the importance of distance from a threat; in *H. sapiens*, it is possible to experience fear and anxiety even when threats are temporally and spatially distant.

There have been important advances in research on fear, anxiety and anxiety disorders over the past few decades. Numerous questions have been investigated ranging from the psychobiology of fear and anxiety to the optimal interventions for anxiety disorders. Less work has, however, been undertaken on the evolutionary basis of these constructs. This chapter will review the existing literature in this area.

From an evolutionary perspective, fear and anxiety are both emotional processes that help organisms cope with threats or danger. Indeed, they are responses that have evolved due to their adaptive value [1]. Distinct stimuli can provoke fear and anxiety, which may differ in underlying mechanisms and overt behavior [2].

Fear is provoked by stimuli which point to possible harm [1], or by perceptible threat [3]. Three forms of response may occur in the presence of a stimulus: freezing, fleeing or fighting. Freezing is helpful to distract the threat's attention, fleeing increases the distance to a threat, and fighting back attempts to defeat the threat [2, 3]. Due to these responses to fear, the chance of getting injured decreases.

Anxiety on the other hand is provoked by more abstract stimuli. The trait of anxiousness is useful for anticipating such theoretical or inexplicit stimuli. The extent of anxiety symptoms is determined by the current risk estimation, and differs among individuals. The main characteristic of anxiety is 'worry'. Worrying focuses on a range of future problems. Examples are: worrying about the weather on a future holiday, or, worrying about the prospects of being fired without a particular reason.

Anxiety and worry may be useful in that they protect the organism from future danger [1]. If fear focuses on particular and determinate matters, then anxiety focuses on less particular and more indeterminate matters. Although fear and anxiety are different processes, both appear to be adaptive.

Two questions arise at this point; first, why do fear and anxiety manifest even when not needed? For example, an unfamiliar noise may cause fear, despite very often being caused by harmless stimuli such as the wind. Second, what is the optimal 'set-point' for fear and anxiety?

Evolutionary principles help explain the high prevalence of fear and anxiety. Natural selection is based on reproductive success [1]. Anxiety, on the one hand, helps extend our survival, thus creating more opportunities to reproduce [1, 4]. On the other hand, anxiety requires the expenditure of energy [1]. Thus, the optimal set level for anxiety involves a trade-off. In this explanation, anxiety symptoms are the result of an adaptive natural development or process, and do not necessarily comprise anxiety disorders.

Variation in the amount of fear and anxiety in humans can be understood by using the concept of a smoke detector. Although many alarms may be false, if the threshold for setting an alarm is too high, then it is likely that real dangers will be missed. On the other hand, if an individual interprets every sound as a threat, the threshold is too low and the rate of false alarms and consequent wasted energy is overly high [1].

Why is there a marked variation in the set point for fear and anxiety alarms across individuals? Perhaps different set points are better suited for different environments. In dangerous contexts, it may be adaptive to have the alarm threshold set lower. On the other hand, in a context where there is little danger, such a high false alarm rate can be conceptualized as an anxiety disorder [1].

As the brain complexity of animal species increases, additional forms of fear and anxiety arise [4]. We will examine this subject in the next paragraphs, together with the specific brain parts that are involved in anxiety disorders. Finally, we will argue that distance to a threat also evokes distinct forms of fear and anxiety.

The Brain: Evolution and Complexity

Analogues of fear and anxiety can be seen in simple species that lived hundreds of million years ago. On the other hand, in the animal kingdom, modern human beings have the most complex brains of all. Here, we review the argument that as the complexity of the brain has increased, so additional forms of fear and anxiety become apparent [4].

Motile bacteria have been in existence for around 2 billion years. These organisms arguably have anxiety-like states insofar as they avoid noxious stimuli [4]. Nevertheless, this response is not a persistent one, since such organisms have very short 'memories' and do not demonstrate fear conditioning.

Five hundred million years ago, marine invertebrates evolved. These animals display anticipatory anxiety, and arguably sometimes even a form of chronic diffuse anxiety. Experiments with sea hares, for example, demonstrate persistent avoidance of stimuli that they have learned are harmful [4].

A fear response, and conditioned avoidance are found in all vertebrates. These phenomena are mediated by the midbrain, or mesencephalon, and do not necessarily require higher cortical processes [5]. Proximal threats activate the periaqueductal gray (PAG) within the midbrain, in turn leading to a fear response [6, 7]. The PAG can be divided into two parts, the ventrolateral and the dorsolateral part. In rats, the ventrolateral part is thought to be responsible for freezing, a passive reaction to fear, while the dorsolateral part is thought to be responsible for an active reaction of escape [8, 9].

A hundred to two hundred million years ago, brain evolution resulted in the development of more complex limbic systems in small mammals. This system mediated more sophisticated emotional states, including different types of fear and anxiety, such as separation anxiety [4].

Further brain evolution in higher mammals resulted in the development of a more complex neocortex. The neocortex allowed more sophisticated cognitive functions such as learning, and planning capacities [4, 10]. Such functions in turn allow more differentiated kinds of anxiety, such as anticipatory anxiety [1].

Among mammals, the brain and cortex of primates is the largest [11]. The first to demonstrate anxiety in primates in the laboratory was Harlow, now famous for his work with rhesus monkeys on maternal separation [12]. In later work in a more natural setting in the Caribbean, Suomi [13] found that rhesus monkey infants that had been left by their mothers during the breeding period also displayed symptoms consistent with anxiety.

In dogs, cats, and other mammals, stereotypic behaviors, arguably analogous to obsessive-compulsive symptoms in humans, may also be found [14]. Examples include acral lick dermatitis, and tail biting. However, more complex cognitive symptoms in obsessive-compulsive disorder (OCD) in humans cannot easily be found in animal models.

Indeed, more complex cognitive-affective phenomena in humans, including worry, are likely mediated in part by the prefrontal cortex (PFC). The PFC in humans is larger than in other animals, and is the part of the brain that is most characteristic of the human brain [11]. Other characteristics that separate the human brain from that of non-human primates include the extent to which development continues after birth, and the larger number of genes expressed in the PFC [1, 4]. The self-awareness that such a brain allows may mediate more complex feelings of existential anxiety that are seen solely in humans [4].

In summary, increasing complexity of the brain may be associated with differences in the nature of fear and anxiety responses. In higher mammals, it is relevant to note that evolutionary newer structures, such as PFC, play a role in controlling older structures such as the amygdala [15]. This can help explain how the engagement of more complex cognitive processes during psychotherapy can be useful in fear extinction. It is also consistent with a social brain hypothesis which emphasizes the adaptive value of neocortex for surviving in complex primate communities [16].

Neurocircuitry of Anxiety Disorders

Brain imaging provides information on the neuronal underpinnings of anxiety. In this section, the following anxiety disorders will be highlighted: posttraumatic stress disorder (PTSD), panic disorder (PD), various forms of phobia, generalized anxiety disorder (GAD) and OCD. Both different and similar aspects of neurobiology in these disorders will be pointed out, with a focus on the functioning of the amygdala and cortex (see also the chapter on Neuroimaging in Anxiety Disorders, pp. 47–66).

Posttraumatic Stress Disorder
If people have experienced a life-threatening situation, PTSD can develop. Symptoms include re-living the experience, avoidance of stimuli that may trigger or resemble the situation, and hyperarousal [17]. Meta-analyses of PTSD show evidence for increased activity in the amygdala and insula compared to healthy subjects. Hypoactivation in the dorsal and rostral anterior cingulate cortices and the ventromedial PFC (vmPFC) is also found. Hypoactivation of the frontal regions is correlated with hyperactivation in limbic and perilimbic regions, which appears to be a distinctive element of PTSD [18].

Panic Disorder
PD is characterized by panic attacks, at least some of which are unexpected, in which a person has to deal with an overpowering feeling of anxiety, respiratory symptoms and autonomic nervous system activity. PD is often associated with anticipatory anxiety about further panic attacks and with agoraphobia, in which people are afraid to have a panic attack in public, or during a situation where no help is available [17]. Meta-analysis of imaging studies shows that panic attacks are associated with increased activity in the amygdala and insula compared to healthy subjects [18].

Phobia
A phobia can develop for specific objects or a social situation (the stimuli). The existence or anticipation of these stimuli will provoke fear. Subtypes of specific phobia are the animal type, the natural environment type, the blood-injection-injury type, and the situational type. For patients with social phobia, social situations lead to intense

distress and anxiety [17]. Meta-analysis of imaging studies in patients with specific phobia shows, again, evidence of increased activity in the amygdala and insula compared to healthy subjects [18].

Generalized Anxiety Disorder

Patients with GAD are disproportionally anxious and worried about everyday life situations. In GAD, the symptoms concern the anticipation of a possible future risk or threat. Meta-analyses show that the number of imaging studies concerning GAD is still scarce. Amygdala and insula function seem to play a role, and a dysfunction of the ventrolateral PFC is probably of relevance [19].

Obsessive-Compulsive Disorder

The defining features of OCD are obsessions and compulsions. Obsessions are intrusive thoughts or images which are experienced as inappropriate. Compulsions are repetitive behaviors or mental acts, often done in order to neutralize obsessions [17]. Meta-analyses of functional neuroimaging studies in OCD patients, based on the provocation of OCD symptoms, show activation in cortical and subcortical regions of the orbitofrontal and anterior cingulate loops. Significant likelihoods of activation were also found in the left dorsolateral PFC and precuneus, and the left superior temporal gyrus [20]. Orbitofrontal hyperactivity is associated with the appearance of intrusive thoughts, while hyperactivity within the anterior cingulate cortex (ACC) may be associated with non-specific anxiety arising from these thoughts [19].

Although each of these disorders is heterogeneous, the brain mechanisms involved in PTSD, PD and phobias can arguably be distinguished from those which mediate GAD and OCD. Studies of the first three disorders showed hyperactivity in the amygdala and insula, compared to healthy subjects. This pattern has also been seen in healthy subjects feeling anticipatory anxiety during fear conditioning. Amygdala and insula hyperactivity was more generally found in specific phobia and social anxiety disorder than in PTSD [18]. In GAD and OCD, additional structures, such as the PFC, seem to play a key role [19, 20]. Thus, different kinds of false alarms, each with its own adaptive value, and underpinned by a somewhat unique neuronal circuitry, may be important in different anxiety disorders.

The Importance of Distance from a Threat

An important predictor of the nature of fear and anxiety responses in animals and humans is distance to a threat [7]. This distance plays an important role in shaping the elicited fear response: fight, flight, or freeze. Mobbs et al. [7] undertook an fMRI study of humans playing a game in which they were faced with threats at different distances. They showed three distinct states related to the distance from a threat:

a Circa-strike state: the prey has a very close interaction with the threat. The moment the threat came close, a switch from forebrain to midbrain activity occurred, with enhanced PAG activity. The PAG became more active when the chance of getting caught increased and certainty of escape decreased. Conversely, when the chance of getting caught decreased and the certainty of escape increased, the vmPFC and BLA were more active. During the circa-strike state, subjects experienced a higher level of panic, with increased activity in the midbrain and PAG.

b Post-encounter state: a state in which the threat is noticed but far away. During anticipation of the possible attack, an increased activity in the forebrain structures was found; the vmPFC including the subgenual ACC. In the same state, including the knowledge of receiving shocks when caught, activity in the right lateral amygdala, corresponding to the BLA, was increased. This is consistent with prior work showing enhanced activity in the vmPFC, hippocampus and amygdala during exposure to threat [21].

c Pre-encounter state: a situation in which a risk is present, but there is no specific danger. Recognition of threat was accompanied by increased activity in the medial orbitofrontal cortex (OFC) and right ACC. The right ACC may be important in determining the nature of the fear response, while the OFC may play a role in estimating the severity of danger. Precautionary behavior includes behaviors associated with vigilance in animals, and with risk assessment in humans. The aim is to produce an optimal reaction should a threat appear [5].

When danger is estimated to be far away and not life threatening, responses may be more likely to be managed by brain regions such as the PFC and limbic system. When danger is estimated to be life threatening, responses may be more likely to be managed by brain regions such as the PAG of the midbrain. Thus, evolutionary older and more simple brain structures are active in proximal threat, while evolutionary newer and more complex brain structures are involved in responding to more distal threats.

It may also be speculated that some anxiety disorders are related to more proximal threats, while others are related to more distal threats. PAG and BLA activity increase in a circa-strike state, as well as in PD. An increase in PFC and limbic activity can be seen in more distal threats, as well as in GAD. Precautionary behavior and OCD both involve the OFC. As noted earlier, different kinds of anxiety disorders may be characterized by different kinds of evolved false alarm, each of which has a somewhat unique adaptive function.

Conclusion

Evolutionary medicine is a growing field that is based on the premise that we need to understand both the distal (evolutionary) and proximal (physiological) mechanisms that underpin biological phenomena. Evolutionary psychiatry has also made significant strides in recent years, and may be particularly relevant for understanding anxiety and anxiety disorders. There is growing sophistication about how to ask and answer evolutionary questions pertinent to behavior, and models such as that of the smoke detector seem invaluable for understanding the nature of anxiety.

A key unresolved area is the nature of the border between normal and pathological anxiety. From a pragmatic perspective, when anxiety levels are accompanied by distress and dysfunction, then an anxiety disorder can be posited, and it is reasonable to provide a diagnosis and intervention. Each of the anxiety disorders may be understood to be governed by an evolved false alarm, which involves somewhat unique distal and proximal mechanisms. At the same time, there are important similarities across the anxiety disorders, which may help explain why similar sorts of treatment are useful across a number of conditions.

Acknowledgement

We would like to gratefully thank Nicole van Veenendaal for help with editing.

References

1 Nesse RM, Williams GC (eds): Why We Get Sick: The New Science of Darwinian Medicine. New York, Vintage Books, 1996.

2 Blanchard DC: Stimulus and environmental control of defensive behaviors; in Bouton M, Fanselow M (eds): The Functional Behaviorism of Robert C. Bolles: Learning, Motivation and Cognition. Washington, American Psychological Association, 1997, pp 283–305.

3 Blanchard DC, Blanchard RJ, Rogers RJ: Risk assessment and animal models anxiety; in Olivier B, Slangen J (eds): Animal Models in Psychopharmacology. Basel, Birkhauser, 1991, pp 117–134.

4 Hofer MA: Evolutionary Concepts in Anxiety; in Stein DJ, Hollander E, Rothbaum BO (eds): Textbook of Anxiety Disorders, ed 2. Arlington, American Psychiatric Publishing, 2010, pp 129–145.

5 Eilam D, Izhar R, Mort J: Threat detection: behavioral practices in animals and humans. Neurosci Biobehav Rev 2011;35:999–1006.

6 Mobbs D, Marchant JL, Hassabis D, Seymour B, Tan G, Gray M, Petrovic P, Dolan RJ, Frith CD: From threat to fear: the neural organization of defensive fear systems in humans. J Neurosci 2009;29:12236–12243.

7 Mobbs D, Petrovic P, Marchant JL, Hassabis D, Weiskopf N, Seymour B, Dolan RJ, Frith CD: When fear is near: threat imminence elicits prefrontal-periaqueductal gray shifts in humans. Science 2007;317:1079–1083.

8 Bandler R, Keay K, Floyd N, Price J: Central circuits mediating patterned autonomic activity during active vs passive emotional coping. Brain Res Bull 2000; 53:95–104.

9 Vianna MRM, Izquierdo LA, Barros DM, et al: Pharmacological differences between memory consolidation of habituation to an open field and inhibitory avoidance learning. Braz J Med Biol Res 2001;34: 233–240.

10 Roth G, Dicke U: Evolution of the brain and intelligence in primates. Prog Brain Res 2012;195:413–430.

11 Berkowitz LR, Coplan JD, Reddy DP, Gorman JM: The human dimension: how the prefrontal cortex modulates the subcortical fear response. Rev Neurosci 2007;18:191–207.

12 Harlow HF: Early social deprivation and later behavior in the monkey; in Abrams A, Gurner HH, Tomal JEP (eds): Unfinished Tasks in the Behavioral Sciences. Baltimore, Williams & Wilkins, 1964, pp 154–173.

13 Suomi SJ: Early determinants of behaviour: evidence from primate studies. Br Med Bull 1997;53:170–184.

14 Luescher UA, McKeown DB, Halip J: Stereotypic or obsessive-compulsive disorder in dogs and cats. Vet Clin North Am Small Anim Pract 1991;21:401–413.

15 Rosenkranz JA, Grace AA: Dopamine attenuates prefrontal cortical suppression of sensory inputs to the basolateral amygdala of rats. J Neurosci 2001;21: 4090–4103.

16 Dunbar RIM: The social brain meets neuroimaging. Trends Cogn Sci 2011;1027:1–2.

17 American Psychiatric Association: Diagnostic and Statistical Manual of Mental Disorders, ed 4. Washington, American Psychiatric Association, 2000.

18 Etkin A, Wager TD: Functional neuroimaging of anxiety: a meta-analysis of emotional processing in PTSD, social anxiety disorder, and specific phobia. Am J Psychiatry 2007;164:1476–1488.

19 Holzschneider K, Mulert C: Neuroimaging in anxiety disorders. Dialogues Clin Neurosci 2011;13:453–461.

20 Rotge JY, Guehl D, Dilharreguy B, Cuny E, Tignol J, Bioulac B, Allard M, Burbaud P, Aouizerate BJ: Provocation of obsessive-compulsive symptoms: a quantitative voxel-based meta-analysis of functional neuroimaging studies. J Psychiatry Neurosci 2008; 33:405–412.

21 Amat J, Baratta MV, Paul E, Bland ST, Watkins LR, Maier SF: Medial prefrontal cortex determines how stressor controllability affects behavior and dorsal raphe nucleus. Nat Neurosci 2005;8:365–371.

Lisette E.W.G. Willers
AMC Psychiatrie
Meibergdreef 5, PA0-154
NL–1105 AZ Amsterdam (The Netherlands)
E-Mail l.e.willers@amc.uva.nl

Baldwin DS, Leonard BE (eds): Anxiety Disorders.
Mod Trends Pharmacopsychiatry. Basel, Karger, 2013, vol 29, pp 24–46 (DOI: 10.1159/000351932)

Genetic Factors in Anxiety Disorders

Katharina Domschke[a] · Eduard Maron[b, c]

[a]Department of Psychiatry, Psychosomatics and Psychotherapy, University of Würzburg, Würzburg, Germany;
[b]Department of Neuropsychopharmacology and Molecular Imaging, Imperial College London, London, UK;
[c]Department of Psychiatry, University of Tartu, Tartu, Estonia

Abstract

Presently available clinical genetic studies point to a considerable heritability of anxiety disorders (30–67%), with multiple vulnerability genes such as $5\text{-}HT_{1A}$, 5-HTT, MAO-A, COMT, CCK-B, ADORA2A, CRHR1, FKBP5, ACE, RGS2/7 and NPSR1 suggested by molecular genetic association studies. These genes have been shown to partially interact with each other as well as with environmental factors to shape the overall disease risk in a complex genetic model. Additionally, recent studies have pointed out the crucial role of epigenetic signatures such as methylation patterns in modifying environmental influences as well as in driving the functional impact of anxiety disorder risk genes. On a systems level, vulnerability genes of anxiety disorders seem to confer some of the disease risk via intermediate phenotypes like behavioral inhibition, anxiety sensitivity or several neurobiological traits such as increased startle reactivity or dysfunctional corticolimbic activity during emotional processing. Finally, first pharmaco- and psychotherapy-genetic studies provide evidence for certain risk genes to confer interindividual variability in response to a pharmacological or psychotherapeutic intervention in anxiety disorders. Genetic research in anxiety disorders will be discussed regarding its potential to foster innovative and individually tailored therapeutic approaches for patients with anxiety disorders.

The etiology of anxiety disorders has been proposed to be multifactorial with a complex interaction of neurobiological and environmental factors. Within the neurobiological pathomechanism of anxiety disorders, the role of genetic factors deserves particular attention. A significant contribution of genetic risk variants to the development of anxiety disorders has been suggested by clinical genetic studies such as family and twin studies.

Clinical Genetic Studies

Family studies report an up to 3-times increased disease risk in first-degree relatives of patients with panic disorder [1], generalized anxiety disorder and specific phobias [2] as well as posttraumatic stress disorder (PTSD) [3]. An increased familial risk seems to particularly apply to early-onset panic disorder with a 17-fold increased risk of panic disorder in relatives of patients with panic disorder onset at or before the age of 20 years [4]. This aggregation of anxiety disorders in families ('familiality') suggests genetic factors and/or shared environmental factors to contribute to the disease risk. To further disentangle genetic and environmental risk factors, twin studies compare concordance rates in monozygotic (100% genetic identity) and dizygotic (50% genetic identity) twins, which allows for an estimation of the actual contribution of genetic factors to a disease ('heritability'). Heritability estimates for anxiety disorders range from ~30% for generalized anxiety disorder, simple phobias and PTSD over 48% (panic disorder), 51% (social phobia) and 59% (blood-injection phobia) to 67% for agoraphobia [2, 5, 6]. The genetic vulnerability towards anxiety disorders, however, does not follow a specific pattern of inheritance according to mendelian rules (e.g. dominant, recessive). Rather, anxiety disorders have been shown to belong to the group of so-called 'complex-genetic' disorders, where multiple susceptibility genes of only a small individual effect interact with each other as well as with environmental factors to constitute the overall disease risk [7].

Within the past ~20 years, much effort has been put into the search for specific genetic variants, which confer this increased genetic risk of anxiety disorders. Molecular genetic approaches such as linkage studies, cytogenetic studies and (genome-wide) association studies have yielded several promising results with respect to potential anxiety risk loci and risk alleles, respectively.

Molecular Genetic Studies

Linkage Studies

Linkage studies analyzing the coinheritance of particular genetic markers with the disease of interest in affected families have revealed several potential risk loci for panic disorder (chromosomes 1p, 4q, 7p, 9q, 11p, 15q and 20p) [8–16] as well as for agoraphobia, specific phobias and social phobia (chromosomes 3q, 14p and 16q) [11, 17, 18]. A genome-wide linkage study of a broad anxiety phenotype yielded evidence for a risk locus on chromosome 14 [19]. Specific risk loci were identified for panic disorder with comorbid bipolar disorder (chromosomes 2, 12 and 18) [20, 21], for a 'panic syndrome' with concomitant interstitial cystitis, kidney/bladder dysfunction, migraine, mitral valve prolapse or thyroid conditions (chromosome 13q) [12, 22–24] and for panic disorder with early-onset susceptibility to anxiety (chromosome 1q) [25, for review see 26].

Cytogenetic Studies

In a cytogenetic study, duplication of a 17-Mb region on chromosome 15q24–26 (DUP25) spanning about 60 genes has been reported to be linked to a panic disorder subtype with joint laxity and mitral valve prolapse [27]. Additionally, a single nucleotide polymorphism in the 5′ untranslated region of the neurotrophin 3 gene located in this duplicated chromosomal region was found to be significantly associated with panic disorder [28]. However, the initial duplication finding could not be replicated in independent samples so far [29–32].

Association Studies

Association studies in anxiety disorders have investigated several hundred candidate genes so far, mostly selected based on results from animal studies, challenge experiments or psychopharmacological interventions in anxiety-related phenotypes or anxiety disorders. These 'usual suspects' comprise genes involved in the serotonergic, noradrenergic, dopaminergic, cholecystokininergic, adenosinergic, GABAergic and hypothalamus-pituitary-adrenal axis-related systems.

Serotonin/Norepinephrine System Genes

Serotonin function has been crucially implied in the pathogenesis and pharmacotherapy of anxiety disorders [33]. Consequently, genes coding for the serotonergic system have been considered prime candidate genes in the molecular genetic investigation of anxiety disorders. Most evidence has accumulated for the monoamine oxidase A (MAO-A) gene to be associated with panic disorder, particularly in female patients [34–36]. Furthermore, the serotonin 1A receptor (5-HT_{1A}) gene [37, 38], the serotonin 2A receptor (5-HT_{2A}) gene [39–42] and the tryptophan hydroxylase 2 (TPH2) gene [43, 44] have been suggested to contribute to the pathogenesis of panic disorder. The role of the serotonin transporter (5-HTT) gene is controversial with evidence for [36, 39, 45–47] as well as against association with panic disorder [48–51]. Social phobia has been found to be associated with variation in the 5-HT_{2A} gene [52], generalized anxiety disorder with a functional MAO-A gene polymorphism [53]. In PTSD, evidence has been provided for the 5-HTT [54–56] and the 5-HT_{2A} gene [57] to constitute potential risk factors. Finally, there is some support for variation in the norepinephrine transporter gene to be associated with panic disorder [58–60].

Dopamine System Genes

The probably best replicated vulnerability gene for panic disorder is the gene coding for the catechol-O-methyltransferase (COMT). Mostly in the subgroup of female patients, the functional val158met polymorphism has been found to be associated with the disease, potentially in an ethnically specific manner [61–66]. Association of COMT gene variation has also been reported in specific phobias [67]. Furthermore, the dopamine D1 receptor has been discerned to confer some vulnerability to panic disorder [39]. In social phobia and generalized anxiety disorder, variants in the dopamine transporter (DAT1) have been proposed to contribute to the disease risk [68]. In PTSD, association has been reported again for the COMT gene [69] and the dopamine D_2 receptor (DRD2) gene [70], with some support for DRD2 to specifically mediate severe comorbid psychopathology (anxiety, depression) and social dysfunction in PTSD subjects [71]. The DAT1 gene has also been found to be associated with PTSD, with, however, also contradictory reports of no association [72–75].

Cholecystokinin System Genes
Given accumulating evidence for cholecystokinin (CCK) in playing an important role with regard to neuroanatomical circuits and neurotransmitters involved in the pathophysiology of panic and anxiety [see 76, 77], molecular genetic studies have focused on several CCK-related gene loci such as the CCK gene itself, the CCK receptor 1 (CCKAR) gene and the CCK receptor 2 (CCKBR) gene. Association has been reported for the CCK gene in panic disorder [78–80] as well as in a broader panic disorder phenotype [39]. Also, variation in the CCKAR [81, 82] and CCKBR [39, 83–86] (but [87]) genes seems to contribute to the genetic susceptibility to panic disorder, potentially particularly to panic disorder with comorbid bipolar disorder [85].

Adenosine System Genes
The adenosinergic system has been implied in the pathogenesis of anxiety in animal models, and the adenosine A2A receptor antagonist caffeine is a potent anxiogenic and arousal-increasing substance [88–90]. Accordingly, variation in the adenosine A2A receptor *(ADORA2A)* gene has been found to be associated with panic disorder [88, 91–93] and to influence anxiety levels also in other psychiatric phenotypes such as autism spectrum disorder [94] and in healthy individuals [91].

GABAergic System Genes
Given the highly potent anxiolytic effect of benzodiazepines acting at the γ-aminobutyric acid (GABA) receptor, the GABAergic system has been proposed to be crucially involved in the pathogenesis of anxiety disorders [95]. However, there is only sparse and not robustly replicated evidence from molecular genetic studies for a potential role of genes coding for the glutamate decarboxylase, GABA receptors, GABA transporters, the peripheral benzodiazepine receptor or the diazepam binding inhibitor in panic disorder or PTSD [96–103].

Hypothalamus-Pituitary-Adrenal Axis-Related Genes
Genes related to the hypothalamus-pituitary-adrenal axis and therefore supposed to be involved in the mediation of stress response have constituted another major focus in molecular genetic association analyses of anxiety disorders: the corticotropin-releasing

hormone and the corticotropin releasing hormone 1 receptor (CRHR1) genes have been found to be associated with panic disorder and behavioral inhibition as an anxiety trait predisposing to panic [104–106]. Furthermore, CRHR1 gene variants were observed to predict PTSD onset and course in pediatric injury patients [107]. The FKBP5 gene – coding for a cochaperone protein influencing glucocorticoid receptor sensitivity – has been found to be associated with PTSD [69, 108], plasma cortisol and PTSD severity [109] as well as specific types of hypothalamic-pituitary-adrenal axis dysfunction within PTSD [110]. Finally, a variant in a putative estrogen response element within the ADCYAP1R1 gene, coding for the receptor of the pituitary adenylate cyclase-activating polypeptide, was associated with PTSD particularly in female patients [111].

Other Candidate Genes

Apart from support for the 'prime suspect' candidate genes in anxiety disorders as detailed above, there is accumulating evidence for other systems to also contribute to the genetic vulnerability toward anxiety disorders: robust association with panic disorder has for instance been reported for the angiotensin converting enzyme (ACE) gene [112–115], the genes for the regulator of G-protein signaling proteins RGS2 and RGS7 [116–118] and the neuropeptide S receptor (NPSR1) gene [119–121]. Single studies provide additional, however, not unequivocally replicated support for the following genes to potentially contribute to panic disorder susceptibility: cyclo-AMP responsive element modulator' gene [122, 123], galanin gene [124], neuropeptide Y 5 receptor gene [125] and genes coding for several hormone receptors [126–128]. The endocannabinoid system has been in the focus of attention with association of variation in the cannabinoid receptor gene observed in PTSD [129]. Finally, the RGS2 gene has been found to be associated with generalized anxiety disorder in a sample of hurricane-exposed individuals [130].

Gene-Gene Interaction Studies

Epistatic effects in the pathogenesis of anxiety disorders as expected in a polygenetic disease model have been explored in only few studies so far: gene-gene interaction has been reported for the 5-HT$_{1A}$ and the COMT genes [131], while no epistasis could be discerned for the 5-HTT gene and the MAO-A gene [132].

In summary, molecular genetic association studies have yielded evidence for several vulnerability genes of anxiety disorder with most robust evidence for the 5-HT$_{1A}$, 5-HTT, MAO-A, COMT, CCK-B, ADORA2A, CRHR1, FKBP5, ACE, RGS2/7 and NPSR1 genes. It has to be noted, though, that for all association findings in anxiety disorders there are also reports of nonreplication or association of the opposite allele, rendering most findings to be subject to reevaluation in larger, better defined samples of patients (for a comprehensive overview of association studies, see Maron et al. [133] and Hamilton [134]).

Genome-Wide Association Studies

Genome-wide association studies (GWAS), interrogating the entire genome for association applying a hypothesis-free approach, have been suggested to aid in the more robust identification of risk variants and at the same time in discerning novel vulnerability genes for complex-genetic disorders. To date, four GWAS have been published in panic disorder: a Japanese group reported evidence for markers in novel candidate genes to increase the disease risk (PKP1, PLEKHG1, TMEM16B, CALCOCO1, SDK2 and CLU), which, however, could not be replicated in an independent sample [135, 136]. A potential role of variation in the TMEM132D gene in the pathogenesis of panic disorder has been reported in a GWAS analyzing a German sample, which could be further corroborated by functional expression analyses and in an animal model of anxiety [137]. In an isolated population of the Faroe Islands, a recent GWAS suggested the amiloride-sensitive cation channel 1 (ACCN1) as a novel candidate gene for panic disorder [138].

Gene-Environment Interaction Studies

Heritability estimates for anxiety disorders ranging from 30 to 67% point to a considerable contribution of genetic factors to the pathogenesis of the disorders; however, at the same time they imply that the remainder of the variance (~30–70%) can be attributed to environmental factors such as abuse [139, 140], loss/separation experiences in childhood [141, 142] or recent stressful life events [143, for review see 144]. Thus, in order to disentangle the complex genetic nature of anxiety disorders, the search for vulnerability genes applying molecular genetic approaches has to be complemented by so-called gene-environment interaction (G × E) studies investigating the interplay of genetic factors and environmental factors.

Anxiety sensitivity, a trait predisposing to anxiety disorders, has been found to be interactively influenced by e.g. serotonin transporter gene (5-HTTLPR) variation and childhood traumata [145, 146] as well as by variation in the NPSR1 gene and proximal/distal stressful life events [147]. The functional 5-HTTLPR variant was furthermore reported to increase the overall risk for anxiety disorders in interaction with high family adversity [148]. Generalized anxiety disorder has been observed to be interactively influenced by neuropeptide Y gene variation and hurricane exposure [149]. PTSD – obviously being influenced by traumatic environmental factors in addition to a genetic vulnerability – has been subject to most G × E studies published in the field of anxiety disorders so far: the risk for PTSD has been found to be interactively increased by variation in the 5-HTT gene and traumatic events [150–153] as well as genetic variation in FKBP5 and child abuse severity [108, 154]. Further G × E interaction in PTSD has been observed for variation in the genes for RGS2 [155], GABRA2 [96], DBH [156] and COMT [157, for review see 158].

Epigenetic Studies

Epigenetic mechanisms such as methylation of the cytosine pyrimidine ring in CpG dinucleotides mainly 'silencing' DNA transcription [159] have been shown to critically influence gene regulation and to constitute biological correlates of adjustment to stressful environmental influences [160, 161]. Thus, the investigation of epigenetic markers is essential for a more comprehensive understanding of G × E interaction in the pathogenesis of complex genetic, temporally dynamic nosological entities such as anxiety disorders [162, 163]. To date, most epigenetic studies in anxiety have been conducted with respect to the categorical phenotype of PTSD: here, a differential methylation status in genes involved in the immune system has been reported to be associated with the disorder [164, 165]. Also, higher methylation in the MAN2C1 gene [166] or lower 5-HTT methylation, respectively [167], and greater exposure to potentially traumatic events have been shown to interactively increase the risk for PTSD. In panic disorder, a recent pilot study identified DNA hypomethylation of the MAO-A gene to be associated with the disease particularly in female patients. Furthermore, MAO-A gene hypomethylation in female subjects seemed to correlate with the occurrence of negative life events prior to inclusion in the study, while positive life events were rather associated with increased methylation [168]. In summary, these first epigenetic studies point to a crucial role of epigenetic processes in the mediation of environmental influences in anxiety disorders. However, since peripheral methylation patterns as investigated in most presently available studies might not necessarily reflect cerebral or even region-specific cerebral patterns of methylation, future studies will have to apply translational as well as functional approaches in animal and human studies to further investigate the role of epigenetic mechanisms in the pathogenesis of anxiety disorders.

Genetic Studies in Intermediate Phenotypes

The influence of genetic factors on complex traits or diseases can be further specified by investigation of so-called intermediate phenotypes, which due to a more narrow definition have been proposed to be closer to the underlying genetic risk factors [169]. Several neuropsychological traits such as behavioral inhibition [104, 105, 170] or anxiety sensitivity [171–173] as well as a variety of neurobiological markers (e.g. peripheral sympathetic activity, carbon dioxide reactivity, response to CCK challenge, startle reflex, neural activation correlates of emotional processing) have been suggested as valid intermediate phenotypes of anxiety disorders. Genetic association studies with respect to neurobiological intermediate phenotypes of anxiety disorders will be reviewed in more detail below.

Peripheral Sympathetic Activity

Regarding neurophysiological measures as intermediate phenotypes of anxiety disorders, an altered sympathovagal balance with relatively decreased parasympathetic activity based on heart rate variability analysis has been reported to be influenced by the functional brain-derived neurotrophic factor (BDNF) val66met polymorphism [174]. In blood-injury phobia, sympathetic activity reflected by an increased respiratory rate and a trend towards elevated measures of systolic/diastolic blood pressure and respiratory minute volume was associated with variation in the ADORA2A gene [175]. The functional 5-HTTLPR serotonin transporter gene variant has been found to drive blushing propensity as measured by the blushing propensity scale in patients with social anxiety disorder [176]. Finally, increased heart rate during a behavioral avoidance test was reported to be associated with the risk allele of a functional NPSR1 gene variant [121].

Carbon Dioxide Reactivity

Laboratory panic challenge models used in the investigation of panic phenomenology may help in testing the premises of genetic predisposition to panic. At least one third of control subjects with no mental disorder show a panic-like response to challenge agents, suggesting endophenotypic markers for vulnerability to panic behavior. One of the well-established panicogenic laboratory tests is a challenge test with 35% carbon dioxide challenge, which has been proposed to constitute a valid intermediate phenotype of anxiety disorders such as panic disorder, social anxiety disorder or PTSD with a considerable familiality/heritability [177–183]. There is preliminary support for functional variation in the 5-HTT gene to drive interindividual differences in CO_2 reactivity [184], with, however, several studies failing to detect this effect [185, 186].

Cholecystokinin Challenge

Another anxiety-relevant challenge test uses an agonist at the central subtype of CCK receptor, CCK-4, that produces panic attacks in up to 100% of patients with panic disorder and, depending on the dose, in up to 50% of healthy subjects [76, 77]. Initial findings on the associations between 5-HTTLPR, MAO-A uVNTR and panic responses to a CCK-4 challenge test in a small sample (n = 32) were not confirmed in a consequent larger sample (n = 110) of healthy subjects [187, 188]. In the latter study, only one of the 9 gene candidates previously implicated in panic disorder showed effects on the susceptibility to CCK-4 challenge. Specifically, the TPH2 gene variant rs1386494 was associated with panic attack rates in healthy females [188], supporting a previous finding of association between this polymorphism and panic disorder in female patients [43]. Furthermore, analysis of peripheral gene expression markers seems very promising as it may provide further insight into genetic substrates of panic response. In a recent study, the microarray Illumina platform was applied for whole genome expression profiling in healthy subjects participating in a CCK-4 challenge test [189]. In the first stage of this study, at least 61 genes were found to be differentially expressed between the CCK-4 panickers (n = 18) and nonpanickers (n = 13), a substantial fraction of which belonged to the mRNA transcripts of the interferon gene group or to genes involved in immune response, whereas others were related to clinical phenotypes of asthma (PHF11), diabetes (OAS1), and coronary artery disease (CCL2). Notably, all these medical conditions are associated with the occurrence of panic attacks. In the second stage, the transcriptional levels of 226 genes showed changes 2 h after CCK-4 challenge. Most of these transcripts could be grouped as related to immune, enzymatic or stress regulation systems. Such a broad physiological response seems plausible considering the acute and stressful nature of panic attacks. Importantly, both Maron et al. [189] and Philibert et al. [190] detected changes in the expression level of sterol regulatory element-binding transcription factor 2 (SREBF2) gene, which is located on the chromosome region 22q13 and is known to regulate cholesterol homeostasis. Alterations in cholesterol levels have been implicated in both panic disorder and pentagastrin-induced panic attacks [191–193], suggesting that SREBF2 gene could be a target for association studies in panic disorder. Interestingly, some markers of SREBF2 gene were associated with schizophrenia in a German as well as in a Scandinavian sample [194], whereas the somatostatin receptor 3 gene, which is also located in the 22q13 region, recently showed at least nominal association with panic disorder [86]. Taken together, the analysis of peripheral gene expression may extend our knowledge of the genetic basis underlying panic phenomenology and point to the biological proximity between panicogenesis and several medical conditions, which may be important in the search for new research and treatment targets.

Startle Reflex

The acoustic startle reflex has been proposed to constitute a neurobiologically founded defensive response potentially intermediately related to anxiety-related states [195]. Several hundred studies in animals and humans have investigated the genetic underpinnings of the startle reflex so far [for reviews see 196, 197]. For example, greater acoustic startle responses – partly in response to unpleasant emotional stimuli in an affect-modulated startle or fear-potentiated startle paradigm – were found to be influenced by the functional COMT val158met polymorphism [198] and a functional variant in the serotonin transporter gene (5-HTTLPR) [199–202]. The risk genotype of an ADORA2A variant – previously observed to be associated with increased anxiety after caffeine administration in healthy volunteers [203–205] – potentiated the acoustic startle reflex in interaction with caffeine administration and processing of stressful emotional stimuli [206].

Neural activation correlates of emotional processing as captured by functional imaging techniques such as functional magnetic resonance imaging have been proposed as another interesting intermediate phenotype of mental disorders viable to genetic analyses applying an imaging genetic approach [207]. Imaging genetic studies investigating the genetic underpinnings of the fear circuit in patients with panic disorder have observed variation in the COMT and the NPSR1 genes to increase amygdala activity in response to anxiety-relevant emotional stimuli [121, 208]. NPSR1 and $5-HT_{1A}$ gene variation additionally decreased pre-/orbitofrontal or cingulate responsiveness to fear-relevant stimuli in panic disorder [121, 209]. In social phobia, 5-HTT and TPH gene variation has been reported to drive amygdala excitability during processing of phobia-relevant emotional stimuli [210–212]. Limbic activation during emotional processing was furthermore found to be influenced by variation in the RGS2 gene, a risk factor for behavioral inhibition [117]. In summary, results emerging from these first imaging genetics studies in anxiety disorders or anxiety-related traits may indicate that COMT, NPSR1, $5-HT_{1A}$, 5-HTT, TPH and RGS2 gene variation potentially contributes to the pathogenesis of anxiety disorders by shaping corticolimbic activity during fear-related emotional processing [for review see 213].

Pharmacogenetic and Psychotherapy-Genetic Studies

The relatively high rate of nonresponse to an initial pharmacotherapy with e.g. selective serotonin reuptake inhibitors (SSRI) or serotonin and norepinephrine reuptake inhibitors of about 20–40% has been suggested to be due to several factors such as age, duration of illness, psychiatric and somatic comorbidity as well as personality traits [214], as well as genetic factors as first-degree relative pairs were found to be highly concordant for antidepressant treatment response [215, 216]. Thus, besides the investigation of the genetic underpinnings of the pathogenesis of anxiety disorders, genetic research can also contribute to unraveling interindividual differences in response to pharmaco- or psychotherapeutic interventions by applying a pharmacogenetic approach.

First pharmacogenetic studies in anxiety disorders report evidence for a significant influence of the functional 5-HTTLPR serotonin transporter polymorphism on response to SSRIs in panic disorder as well as in generalized social phobia [217–219]. Response to paroxetine in panic disorder has been shown to be partly driven by functional variation in the $5-HT_{1A}$ gene [220, 221]. In generalized anxiety disorder, there is evidence for a potential role of the $5-HT_{2A}$ [222], the 5-HTT [223] and CRHR1 [224] genes in the mediation of treatment response to venlafaxine, escitalopram or duloxetine, respectively. The first psychotherapy-genetic study in panic disorder reported a significant influence of the functional COMT val158met polymorphism on response to cognitive behavioral therapy [225].

Discussion and Outlook

The presently available clinical genetic studies point to a considerable heritability of anxiety disorders (30–67%), with multiple vulnerability genes such as 5-HT$_{1A}$, 5-HTT, MAO-A, COMT, CCK-B, ADORA2A, CRHR1, FKBP5, ACE, RGS2/7 and NPSR1 emerging from molecular genetic association studies. These genes have been shown to partially interact with each other (COMT/5-HT$_{1A}$) as well as with environmental factors to shape the overall disease risk in a complex-genetic model. Additionally, recent studies have pointed out the crucial role of epigenetic signatures such as methylation patterns in modifying environmental influences as well as in driving the functional impact of anxiety disorder risk genes. On a systems level, vulnerability genes of anxiety disorders seem to confer some of the disease risk via intermediate phenotypes like behavioral inhibition, anxiety sensitivity or several neurobiological susceptibility traits such as increased startle reactivity, CCK-4 challenge response or dysfunctional corticolimbic activity during emotional processing. Finally, emerging pharmaco- and psychotherapy genetic studies provide evidence for certain risk genes to confer inter-individual variability in response to a pharmacological or psychotherapeutic intervention in anxiety disorders.

However, to date the identified genetic risk factors are of no diagnostic or predictive value, as the field is far from having identified the entirety of all genetic and epigenetic risk factors interdependent with environmental factors. Technical advances in genetic research might aid in elucidating the missing heritability of anxiety disorders. For instance, there are first studies providing support for genetic variation in micro-RNA genes miR-22 and miR-339 as well as miR-138-2, miR-488, miR-491 and miR-148a to be associated with panic disorder and to functionally regulate several candidate genes of the disorder such as GABRA6, CCKBR, POMC, BDNF, HTR2C, MAO-A and RGS2 [226]. Furthermore, copy number variations (CNV), i.e. deletions/duplications of large parts of the genome, are presently subject to investigation in neuropsychiatric phenotypes [227], with, however, to date no evidence for an increased genome-wide rare CNV burden in patients with panic disorder [228]. Furthermore, novel methods such as pathway-based analyses [229] or next generation sequencing techniques such as exome sequencing [230, 231] have been proven to be generally applicable to complex-genetic disorders. A first pilot pathway-based study in anxiety and depression phenotypes points to a dysregulation of carbohydrate metabolism, tight junction and phosphatidylinositol signaling pathways in anxiety [232]. Furthermore, more detailed G × E interaction studies are warranted preferably in a genome-wide fashion [233, 234] and taking into account epigenetic factors in order to disentangle the interactive effect of genetic and environmental factors conferring risk or resilience, respectively, to anxiety disorders in a more specific way. Finally, it will be worthwhile to combine epigenetic analyses with intermediate phenotype approaches e.g. to 'imaging epigenetic studies' as successfully demonstrated in a landmark study by Ursini et al. [235], who reported stress-related methylation of the COMT gene to influence human brain physiology related to working memory performance. On a phenotypic level, investigation of more targeted intermediate phenotypes of specific anxiety disorders such as interoceptive sensitivity in panic disorder [236] or conditioning processes in specific phobias [237] might aid in the identification of specific anxiety disorder risk genes and their functional relevance. In parallel, given the common genetic trunk theory of mental disorders, so-called cross-disorders analyses might reveal common variants to confer susceptibility to several related psychiatric disorders, e.g. first evidence has been reported for the bradykinin receptor B2 gene to be associated with three disorders (panic disorder, substance abuse, and bipolar disorder) [86].

This variety of genetic approaches to unravel the pathogenesis of anxiety disorders is hoped to nourish the development of innovative pharmacotherapeutic substances in the treatment of anxiety disorders, e.g. targeting the neuropeptide S system [238] or modulating epigenetic patterns [239]. Additionally, pharmacogenetic and psychotherapy genetic research might eventually aid in the design of personalized and thereby more efficient therapeutic approaches individually tailored to the individual patient's constellation of genetic and environmental risk factors. It has to be noted, though, that these advances in genetic methodology allowing for increasing revelation of the genetic underpinnings of mental disorders has to be accompanied by strict national and international regulations about stigmatization, privacy confidentiality and data protection [240, 241].

Acknowledgements

The present work has been supported by the Deutsche Forschungsgemeinschaft (SFB-TRR-58, project C2; K.D.).

References

1 Maier W, Lichtermann D, Minges J, Oehrlein A, Franke P: A controlled family study in panic disorder. J Psychiatr Res 1993;27:79–87.

2 Hettema JM, Neale MC, Kendler KS: A review and meta-analysis of the genetic epidemiology of anxiety disorders. Am J Psychiatry 2001;158:1568–1578.

3 Yehuda R, Bell A, Bierer LM, Schmeidler J: Maternal, not paternal, PTSD is related to increased risk for PTSD in offspring of Holocaust survivors. J Psychiatr Res 2008;42:1104–1111.

4 Goldstein RB, Wickramaratne PJ, Horwath E, Weissman MM: Familial aggregation and phenomenology of 'early'-onset (at or before age 20 years) panic disorder. Arch Gen Psychiatry 1997;54:271–278.

5 Segman RH, Shalev AY: Genetics of posttraumatic stress disorder. CNS Spectr 2003;8:693–698.

6 Kendler KS, Karkowski LM, Prescott CA: Fears and phobias: reliability and heritability. Psychol Med 1999;29:539–553.

7 Vieland VJ, Goodman DW, Chapman T, Fyer AJ: New segregation analysis of panic disorder. Am J Med Genet 1996;67:147–153.

8 Crowe RR, Noyes R Jr, Wilson AF, Elston RC, Ward LJ: A linkage study of panic disorder. Arch Gen Psychiatry 1987;44:933–937.

9 Crowe RR, Goedken R, Samuelson S, Wilson R, Nelson J, Noyes R Jr: Genomewide survey of panic disorder. Am J Med Genet 2001;105:105–109.

10 Knowles JA, Fyer AJ, Vieland VJ, et al: Results of a genome-wide genetic screen for panic disorder. Am J Med Genet 1998;81:139–147.

11 Gelernter J, Bonvicini K, Page G, Woods SW, Goddard AW, Kruger S, Pauls DL, Goodson S: Linkage genome scan for loci predisposing to panic disorder or agoraphobia. Am J Med Genet 2001;105:548–557.

12 Hamilton SP, Fyer AJ, Durner M, Heiman GA, Baisre de LA, Hodge SE, Knowles JA, Weissman MM: Further genetic evidence for a panic disorder syndrome mapping to chromosome 13q. Proc Natl Acad Sci USA 2003;100:2550–2555.

13 Thorgeirsson TE, Oskarsson H, Desnica N, Kostic JP, Stefansson JG, Kolbeinsson H, Lindal E, Gagunashvili N, Frigge ML, Kong A, Stefansson K, Gulcher JR: Anxiety with panic disorder linked to chromosome 9q in Iceland. Am J Hum Genet 2003; 72:1221–1230.

14 Fyer AJ, Hamilton SP, Durner M, Haghighi F, Heiman GA, Costa R, Evgrafov O, Adams P, De Leon AB, Taveras N, Klein DF, Hodge SE, Weissman MM, Knowles JA: A third-pass genome scan in panic disorder: evidence for multiple susceptibility loci. Biol Psychiatry 2006;60:388–401.

15 Kaabi B, Gelernter J, Woods SW, Goddard A, Page GP, Elston RC: Genome scan for loci predisposing to anxiety disorders using a novel multivariate approach: strong evidence for a chromosome 4 risk locus. Am J Hum Genet 2006;78:543–553.

16 Logue MW, Bauver SR, Knowles JA, Gameroff MJ, Weissman MM, Crowe RR, Fyer AJ, Hamilton SP: Multivariate analysis of anxiety disorders yields further evidence of linkage to chromosomes 4q21 and 7p in panic disorder families. Am J Med Genet B Neuropsychiatr Genet 2012;159B:274–280.

17 Gelernter J, Page GP, Bonvicini K, Woods SW, Pauls DL, Kruger S: A chromosome 14 risk locus for simple phobia: results from a genomewide linkage scan. Mol Psychiatry 2003;8:71–82.

18 Gelernter J, Page GP, Stein MB, Woods SW: Genome-wide linkage scan for loci predisposing to social phobia: evidence for a chromosome 16 risk locus. Am J Psychiatry 2004;161:59–66.

19 Middeldorp CM, Hottenga JJ, Slagboom PE, Sullivan PF, de Geus EJ, Posthuma D, Willemsen G, Boomsma DI: Linkage on chromosome 14 in a genome-wide linkage study of a broad anxiety phenotype. Mol Psychiatry 2008;13:84–89.

20 Logue MW, Durner M, Heiman GA, Hodge SE, Hamilton SP, Knowles JA, Fyer AJ, Weissman MM: A linkage search for joint panic disorder/bipolar genes. Am J Med Genet B Neuropsychiatr Genet 2009;150B:1139–1146.

21 MacKinnon DF, Xu J, McMahon FJ, Simpson SG, Stine OC, McInnis MG, DePaulo JR: Bipolar disorder and panic disorder in families: an analysis of chromosome 18 data. Am J Psychiatry 1998;155: 829–831.

22 Talati A, Ponniah K, Strug LJ, Hodge SE, Fyer AJ, Weissman MM: Panic disorder, social anxiety disorder, and a possible medical syndrome previously linked to chromosome 13. Biol Psychiatry 2008;63: 594–601.

23 Weissman MM, Fyer AJ, Haghighi F, Heiman G, Deng Z, Hen R, Hodge SE, Knowles JA: Potential panic disorder syndrome: clinical and genetic linkage evidence. Am J Med Genet 2000;96:24–35.

24 Weissman MM, Gross R, Fyer A, Heiman GA, Gameroff MJ, Hodge SE, Kaufman D, Kaplan SA, Wickramaratne PJ: Interstitial cystitis and panic disorder: a potential genetic syndrome. Arch Gen Psychiatry 2004;61:273–279.

25 Smoller JW, Acierno JS Jr, Rosenbaum JF, Biederman J, Pollack MH, Meminger S, Pava JA, Chadwick LH, White C, Bulzacchelli M, Slaugenhaupt SA: Targeted genome screen of panic disorder and anxiety disorder proneness using homology to murine QTL regions. Am J Med Genet 2001;105:195–206.

26 Smoller JW, Gardner-Schuster E, Covino J: The genetic basis of panic and phobic anxiety disorders. Am J Med Genet C Semin Med Genet 2008; 148C:118–126.

27 Gratacos M, Nadal M, Martin-Santos R, Pujana MA, Gago J, Peral B, Armengol L, Ponsa I, Miro R, Bulbena A, Estivill X: A polymorphic genomic duplication on human chromosome 15 is a susceptibility factor for panic and phobic disorders. Cell 2001;106: 367–379.

28 Armengol L, Gratacos M, Pujana MA, Ribases M, Martin-Santos R, Estivill X: 5′ UTR-region SNP in the NTRK3 gene is associated with panic disorder. Mol Psychiatry 2002;7:928–930.

29 Henrichsen CN, Delorme R, Boucherie M, Marelli D, Baud P, Bellivier F, Courtet P, Chabane N, Henry C, Leboyer M, Malafosse A, Antonarakis SE, Dahoun S: No association between DUP25 and anxiety disorders. Am J Med Genet B Neuropsychiatr Genet 2004; 128B:80–83.

30 Zhu G, Bartsch O, Skrypnyk C, Rotondo A, Akhtar LA, Harris C, Virkkunen M, Cassano G, Goldman D: Failure to detect DUP25 in lymphoblastoid cells derived from patients with panic disorder and control individuals representing European and American populations. Eur J Hum Genet 2004;12:505–508.

31 Schumacher J, Otte AC, Becker T, Sun Y, Wienker TF, Wirth B, Franke P, Abou JR, Propping P, Deckert J, Nothen MM, Cichon S: No evidence for DUP25 in patients with panic disorder using a quantitative real-time PCR approach. Hum Genet 2003;114:115–117.

32 Tabiner M, Youings S, Dennis N, Baldwin D, Buis C, Mayers A, Jacobs PA, Crolla JA: Failure to find DUP25 in patients with anxiety disorders, in control individuals, or in previously reported positive control cell lines. Am J Hum Genet 2003;72:535–538.

33 Maron E, Shlik J: Serotonin function in panic disorder: important, but why? Neuropsychopharmacology 2006;31:1–11.

34 Deckert J, Catalano M, Syagailo YV, Bosi M, Oklandnova O, Di BD, Nothen MM, Maffei P, Franke P, Fritze J, Maier W, Propping P, Beckmann H, Bellodi L, Lesch KP: Excess of high activity monoamine oxidase A gene promoter alleles in female patients with panic disorder. Hum Mol Genet 1999;8:621–624.

35 Samochowiec J, Hajduk A, Samochowiec A, Horodnicki J, Stepien G, Grzywacz A, Kucharska-Mazur J: Association studies of MAO-A, COMT, and 5-HTT genes polymorphisms in patients with anxiety disorders of the phobic spectrum. Psychiatry Res 2004; 128:21–26.

36 Maron E, Lang A, Tasa G, Liivlaid L, Toru I, Must A, Vasar V, Shlik J: Associations between serotonin-related gene polymorphisms and panic disorder. Int J Neuropsychopharmacol 2005;8:261–266.

37 Rothe C, Gutknecht L, Freitag C, Tauber R, Mossner R, Franke P, Fritze J, Wagner G, Peikert G, Wenda B, Sand P, Jacob C, Rietschel M, Nothen MM, Garritsen H, Fimmers R, Deckert J, Lesch KP: Association of a functional 1019C>G 5-HT1A receptor gene polymorphism with panic disorder with agoraphobia. Int J Neuropsychopharmacol 2004;7:189–192.

38 Huang YY, Battistuzzi C, Oquendo MA, Harkavy-Friedman J, Greenhill L, Zalsman G, Brodsky B, Arango V, Brent DA, Mann JJ: Human 5-HT1A receptor C(-1019)G polymorphism and psychopathology. Int J Neuropsychopharmacol 2004;7:441–451.

39 Maron E, Nikopensius T, Koks S, Altmae S, Heinaste E, Vabrit K, Tammekivi V, Hallast P, Koido K, Kurg A, Metspalu A, Vasar E, Vasar V, Shlik J: Association study of 90 candidate gene polymorphisms in panic disorder. Psychiatr Genet 2005;15:17–24.

40 Inada Y, Yoneda H, Koh J, Sakai J, Himei A, Kinoshita Y, Akabame K, Hiraoka Y, Sakai T: Positive association between panic disorder and polymorphism of the serotonin 2A receptor gene. Psychiatry Res 2003;118:25–31.

41 Unschuld PG, Ising M, Erhardt A, Lucae S, Kloiber S, Kohli M, Salyakina D, Welt T, Kern N, Lieb R, Uhr M, Binder EB, Muller-Myhsok B, Holsboer F, Keck ME: Polymorphisms in the serotonin receptor gene HTR2A are associated with quantitative traits in panic disorder. Am J Med Genet B Neuropsychiatr Genet 2007;144B:424–429.

42 Yoon HK, Yang JC, Lee HJ, Kim YK: The association between serotonin-related gene polymorphisms and panic disorder. J Anxiety Disord 2008;22:1529–1534.

43 Maron E, Toru I, Must A, Tasa G, Toover E, Vasar V, Lang A, Shlik J: Association study of tryptophan hydroxylase 2 gene polymorphisms in panic disorder. Neurosci Lett 2007;411:180–184.

44 Kim YK, Lee HJ, Yang JC, Hwang JA, Yoon HK: A tryptophan hydroxylase 2 gene polymorphism is associated with panic disorder. Behav Genet 2009;39: 170–175.

45 Ohara K, Nagai M, Suzuki Y, Ochiai M, Ohara K: Association between anxiety disorders and a functional polymorphism in the serotonin transporter gene. Psychiatry Res 1998;81:277–279.

46 Strug LJ, Suresh R, Fyer AJ, Talati A, Adams PB, Li W, Hodge SE, Gilliam TC, Weissman MM: Panic disorder is associated with the serotonin transporter gene (SLC6A4) but not the promoter region (5-HTTLPR). Mol Psychiatry 2010;15:166–176.

47 Gyawali S, Subaran R, Weissman MM, Hershkowitz D, McKenna MC, Talati A, Fyer AJ, Wickramaratne P, Adams PB, Hodge SE, Schmidt CJ, Bannon MJ, Glatt CE: Association of a polyadenylation polymorphism in the serotonin transporter and panic disorder. Biol Psychiatry 2010;67:331–338.

48 Deckert J, Catalano M, Heils A, Di BD, Friess F, Politi E, Franke P, Nothen MM, Maier W, Bellodi L, Lesch KP: Functional promoter polymorphism of the human serotonin transporter: lack of association with panic disorder. Psychiatr Genet 1997;7: 45–47.

49 Blaya C, Salum GA, Lima MS, Leistner-Segal S, Manfro GG: Lack of association between the serotonin transporter promoter polymorphism (5-HTTLPR) and panic disorder: a systematic review and meta-analysis. Behav Brain Funct 2007;3:41.

50 Hamilton SP, Heiman GA, Haghighi F, Mick S, Klein DF, Hodge SE, Weissman MM, Fyer AJ, Knowles JA: Lack of genetic linkage or association between a functional serotonin transporter polymorphism and panic disorder. Psychiatr Genet 1999;9:1–6.

51 Schumacher J, Deckert J: Serotonin transporter polymorphisms and panic disorder. Genome Med 2010; 2:40.

52 Lochner C, Hemmings S, Seedat S, Kinnear C, Schoeman R, Annerbrink K, Olsson M, Eriksson E, Moolman-Smook J, Allgulander C, Stein DJ: Genetics and personality traits in patients with social anxiety disorder: a case-control study in South Africa. Eur Neuropsychopharmacol 2007;17:321–327.

53 Tadic A, Rujescu D, Szegedi A, Giegling I, Singer P, Moller HJ, Dahmen N: Association of a MAOA gene variant with generalized anxiety disorder, but not with panic disorder or major depression. Am J Med Genet B Neuropsychiatr Genet 2003;117B:1–6.

54 Lee HJ, Lee MS, Kang RH, Kim H, Kim SD, Kee BS, Kim YH, Kim YK, Kim JB, Yeon BK, Oh KS, Oh BH, Yoon JS, Lee C, Jung HY, Chee IS, Paik IH: Influence of the serotonin transporter promoter gene polymorphism on susceptibility to posttraumatic stress disorder. Depress Anxiety 2005;21: 135–139.

55 Mercer KB, Orcutt HK, Quinn JF, Fitzgerald CA, Conneely KN, Barfield RT, Gillespie CF, Ressler KJ: Acute and posttraumatic stress symptoms in a prospective gene × environment study of a university campus shooting. Arch Gen Psychiatry 2012;69:89–97.

56 Wang Z, Baker DG, Harrer J, Hamner M, Price M, Amstadter A: The relationship between combat-related posttraumatic stress disorder and the 5-HTTLPR/rs25531 polymorphism. Depress Anxiety 2011;28:1067–1073.

57 Mellman TA, Alim T, Brown DD, Gorodetsky E, Buzas B, Lawson WB, Goldman D, Charney DS: Serotonin polymorphisms and posttraumatic stress disorder in a trauma exposed African American population. Depress Anxiety 2009;26:993–997.

58 Lee YJ, Hohoff C, Domschke K, Sand P, Kuhlenbaumer G, Schirmacher A, Freitag CM, Meyer J, Stober G, Franke P, Nothen MM, Fritze J, Fimmers R, Garritsen HS, Stogbauer F, Deckert J: Norepinephrine transporter (NET) promoter and 5′-UTR polymorphisms: association analysis in panic disorder. Neurosci Lett 2005;377:40–43.

59 Sand PG, Mori T, Godau C, Stober G, Flachenecker P, Franke P, Nothen MM, Fritze J, Maier W, Lesch KP, Riederer P, Beckmann H, Deckert J: Norepinephrine transporter gene (NET) variants in patients with panic disorder. Neurosci Lett 2002;333:41–44.

60 Buttenschon HN, Kristensen AS, Buch HN, Andersen JH, Bonde JP, Grynderup M, Hansen AM, Kolstad H, Kaergaard A, Kaerlev L, Mikkelsen S, Thomsen JF, Koefoed P, Erhardt A, Woldbye DP, Borglum AD, Mors O: The norepinephrine transporter gene is a candidate gene for panic disorder. J Neural Transm 2011;118:969–976.

61 Hamilton SP, Slager SL, Heiman GA, Deng Z, Haghighi F, Klein DF, Hodge SE, Weissman MM, Fyer AJ, Knowles JA: Evidence for a susceptibility locus for panic disorder near the catechol-O-methyltransferase gene on chromosome 22. Biol Psychiatry 2002;51:591–601.

62 Domschke K, Freitag CM, Kuhlenbaumer G, Schirmacher A, Sand P, Nyhuis P, Jacob C, Fritze J, Franke P, Rietschel M, Garritsen HS, Fimmers R, Nothen MM, Lesch KP, Stogbauer F, Deckert J: Association of the functional V158M catechol-O-methyl-transferase polymorphism with panic disorder in women. Int J Neuropsychopharmacol 2004;7:183–188.

63 Domschke K, Deckert J, O'donovan MC, Glatt SJ: Meta-analysis of COMT val158met in panic disorder: ethnic heterogeneity and gender specificity. Am J Med Genet B Neuropsychiatr Genet 2007;144B:667–673.

64 Zintzaras E, Sakelaridis N: Is 472G/A catechol-O-methyl-transferase gene polymorphism related to panic disorder? Psychiatr Genet 2007;17:267–273.

65 Woo JM, Yoon KS, Choi YH, Oh KS, Lee YS, Yu BH: The association between panic disorder and the L/L genotype of catechol-O-methyltransferase. J Psychiatr Res 2004;38:365–370.

66 Woo JM, Yoon KS, Yu BH: Catechol O-methyltransferase genetic polymorphism in panic disorder. Am J Psychiatry 2002;159:1785–1787.

67 McGrath M, Kawachi I, Ascherio A, Colditz GA, Hunter DJ, De Vivo I: Association between catechol-O-methyltransferase and phobic anxiety. Am J Psychiatry 2004;161:1703–1705.

68 Rowe DC, Stever C, Gard JM, Cleveland HH, Sanders ML, Abramowitz A, Kozol ST, Mohr JH, Sherman SL, Waldman ID: The relation of the dopamine transporter gene (DAT1) to symptoms of internalizing disorders in children. Behav Genet 1998;28:215–225.

69 Boscarino JA, Erlich PM, Hoffman SN, Rukstalis M, Stewart WF: Association of FKBP5, COMT and CHRNA5 polymorphisms with PTSD among outpatients at risk for PTSD. Psychiatry Res 2011;188:173–174.

70 Voisey J, Swagell CD, Hughes IP, Morris CP, van DA, Noble EP, Kann B, Heslop KA, Young RM, Lawford BR: The DRD2 gene 957C>T polymorphism is associated with posttraumatic stress disorder in war veterans. Depress Anxiety 2009;26:28–33.

71 Lawford BR, Young R, Noble EP, Kann B, Ritchie T: The D2 dopamine receptor (DRD2) gene is associated with co-morbid depression, anxiety and social dysfunction in untreated veterans with post-traumatic stress disorder. Eur Psychiatry 2006;21:180–185.

72 Valente NL, Vallada H, Cordeiro Q, Miguita K, Bressan RA, Andreoli SB, Mari JJ, Mello MF: Candidate-gene approach in posttraumatic stress disorder after urban violence: association analysis of the genes encoding serotonin transporter, dopamine transporter, and BDNF. J Mol Neurosci 2011;44:59–67.

73 Bailey JN, Goenjian AK, Noble EP, Walling DP, Ritchie T, Goenjian HA: PTSD and dopaminergic genes, DRD2 and DAT, in multigenerational families exposed to the Spitak earthquake. Psychiatry Res 2010;178:507–510.

74 Drury SS, Theall KP, Keats BJ, Scheeringa M: The role of the dopamine transporter (DAT) in the development of PTSD in preschool children. J Trauma Stress 2009;22:534–539.

75 Segman RH, Cooper-Kazaz R, Macciardi F, Goltser T, Halfon Y, Dobroborski T, Shalev AY: Association between the dopamine transporter gene and post-traumatic stress disorder. Mol Psychiatry 2002;7:903–907.

76 Zwanzger P, Domschke K, Bradwejn J: The neuronal network of panic: the role of the neuropeptide cholecystokinin. Depress Anxiety 2012;29:762–774.

77 Bradwejn J, Koszycki D: Cholecystokinin and panic disorder: past and future clinical research strategies. Scand J Clin Lab Invest Suppl 2001;234:19–27.

78 Wang Z, Valdes J, Noyes R, Zoega T, Crowe RR: Possible association of a cholecystokinin promotor polymorphism (CCK-36CT) with panic disorder. Am J Med Genet 1998;81:228–234.

79 Hattori E, Ebihara M, Yamada K, Ohba H, Shibuya H, Yoshikawa T: Identification of a compound short tandem repeat stretch in the 5′-upstream region of the cholecystokinin gene, and its association with panic disorder but not with schizophrenia. Mol Psychiatry 2001;6:465–470.

80 Ebihara M, Ohba H, Hattori E, Yamada K, Yoshikawa T: Transcriptional activities of cholecystokinin promoter haplotypes and their relevance to panic disorder susceptibility. Am J Med Genet B Neuropsychiatr Genet 2003;118B:32–35.

81 Miyasaka K, Yoshida Y, Matsushita S, Higuchi S, Shirakawa O, Shimokata H, Funakoshi A: Association of cholecystokinin-A receptor gene polymorphisms and panic disorder in Japanese. Am J Med Genet B Neuropsychiatr Genet 2004;127B:78–80.

82 Koefoed P, Woldbye DP, Hansen TO, Hansen ES, Knudsen GM, Bolwig TG, Rehfeld JF: Gene variations in the cholecystokinin system in patients with panic disorder. Psychiatr Genet 2010;20:59–64.

83 Kennedy JL, Bradwejn J, Koszycki D, King N, Crowe R, Vincent J, Fourie O: Investigation of cholecystokinin system genes in panic disorder. Mol Psychiatry 1999;4:284–285.

84 Hösing VG, Schirmacher A, Kuhlenbäumer G, Freitag C, Sand P, Schlesiger C, Jacob C, Fritze J, Franke P, Rietschel M, Garritsen H, Nöthen MM, Fimmers R, Stögbauer F, Deckert J: Cholecystokinin- and cholecystokinin-B-receptor gene polymorphisms in panic disorder. J Neural Transm Suppl 2004;68:147–156.

85 Wilson J, Markie D, Fitches A: Cholecystokinin system genes: associations with panic and other psychiatric disorders. J Affect Disord 2012;136:902–908.

86 Gratacos M, Costas J, de Cid R, et al: Identification of new putative susceptibility genes for several psychiatric disorders by association analysis of regulatory and non-synonymous SNPs of 306 genes involved in neurotransmission and neurodevelopment. Am J Med Genet B Neuropsychiatr Genet 2009;150B:808–816.

87 Hamilton SP, Slager SL, Helleby L, Heiman GA, Klein DF, Hodge SE, Weissman MM, Fyer AJ, Knowles JA: No association or linkage between polymorphisms in the genes encoding cholecystokinin and the cholecystokinin B receptor and panic disorder. Mol Psychiatry 2001;6:59–65.

88 Deckert J: The adenosine A(2A) receptor knockout mouse: a model for anxiety? Int J Neuropsychopharmacol 1998;1:187–190.

89 Huang ZL, Qu WM, Eguchi N, Chen JF, Schwarzschild MA, Fredholm BB, Urade Y, Hayaishi O: Adenosine A2A, but not A1, receptors mediate the arousal effect of caffeine. Nat Neurosci 2005;8:858–859.

90 Correa M, Font L: Is there a major role for adenosine A2A receptors in anxiety? Front Biosci 2008;13:4058–4070.

91 Hohoff C, Mullings EL, Heatherley SV, Freitag CM, Neumann LC, Domschke K, Krakowitzky P, Rothermundt M, Keck ME, Erhardt A, Unschuld PG, Jacob C, Fritze J, Bandelow B, Maier W, Holsboer F, Rogers PJ, Deckert J: Adenosine A(2A) receptor gene: evidence for association of risk variants with panic disorder and anxious personality. J Psychiatr Res 2010;44:930–937.

92 Lam P, Hong CJ, Tsai SJ: Association study of A2a adenosine receptor genetic polymorphism in panic disorder. Neurosci Lett 2005;378:98–101.

93 Hamilton SP, Slager SL, De Leon AB, Heiman GA, Klein DF, Hodge SE, Weissman MM, Fyer AJ, Knowles JA: Evidence for genetic linkage between a polymorphism in the adenosine 2A receptor and panic disorder. Neuropsychopharmacology 2004;29:558–565.

94 Freitag CM, Agelopoulos K, Huy E, Rothermundt M, Krakowitzky P, Meyer J, Deckert J, von GA, Hohoff C: Adenosine A(2A) receptor gene (ADORA2A) variants may increase autistic symptoms and anxiety in autism spectrum disorder. Eur Child Adolesc Psychiatry 2010;19:67–74.

95 Domschke K, Zwanzger P: GABAergic and endocannabinoid dysfunction in anxiety – future therapeutic targets? Curr Pharm Des 2008;14:3508–3517.

96 Nelson EC, Agrawal A, Pergadia ML, Lynskey MT, Todorov AA, Wang JC, Todd RD, Martin NG, Heath AC, Goate AM, Montgomery GW, Madden PA: Association of childhood trauma exposure and GABRA2 polymorphisms with risk of posttraumatic stress disorder in adults. Mol Psychiatry 2009;14:234–235.

97 Crowe RR, Wang Z, Noyes R Jr, Albrecht BE, Darlison MG, Bailey ME, Johnson KJ, Zoega T: Candidate gene study of eight GABAA receptor subunits in panic disorder. Am J Psychiatry 1997;154:1096–1100.

98 Sand PG, Godau C, Riederer P, Peters C, Franke P, Nothen MM, Stober G, Fritze J, Maier W, Propping P, Lesch KP, Riess O, Sander T, Beckmann H, Deckert J: Exonic variants of the GABA(B) receptor gene and panic disorder. Psychiatr Genet 2000;10:191–194.

99 Thoeringer CK, Ripke S, Unschuld PG, Lucae S, Ising M, Bettecken T, Uhr M, Keck ME, Mueller-Myhsok B, Holsboer F, Binder EB, Erhardt A: The GABA transporter 1 (SLC6A1): a novel candidate gene for anxiety disorders. J Neural Transm 2009;116:649–657.

100 Kobayashi Y, Akiyoshi J, Kanehisa M, Ichioka S, Tanaka Y, Tsuru J, Hanada H, Kodama K, Isogawa K, Tsutsumi T: Lack of polymorphism in genes encoding mGluR 7, mGluR 8, GABA(A) receptor alfa-6 subunit and nociceptin/orphanin FQ receptor and panic disorder. Psychiatr Genet 2007;17:9.

101 Thoeringer CK, Binder EB, Salyakina D, Erhardt A, Ising M, Unschuld PG, Kern N, Lucae S, Brueckl TM, Mueller MB, Fuchs B, Puetz B, Lieb R, Uhr M, Holsboer F, Mueller-Myhsok B, Keck ME: Association of a Met88Val diazepam binding inhibitor (DBI) gene polymorphism and anxiety disorders with panic attacks. J Psychiatr Res 2007;41:579–584.

102 Unschuld PG, Ising M, Specht M, Erhardt A, Ripke S, Heck A, Kloiber S, Straub V, Brueckl T, Muller-Myhsok B, Holsboer F, Binder EB: Polymorphisms in the GAD2 gene-region are associated with susceptibility for unipolar depression and with a risk factor for anxiety disorders. Am J Med Genet B Neuropsychiatr Genet 2009;150B:1100–1109.

103 Hettema JM, An SS, Neale MC, Bukszar J, van den Oord EJ, Kendler KS, Chen X: Association between glutamic acid decarboxylase genes and anxiety disorders, major depression, and neuroticism. Mol Psychiatry 2006;11:752–762.

104 Smoller JW, Rosenbaum JF, Biederman J, Kennedy J, Dai D, Racette SR, Laird NM, Kagan J, Snidman N, Hirshfeld-Becker D, Tsuang MT, Sklar PB, Slaugenhaupt SA: Association of a genetic marker at the corticotropin-releasing hormone locus with behavioral inhibition. Biol Psychiatry 2003;54:1376–1381.

105 Smoller JW, Yamaki LH, Fagerness JA, Biederman J, Racette S, Laird NM, Kagan J, Snidman N, Faraone SV, Hirshfeld-Becker D, Tsuang MT, Slaugenhaupt SA, Rosenbaum JF, Sklar PB: The corticotropin-releasing hormone gene and behavioral inhibition in children at risk for panic disorder. Biol Psychiatry 2005;57:1485–1492.

106 Keck ME, Kern N, Erhardt A, Unschuld PG, Ising M, Salyakina D, Muller MB, Knorr CC, Lieb R, Hohoff C, Krakowitzky P, Maier W, Bandelow B, Fritze J, Deckert J, Holsboer F, Muller-Myhsok B, Binder EB: Combined effects of exonic polymorphisms in CRHR1 and AVPR1B genes in a case/control study for panic disorder. Am J Med Genet B Neuropsychiatr Genet 2008;147B:1196–1204.

107 Amstadter AB, Nugent NR, Yang BZ, Miller A, Siburian R, Moorjani P, Haddad S, Basu A, Fagerness J, Saxe G, Smoller JW, Koenen KC: Corticotrophin-releasing hormone type 1 receptor gene (CRHR1) variants predict posttraumatic stress disorder onset and course in pediatric injury patients. Dis Markers 2011;30:89–99.

108 Binder EB, Bradley RG, Liu W, Epstein MP, Deveau TC, Mercer KB, Tang Y, Gillespie CF, Heim CM, Nemeroff CB, Schwartz AC, Cubells JF, Ressler KJ: Association of FKBP5 polymorphisms and childhood abuse with risk of posttraumatic stress disorder symptoms in adults. JAMA 2008;299:1291–1305.

109 Sarapas C, Cai G, Bierer LM, Golier JA, Galea S, Ising M, Rein T, Schmeidler J, Muller-Myhsok B, Uhr M, Holsboer F, Buxbaum JD, Yehuda R: Genetic markers for PTSD risk and resilience among survivors of the World Trade Center attacks. Dis Markers 2011;30:101–110.

110 Mehta D, Gonik M, Klengel T, Rex-Haffner M, Menke A, Rubel J, Mercer KB, Putz B, Bradley B, Holsboer F, Ressler KJ, Muller-Myhsok B, Binder EB: Using polymorphisms in FKBP5 to define biologically distinct subtypes of posttraumatic stress disorder: evidence from endocrine and gene expression studies. Arch Gen Psychiatry 2011;68:901–910.

111 Ressler KJ, Mercer KB, Bradley B, Jovanovic T, Mahan A, Kerley K, Norrholm SD, Kilaru V, Smith AK, Myers AJ, Ramirez M, Engel A, Hammack SE, Toufexis D, Braas KM, Binder EB, May V: Posttraumatic stress disorder is associated with PACAP and the PAC1 receptor. Nature 2011;470:492–497.

112 Olsson M, Annerbrink K, Westberg L, Melke J, Baghaei F, Rosmond R, Holm G, Andersch S, Allgulander C, Eriksson E: Angiotensin-related genes in patients with panic disorder. Am J Med Genet B Neuropsychiatr Genet 2004;127B:81–84.

113 Erhardt A, Lucae S, Kern N, Unschuld PG, Ising M, Lieb R, Uhr M, Hohoff C, Deckert J, Bandelow B, Maier W, Binder EB, Muller-Myhsok B, Keck ME, Holsboer F: Association of polymorphisms in the angiotensin-converting enzyme gene with syndromal panic attacks. Mol Psychiatry 2008;13:242–243.

114 Bandelow B, Saleh K, Pauls J, Domschke K, Wedekind D, Falkai P: Insertion/deletion polymorphism in the gene for angiotensin converting enzyme (ACE) in panic disorder: a gender-specific effect? World J Biol Psychiatry 2010;11:66–70.

115 Shimizu E, Hashimoto K, Kobayashi K, Mitsumori M, Ohgake S, Koizumi H, Okamura N, Koike K, Kumakiri C, Nakazato M, Komatsu N, Iyo M: Lack of association between angiotensin I-converting enzyme insertion/deletion gene functional polymorphism and panic disorder in humans. Neurosci Lett 2004;363:81–83.

116 Hohoff C, Neumann A, Domschke K, Jacob C, Maier W, Fritze J, Bandelow B, Krakowitzky P, Rothermundt M, Arolt V, Deckert J: Association analysis of Rgs7 variants with panic disorder. J Neural Transm 2009;116:1523–1528.

117 Smoller JW, Paulus MP, Fagerness JA, Purcell S, Yamaki LH, Hirshfeld-Becker D, Biederman J, Rosenbaum JF, Gelernter J, Stein MB: Influence of RGS2 on anxiety-related temperament, personality, and brain function. Arch Gen Psychiatry 2008; 65:298–308.

118 Leygraf A, Hohoff C, Freitag C, Willis-Owen SA, Krakowitzky P, Fritze J, Franke P, Bandelow B, Fimmers R, Flint J, Deckert J: Rgs 2 gene polymorphisms as modulators of anxiety in humans? J Neural Transm 2006;113:1921–1925.

119 Donner J, Haapakoski R, Ezer S, et al: Assessment of the neuropeptide S system in anxiety disorders. Biol Psychiatry 2010;68:474–483.

120 Okamura N, Hashimoto K, Iyo M, Shimizu E, Dempfle A, Friedel S, Reinscheid RK: Gender-specific association of a functional coding polymorphism in the Neuropeptide S receptor gene with panic disorder but not with schizophrenia or attention-deficit/hyperactivity disorder. Prog Neuropsychopharmacol Biol Psychiatry 2007;31:1444–1448.

121 Domschke K, Reif A, Weber H, et al: Neuropeptide S receptor gene – converging evidence for a role in panic disorder. Mol Psychiatry 2011;16: 938–948.

122 Domschke K, Kuhlenbaumer G, Schirmacher A, et al: Human nuclear transcription factor gene CREM: genomic organization, mutation screening, and association analysis in panic disorder. Am J Med Genet B Neuropsychiatr Genet 2003;117B:70–78.

123 Hamilton SP, Slager SL, Mayo D, Heiman GA, Klein DF, Hodge SE, Fyer AJ, Weissman MM, Knowles JA: Investigation of polymorphisms in the CREM gene in panic disorder. Am J Med Genet B Neuropsychiatr Genet 2004;126B:111–115.

124 Unschuld PG, Ising M, Erhardt A, Lucae S, Kohli M, Kloiber S, Salyakina D, Thoeringer CK, Kern N, Lieb R, Uhr M, Binder EB, Muller-Myhsok B, Holsboer F, Keck ME: Polymorphisms in the galanin gene are associated with symptom-severity in female patients suffering from panic disorder. J Affect Disord 2008;105:177–184.

125 Domschke K, Dannlowski U, Hohoff C, Ohrmann P, Bauer J, Kugel H, Zwanzger P, Heindel W, Deckert J, Arolt V, Suslow T, Baune BT: Neuropeptide Y (NPY) gene: Impact on emotional processing and treatment response in anxious depression. Eur Neuropsychopharmacol 2010;20:301–309.

126 Sand PG, Schlurmann K, Luckhaus C, Gotz M, Stober G, Lesch KP, Riederer P, Franke P, Maier W, Nothen MM, Propping P, Fritze J, Deckert J: Estrogen receptor 1 gene (ESR1) variants in panic disorder. Am J Med Genet 2002;114:426–428.

127 Hodges LM, Weissman MM, Haghighi F, Costa R, Bravo O, Evgrafov O, Knowles JA, Fyer AJ, Hamilton SP: Association and linkage analysis of candidate genes GRP, GRPR, CRHR1, and TACR1 in panic disorder. Am J Med Genet B Neuropsychiatr Genet 2009;150B:65–73.

128 Ho HP, Westberg L, Annerbrink K, Olsson M, Melke J, Nilsson S, Baghaei F, Rosmond R, Holm G, Bjorntorp P, Andersch S, Allgulander C, Eriksson E: Association between a functional polymorphism in the progesterone receptor gene and panic disorder in women. Psychoneuroendocrinology 2004; 29:1138–1141.

129 Lu AT, Ogdie MN, Jarvelin MR, Moilanen IK, Loo SK, McCracken JT, McGough JJ, Yang MH, Peltonen L, Nelson SF, Cantor RM, Smalley SL: Association of the cannabinoid receptor gene (CNR1) with ADHD and post-traumatic stress disorder. Am J Med Genet B Neuropsychiatr Genet 2008; 147B:1488–1494.

130 Koenen KC, Amstadter AB, Ruggiero KJ, Acierno R, Galea S, Kilpatrick DG, Gelernter J: RGS2 and generalized anxiety disorder in an epidemiologic sample of hurricane-exposed adults. Depress Anxiety 2009;26:309–315.

131 Freitag CM, Domschke K, Rothe C, Lee YJ, Hohoff C, Gutknecht L, Sand P, Fimmers R, Lesch KP, Deckert J: Interaction of serotonergic and noradrenergic gene variants in panic disorder. Psychiatr Genet 2006;16:59–65.

132 Sand P, Lesch KP, Catalano M, Bosi M, Syagailo YV, Okladnova O, Di BD, Maffei P, Heils A, Friess F, Politi E, Nothen MM, Franke P, Stober G, Fritze J, Maier W, Propping P, Beckmann H, Bellodi L, Riederer P, Deckert J: Polymorphic MAO-A and 5-HT-transporter genes: analysis of interactions in panic disorder. World J Biol Psychiatry 2000;1: 147–150.

133 Maron E, Hettema JM, Shlik J: Advances in molecular genetics of panic disorder. Mol Psychiatry 2010;15:681–701.

134 Hamilton SP: Linkage and association studies of anxiety disorders. Depress Anxiety 2009;26:976–983.

135 Otowa T, Yoshida E, Sugaya N, Yasuda S, Nishimura Y, Inoue K, Tochigi M, Umekage T, Miyagawa T, Nishida N, Tokunaga K, Tanii H, Sasaki T, Kaiya H, Okazaki Y: Genome-wide association study of panic disorder in the Japanese population. J Hum Genet 2009;54:122–126.

136 Otowa T, Tanii H, Sugaya N, Yoshida E, Inoue K, Yasuda S, Shimada T, Kawamura Y, Tochigi M, Minato T, Umekage T, Miyagawa T, Nishida N, Tokunaga K, Okazaki Y, Kaiya H, Sasaki T: Replication of a genome-wide association study of panic disorder in a Japanese population. J Hum Genet 2010;55: 91–96.

137 Erhardt A, Czibere L, Roeske D, et al: TMEM132D, a new candidate for anxiety phenotypes: evidence from human and mouse studies. Mol Psychiatry 2011;16:647–663.

138 Gregersen N, Dahl HA, Buttenschon HN, Nyegaard M, Hedemand A, Als TD, Wang AG, Joensen S, Woldbye DP, Koefoed P, Kristensen AS, Kruse TA, Borglum AD, Mors O: A genome-wide study of panic disorder suggests the amiloride-sensitive cation channel 1 as a candidate gene. Eur J Hum Genet 2012;20:84–90.

139 Bandelow B, Spath C, Tichauer GA, Broocks A, Hajak G, Ruther E: Early traumatic life events, parental attitudes, family history, and birth risk factors in patients with panic disorder. Compr Psychiatry 2002;43:269–278.

140 Stein MB, Walker JR, Anderson G, Hazen AL, Ross CA, Eldridge G, Forde DR: Childhood physical and sexual abuse in patients with anxiety disorders and in a community sample. Am J Psychiatry 1996;153: 275–277.

141 Kendler KS, Neale MC, Kessler RC, Heath AC, Eaves LJ: Childhood parental loss and adult psychopathology in women. A twin study perspective. Arch Gen Psychiatry 1992;49:109–116.

142 Bandelow B, Alvarez TG, Spath C, Broocks A, Hajak G, Bleich S, Ruther E: Separation anxiety and actual separation experiences during childhood in patients with panic disorder. Can J Psychiatry 2001; 46:948–952.

143 Faravelli C: Life events preceding the onset of panic disorder. J Affect Disord 1985;9:103–105.

144 Klauke B, Deckert J, Reif A, Pauli P, Domschke K: Life events in panic disorder-an update on 'candidate stressors'. Depress Anxiety 2010;27:716–730.

145 Klauke B, Deckert J, Reif A, Pauli P, Zwanzger P, Baumann C, Arolt V, Glockner-Rist A, Domschke K: Serotonin transporter gene and childhood trauma – a G × E effect on anxiety sensitivity. Depress Anxiety 2011;28:1048–1057.

146 Stein MB, Schork NJ, Gelernter J: Gene-by-environment (serotonin transporter and childhood maltreatment) interaction for anxiety sensitivity, an intermediate phenotype for anxiety disorders. Neuropsychopharmacology 2008;33:312–319.

147 Klauke B, Deckert J, Zwanzger P, Baumann C, Arolt V, Pauli P, Reif A, Domschke K: Neuropeptide S receptor gene (NPSR1) and life events: G × E effects on anxiety sensitivity and its subdimensions. World J Biol Psychiatry, in press.

148 Laucht M, Treutlein J, Blomeyer D, Buchmann AF, Schmid B, Becker K, Zimmermann US, Schmidt MH, Esser G, Rietschel M, Banaschewski T: Interaction between the 5-HTTLPR serotonin transporter polymorphism and environmental adversity for mood and anxiety psychopathology: evidence from a high-risk community sample of young adults. Int J Neuropsychopharmacol 2009;12:737–747.

149 Amstadter AB, Koenen KC, Ruggiero KJ, Acierno R, Galea S, Kilpatrick DG, Gelernter J: NPY moderates the relation between hurricane exposure and generalized anxiety disorder in an epidemiologic sample of hurricane-exposed adults. Depress Anxiety 2010;27:270–275.

150 Kolassa IT, Ertl V, Eckart C, Glockner F, Kolassa S, Papassotiropoulos A, de Quervain DJ, Elbert T: Association study of trauma load and SLC6A4 promoter polymorphism in posttraumatic stress disorder: evidence from survivors of the Rwandan genocide. J Clin Psychiatry 2010;71:543–547.

151 Koenen KC, Aiello AE, Bakshis E, Amstadter AB, Ruggiero KJ, Acierno R, Kilpatrick DG, Gelernter J, Galea S: Modification of the association between serotonin transporter genotype and risk of posttraumatic stress disorder in adults by county-level social environment. Am J Epidemiol 2009;169: 704–711.

152 Kilpatrick DG, Koenen KC, Ruggiero KJ, Acierno R, Galea S, Resnick HS, Roitzsch J, Boyle J, Gelernter J: The serotonin transporter genotype and social support and moderation of posttraumatic stress disorder and depression in hurricane-exposed adults. Am J Psychiatry 2007;164:1693–1699.

153 Grabe HJ, Spitzer C, Schwahn C, Marcinek A, Frahnow A, Barnow S, Lucht M, Freyberger HJ, John U, Wallaschofski H, Volzke H, Rosskopf D: Serotonin transporter gene (SLC6A4) promoter polymorphisms and the susceptibility to posttraumatic stress disorder in the general population. Am J Psychiatry 2009;166:926–933.

154 Xie P, Kranzler HR, Poling J, Stein MB, Anton RF, Farrer LA, Gelernter J: Interaction of FKBP5 with childhood adversity on risk for post-traumatic stress disorder. Neuropsychopharmacology 2010; 35:1684–1692.

155 Amstadter AB, Koenen KC, Ruggiero KJ, Acierno R, Galea S, Kilpatrick DG, Gelernter J: Variant in RGS2 moderates posttraumatic stress symptoms following potentially traumatic event exposure. J Anxiety Disord 2009;23:369–373.

156 Mustapic M, Pivac N, Kozaric-Kovacic D, Dezeljin M, Cubells JF, Muck-Seler D: Dopamine beta-hydroxylase (DBH) activity and -1021C/T polymorphism of DBH gene in combat-related post-traumatic stress disorder. Am J Med Genet B Neuropsychiatr Genet 2007;144B:1087–1089.

157 Kolassa IT, Kolassa S, Ertl V, Papassotiropoulos A, de Quervain DJ: The risk of posttraumatic stress disorder after trauma depends on traumatic load and the catechol-o-methyltransferase Val(158)Met polymorphism. Biol Psychiatry 2010;67:304–308.

158 Nugent NR, Tyrka AR, Carpenter LL, Price LH: Gene-environment interactions: early life stress and risk for depressive and anxiety disorders. Psychopharmacology (Berl) 2011;214:175–196.

159 Jaenisch R, Bird A: Epigenetic regulation of gene expression: how the genome integrates intrinsic and environmental signals. Nat Genet 2003;33: 245–254.

160 Chertkow-Deutsher Y, Cohen H, Klein E, Ben-Shachar D: DNA methylation in vulnerability to post-traumatic stress in rats: evidence for the role of the post-synaptic density protein Dlgap2. Int J Neuropsychopharmacol 2010;13:347–359.

161 Lesch KP: When the serotonin transporter gene meets adversity: the contribution of animal models to understanding epigenetic mechanisms in affective disorders and resilience. Curr Top Behav Neurosci 2011;7:251–280.

162 Fraga MF, Ballestar E, Paz MF, et al: Epigenetic differences arise during the lifetime of monozygotic twins. Proc Natl Acad Sci USA 2005;102:10604–10609.

163 Diemer J, Vennewald N, Domschke K, Zwanzger P: Therapy-refractory panic: current research areas as possible perspectives in the treatment of anxiety. Eur Arch Psychiatry Clin Neurosci 2010;260:127–131.

164 Smith AK, Conneely KN, Kilaru V, Mercer KB, Weiss TE, Bradley B, Tang Y, Gillespie CF, Cubells JF, Ressler KJ: Differential immune system DNA methylation and cytokine regulation in post-traumatic stress disorder. Am J Med Genet B Neuropsychiatr Genet 2011;156B:700–708.

165 Uddin M, Aiello AE, Wildman DE, Koenen KC, Pawelec G, de Los SR, Goldmann E, Galea S: Epigenetic and immune function profiles associated with posttraumatic stress disorder. Proc Natl Acad Sci USA 2010;107:9470–9475.

166 Uddin M, Galea S, Chang SC, Aiello AE, Wildman DE, de Los SR, Koenen KC: Gene expression and methylation signatures of MAN2C1 are associated with PTSD. Dis Markers 2011;30:111–121.

167 Koenen KC, Uddin M, Chang SC, Aiello AE, Wildman DE, Goldmann E, Galea S: SLC6A4 methylation modifies the effect of the number of traumatic events on risk for posttraumatic stress disorder. Depress Anxiety 2011;28:639–647.

168 Domschke K, Tidow N, Kuithan H, Schwarte K, Klauke B, Ambrée O, Reif A, Schmidt H, Arolt V, Kersting A, Zwanzger P, Deckert J: Monoamine oxidase A gene hypomethylation – a risk factor for panic disorder? Int J Neuropsychopharmacol 2012; 15:1217–1228.

169 Gottesman II, Gould TD: The endophenotype concept in psychiatry: etymology and strategic intentions. Am J Psychiatry 2003;160:636–645.

170 Smoller JW, Rosenbaum JF, Biederman J, Susswein LS, Kennedy J, Kagan J, Snidman N, Laird N, Tsuang MT, Faraone SV, Schwarz A, Slaugenhaupt SA: Genetic association analysis of behavioral inhibition using candidate loci from mouse models. Am J Med Genet 2001;105:226–235.

171 Schmidt NB, Mitchell MA, Richey JA: Anxiety sensitivity as an incremental predictor of later anxiety symptoms and syndromes. Compr Psychiatry 2008;49:407–412.

172 Schmidt NB, Zvolensky MJ, Maner JK: Anxiety sensitivity: prospective prediction of panic attacks and Axis I pathology. J Psychiatr Res 2006;40:691–699.

173 Schmidt NB, Lerew DR, Jackson RJ: The role of anxiety sensitivity in the pathogenesis of panic: prospective evaluation of spontaneous panic attacks during acute stress. J Abnorm Psychol 1997; 106:355–364.

174 Yang AC, Chen TJ, Tsai SJ, Hong CJ, Kuo CH, Yang CH, Kao KP: BDNF Val66Met polymorphism alters sympathovagal balance in healthy subjects. Am J Med Genet B Neuropsychiatr Genet 2010;153B:1024–1030.

175 Hohoff C, Domschke K, Schwarte K, Spellmeyer G, Vogele C, Hetzel G, Deckert J, Gerlach AL: Sympathetic activity relates to adenosine A(2A) receptor gene variation in blood-injury phobia. J Neural Transm 2009;116:659–662.

176 Domschke K, Stevens S, Beck B, Baffa A, Hohoff C, Deckert J, Gerlach AL: Blushing propensity in social anxiety disorder: influence of serotonin transporter gene variation. J Neural Transm 2009;116: 663–666.

177 Coryell W, Fyer A, Pine D, Martinez J, Arndt S: Aberrant respiratory sensitivity to CO(2) as a trait of familial panic disorder. Biol Psychiatry 2001;49: 582–587.

178 Bellodi L, Perna G, Caldirola D, Arancio C, Bertani A, Di BD: CO2-induced panic attacks: a twin study. Am J Psychiatry 1998;155:1184–1188.

179 Schmidt NB, Maner JK, Zvolensky MJ: Reactivity to challenge with carbon dioxide as a prospective predictor of panic attacks. Psychiatry Res 2007;151: 173–176.

180 Battaglia M, Pesenti-Gritti P, Spatola CA, Ogliari A, Tambs K: A twin study of the common vulnerability between heightened sensitivity to hypercapnia and panic disorder. Am J Med Genet B Neuropsychiatr Genet 2008;147B:586–593.

181 Battaglia M, Ogliari A, Harris J, Spatola CA, Pesenti-Gritti P, Reichborn-Kjennerud T, Torgersen S, Kringlen E, Tambs K: A genetic study of the acute anxious response to carbon dioxide stimulation in man. J Psychiatr Res 2007;41:906–917.

182 Schutters SI, Viechtbauer W, Knuts IJ, Griez EJ, Schruers KR: 35% CO_2 sensitivity in social anxiety disorder. J Psychopharmacol 2012;26:479–486.

183 Muhtz C, Yassouridis A, Daneshi J, Braun M, Kellner M: Acute panicogenic, anxiogenic and dissociative effects of carbon dioxide inhalation in patients with post-traumatic stress disorder (PTSD). J Psychiatr Res 2011;45:989–993.

184 Schruers K, Esquivel G, van DM, Wichers M, Kenis G, Colasanti A, Knuts I, Goossens L, Jacobs N, van RJ, Smeets H, van OJ, Griez E: Genetic moderation of CO2-induced fear by 5-HTTLPR genotype. J Psychopharmacol 2011;25:37–42.

185 Perna G, Di BD, Favaron E, Cucchi M, Liperi L, Bellodi L: Lack of relationship between CO2 reactivity and serotonin transporter gene regulatory region polymorphism in panic disorder. Am J Med Genet B Neuropsychiatr Genet 2004;129B:41–43.

186 Verschoor E, Markus CR: Physiological and affective reactivity to a 35% CO_2 inhalation challenge in individuals differing in the 5-HTTLPR genotype and trait neuroticism. Eur Neuropsychopharmacol 2012;22:546–554.

187 Maron E, Tasa G, Toru I, Lang A, Vasar V, Shlik J: Association between serotonin-related genetic polymorphisms and CCK-4-induced panic attacks with or without 5-hydroxytryptophan pretreatment in healthy volunteers. World J Biol Psychiatry 2004;5:149–154.

188 Maron E, Toru I, Tasa G, Must A, Toover E, Lang A, Vasar V, Shlik J: Association testing of panic disorder candidate genes using CCK-4 challenge in healthy volunteers. Neurosci Lett 2008;446:88–92.

189 Maron E, Kallassalu K, Tammiste A, Kolde R, Vilo J, Toru I, Vasar V, Shlik J, Metspalu A: Peripheral gene expression profiling of CCK-4-induced panic in healthy subjects. Am J Med Genet B Neuropsychiatr Genet 2010;153B:269–274.

190 Philibert RA, Crowe R, Ryu GY, Yoon JG, Secrest D, Sandhu H, Madan A: Transcriptional profiling of lymphoblast lines from subjects with panic disorder. Am J Med Genet B Neuropsychiatr Genet 2007;144B:674–682.

191 Perez-Parada J, Jhangri GS, Lara N, Chrapko W, Castillo Abadia MP, Gil L, Le Melledo JM: Delayed increase in LDL cholesterol following pentagastrin-induced panic attacks. Psychopharmacology (Berl) 2007;193:333–340.

192 Bajwa WK, Asnis GM, Sanderson WC, Irfan A, van Praag HM: High cholesterol levels in patients with panic disorder. Am J Psychiatry 1992;149:376–378.

193 Agargun MY, Kara H, Algun E, Sekeroglu R, Tarakcioglu M: High cholesterol levels in patients with sleep panic. Biol Psychiatry 1996;40:1064–1065.

194 Le HS, Muhleisen TW, Djurovic S, et al: Polymorphisms in SREBF1 and SREBF2, two antipsychotic-activated transcription factors controlling cellular lipogenesis, are associated with schizophrenia in German and Scandinavian samples. Mol Psychiatry 2010;15:463–472.

195 Grillon C, Baas J: A review of the modulation of the startle reflex by affective states and its application in psychiatry. Clin Neurophysiol 2003;114:1557–1579.

196 Plappert CF, Pilz PK: The acoustic startle response as an effective model for elucidating the effect of genes on the neural mechanism of behavior in mice. Behav Brain Res 2001;125:183–188.

197 Zhang L, Hu XZ, Li H, Li X, Smerin S, Benedek DM, Ursano R: Startle response related genes. Med Hypotheses 2011;77:685–691.

198 Montag C, Buckholtz JW, Hartmann P, Merz M, Burk C, Hennig J, Reuter M: COMT genetic variation affects fear processing: psychophysiological evidence. Behav Neurosci 2008;122:901–909.

199 Armbruster D, Moser DA, Strobel A, Hensch T, Kirschbaum C, Lesch KP, Brocke B: Serotonin transporter gene variation and stressful life events impact processing of fear and anxiety. Int J Neuropsychopharmacol 2009;12:393–401.

200 Brocke B, Armbruster D, Muller J, Hensch T, Jacob CP, Lesch KP, Kirschbaum C, Strobel A: Serotonin transporter gene variation impacts innate fear processing: Acoustic startle response and emotional startle. Mol Psychiatry 2006;11:1106–1112.

201 Klumpers F, Heitland I, Oosting RS, Kenemans JL, Baas JM: Genetic variation in serotonin transporter function affects human fear expression indexed by fear-potentiated startle. Biol Psychol 2012;89:277–282.

202 Lonsdorf TB, Ruck C, Bergstrom J, Andersson G, Ohman A, Schalling M, Lindefors N: The symptomatic profile of panic disorder is shaped by the 5-HTTLPR polymorphism. Prog Neuropsychopharmacol Biol Psychiatry 2009;33:1479–1483.

203 Alsene K, Deckert J, Sand P, de WH: Association between A2a receptor gene polymorphisms and caffeine-induced anxiety. Neuropsychopharmacology 2003;28:1694–1702.

204 Childs E, Hohoff C, Deckert J, Xu K, Badner J, de WH: Association between ADORA2A and DRD2 polymorphisms and caffeine-induced anxiety. Neuropsychopharmacology 2008;33:2791–2800.

205 Rogers PJ, Hohoff C, Heatherley SV, Mullings EL, Maxfield PJ, Evershed RP, Deckert J, Nutt DJ: Association of the anxiogenic and alerting effects of caffeine with ADORA2A and ADORA1 polymorphisms and habitual level of caffeine consumption. Neuropsychopharmacology 2010;35:1973–1983.

206 Domschke K, Gajewska A, Winter B, Herrmann MJ, Warrings B, Muhlberger A, Wosnitza K, Glotzbach E, Conzelmann A, Dlugos A, Fobker M, Jacob C, Arolt V, Reif A, Pauli P, Zwanzger P, Deckert J: ADORA2A gene variation, caffeine, and emotional processing: a multi-level interaction on startle reflex. Neuropsychopharmacology 2012;37:759–769.

207 Hariri AR, Mattay VS, Tessitore A, Kolachana B, Fera F, Goldman D, Egan MF, Weinberger DR: Serotonin transporter genetic variation and the response of the human amygdala. Science 2002;297:400–403.

208 Domschke K, Ohrmann P, Braun M, Suslow T, Bauer J, Hohoff C, Kersting A, Engelien A, Arolt V, Heindel W, Deckert J, Kugel H: Influence of the catechol-O-methyltransferase val158met genotype on amygdala and prefrontal cortex emotional processing in panic disorder. Psychiatry Res 2008;163: 13–20.

209 Domschke K, Braun M, Ohrmann P, Suslow T, Kugel H, Bauer J, Hohoff C, Kersting A, Engelien A, Arolt V, Heindel W, Deckert J: Association of the functional –1019C/G 5-HT1A polymorphism with prefrontal cortex and amygdala activation measured with 3 T fMRI in panic disorder. Int J Neuropsychopharmacol 2006;9:349–355.

210 Furmark T, Henningsson S, Appel L, Ahs F, Linnman C, Pissiota A, Faria V, Oreland L, Bani M, Pich EM, Eriksson E, Fredrikson M: Genotype over-diagnosis in amygdala responsiveness: affective processing in social anxiety disorder. J Psychiatry Neurosci 2009;34:30–40.

211 Furmark T, Appel L, Henningsson S, Ahs F, Faria V, Linnman C, Pissiota A, Frans O, Bani M, Bettica P, Pich EM, Jacobsson E, Wahlstedt K, Oreland L, Langstrom B, Eriksson E, Fredrikson M: A link between serotonin-related gene polymorphisms, amygdala activity, and placebo-induced relief from social anxiety. J Neurosci 2008;28:13066–13074.

212 Furmark T, Tillfors M, Garpenstrand H, Marteinsdottir I, Langstrom B, Oreland L, Fredrikson M: Serotonin transporter polymorphism related to amygdala excitability and symptom severity in patients with social phobia. Neurosci Lett 2004;362: 189–192.

213 Domschke K, Dannlowski U: Imaging genetics of anxiety disorders. Neuroimage 2010;53:822–831.

214 Slaap BR, den Boer JA: The prediction of nonresponse to pharmacotherapy in panic disorder: a review. Depress Anxiety 2001;14:112–122.

215 O'Reilly RL, Bogue L, Singh SM: Pharmacogenetic response to antidepressants in a multicase family with affective disorder. Biol Psychiatry 1994;36: 467–471.

216 Franchini L, Serretti A, Gasperini M, Smeraldi E: Familial concordance of fluvoxamine response as a tool for differentiating mood disorder pedigrees. J Psychiatr Res 1998;32:255–259.

217 Saeki Y, Watanabe T, Ueda M, Saito A, Akiyama K, Inoue Y, Hirokane G, Morita S, Yamada N, Shimoda K: Genetic and pharmacokinetic factors affecting the initial pharmacotherapeutic effect of paroxetine in Japanese patients with panic disorder. Eur J Clin Pharmacol 2009;65:685–691.

218 Perna G, Favaron E, Di BD, Bussi R, Bellodi L: Antipanic efficacy of paroxetine and polymorphism within the promoter of the serotonin transporter gene. Neuropsychopharmacology 2005;30:2230–2235.

219 Stein MB, Seedat S, Gelernter J: Serotonin transporter gene promoter polymorphism predicts SSRI response in generalized social anxiety disorder. Psychopharmacology (Berl) 2006;187:68–72.

220 Yevtushenko OO, Oros MM, Reynolds GP: Early response to selective serotonin reuptake inhibitors in panic disorder is associated with a functional 5-HT1A receptor gene polymorphism. J Affect Disord 2010;123:308–311.

221 Ishiguro S, Watanabe T, Ueda M, Saeki Y, Hayashi Y, Akiyama K, Saito A, Kato K, Inoue Y, Shimoda K: Determinants of pharmacodynamic trajectory of the therapeutic response to paroxetine in Japanese patients with panic disorder. Eur J Clin Pharmacol 2011;67:1213–1221.

222 Lohoff FW, Aquino TD, Narasimhan S, Multani PK, Etemad B, Rickels K: Serotonin receptor 2A (HTR2A) gene polymorphism predicts treatment response to venlafaxine XR in generalized anxiety disorder. Pharmacogenomics J 2013;13:21–26.

223 Lenze EJ, Goate AM, Nowotny P, Dixon D, Shi P, Bies RR, Lotrich FK, Rollman BL, Shear MK, Thompson PA, Andreescu C, Pollock BG: Relation of serotonin transporter genetic variation to efficacy of escitalopram for generalized anxiety disorder in older adults. J Clin Psychopharmacol 2010; 30:672–677.

224 Perlis RH, Fijal B, Dharia S, Houston JP: Pharmacogenetic investigation of response to duloxetine treatment in generalized anxiety disorder. Pharmacogenomics J 2013;13:280–285.

225 Lonsdorf TB, Ruck C, Bergstrom J, Andersson G, Ohman A, Lindefors N, Schalling M: The COMTval158met polymorphism is associated with symptom relief during exposure-based cognitive-behavioral treatment in panic disorder. BMC Psychiatry 2010;10:99.

226 Muinos-Gimeno M, Espinosa-Parrilla Y, Guidi M, Kagerbauer B, Sipila T, Maron E, Pettai K, Kananen L, Navines R, Martin-Santos R, Gratacos M, Metspalu A, Hovatta I, Estivill X: Human microRNAs miR-22, miR-138–2, miR-148a, and miR-488 are associated with panic disorder and regulate several anxiety candidate genes and related pathways. Biol Psychiatry 2011;69:526–533.

227 Saus E, Brunet A, Armengol L, Alonso P, Crespo JM, Fernandez-Aranda F, Guitart M, Martin-Santos R, Menchon JM, Navines R, Soria V, Torrens M, Urretavizcaya M, Valles V, Gratacos M, Estivill X: Comprehensive copy number variant (CNV) analysis of neuronal pathways genes in psychiatric disorders identifies rare variants within patients. J Psychiatr Res 2010;44:971–978.

228 Kawamura Y, Otowa T, Koike A, Sugaya N, Yoshida E, Yasuda S, Inoue K, Takei K, Konishi Y, Tanii H, Shimada T, Tochigi M, Kakiuchi C, Umekage T, Liu X, Nishida N, Tokunaga K, Kuwano R, Okazaki Y, Kaiya H, Sasaki T: A genome-wide CNV association study on panic disorder in a Japanese population. J Hum Genet 2011;56:852–856.

229 Jia P, Wang L, Meltzer HY, Zhao Z: Pathway-based analysis of GWAS datasets: effective but caution required. Int J Neuropsychopharmacol 2011;14:567–572.

230 Xu B, Roos JL, Dexheimer P, Boone B, Plummer B, Levy S, Gogos JA, Karayiorgou M: Exome sequencing supports a de novo mutational paradigm for schizophrenia. Nat Genet 2011;43:864–868.

231 Lyon GJ, Jiang T, Van WR, et al: Exome sequencing and unrelated findings in the context of complex disease research: ethical and clinical implications. Discov Med 2011;12:41–55.

232 Gormanns P, Mueller NS, Ditzen C, Wolf S, Holsboer F, Turck CW: Phenome-transcriptome correlation unravels anxiety and depression related pathways. J Psychiatr Res 2011;45:973–979.

233 Thomas D: Gene-environment-wide association studies: emerging approaches. Nat Rev Genet 2010; 11:259–272.

234 Poulton R, Andrews G, Millichamp J: Gene-environment interaction and the anxiety disorders. Eur Arch Psychiatry Clin Neurosci 2008;258:65–68.

235 Ursini G, Bollati V, Fazio L, Porcelli A, Iacovelli L, Catalani A, Sinibaldi L, Gelao B, Romano R, Rampino A, Taurisano P, Mancini M, Di GA, Popolizio T, Baccarelli A, De BA, Blasi G, Bertolino A: Stress-related methylation of the catechol-O-methyltransferase Val 158 allele predicts human prefrontal cognition and activity. J Neurosci 2011; 31:6692–6698.

236 Domschke K, Stevens S, Pfleiderer B, Gerlach AL: Interoceptive sensitivity in anxiety and anxiety disorders: an overview and integration of neurobiological findings. Clin Psychol Rev 2010;30:1–11.

237 Stein DJ, Matsunaga H: Specific phobia: a disorder of fear conditioning and extinction. CNS Spectr 2006;11:248–251.

238 Lukas M, Neumann ID: Nasal application of neuropeptide S reduces anxiety and prolongs memory in rats: social versus non-social effects. Neuropharmacology 2012;62:398–405.

239 Hamm CA, Costa FF: The impact of epigenomics on future drug design and new therapies. Drug Discov Today 2011;16:626–635.

240 Serretti A, Artioli P: Ethical problems in pharmacogenetic studies of psychiatric disorders. Pharmacogenomics J 2006;6:289–295.

241 Deckert J, Arolt V: Genetische Forschung in der Psychiatrie: Fortschritt und Ethische Verantwortung; in Raem A, Braun R, Fenger H, Michaelis W, Nikol S, Winter S (eds): Genmedizin. Berlin, Springer, 2000, pp 477–491.

Prof. Katharina Domschke, MA, MD, PhD
Department of Psychiatry, University of Würzburg
Füchsleinstrasse 15
DE–97080 Würzburg (Germany)
E-Mail Domschke_K@klinik.uni-wuerzburg.de

Baldwin DS, Leonard BE (eds): Anxiety Disorders.
Mod Trends Pharmacopsychiatry. Basel, Karger, 2013, vol 29, pp 47–66 (DOI: 10.1159/000351938)

Neuroimaging in Anxiety Disorders

Mats Fredrikson · Vanda Faria

Department of Psychology, Uppsala University, Uppsala, Sweden

Abstract

Neuroimaging studies using functional magnetic resonance imaging (fMRI), positron emission to-mography (PET) and single-photon emission computed tomography (SPECT) to evaluate neurofunc-tional and neurochemical alterations related to the generation and control of affect in patients with anxiety disorders are reviewed. We performed a meta-analysis of symptom provocation studies, where neural activity was measured using fMRI, PET or SPECT to test the hypothesis that prefrontal regions modulate amygdala activity. Data revealed that reactivity in the amygdala was enhanced in patients with phobia as well as posttraumatic stress disorder (PTSD). The dorsal anterior cingulate cortex was activated in concert with the amygdala, both in PTSD and in phobic states, suggesting a role in fear expression, rather than emotional control. Activity in emotion-regulating areas in the ventromedial prefrontal cortex including the subgenual anterior cingulate cortex and the medial orbitofrontal cortex was compromised in the symptomatic state in PTSD and phobic disorders, re-spectively. Increased amygdala reactivity was restored with psychological treatment. Treatment ef-fects across different modalities including pharmacological and psychological interventions as well as with placebo regimens support that reduction of neural activity in the amygdala may be a final common pathway for successful therapeutic interventions irrespective of method, thereby linking neurotransmission to plasticity in a pivotal node of the core fear network of the brain.

Diagnosis and Prevalence

Anxiety involves the subjective experience of fear and apprehension and is associated with bodily reactions and avoidance or escape behavior. When the intensity or the frequency of anxiety experiences compromises quality of life, an anxiety disorder may be diagnosed. Anxiety can come 'out of the blue' as in panic disorder (PD), result from memory reminders as in posttraumatic stress disorder (PTSD), be elicited by environ-mental triggers as in social anxiety disorder (SAD) and specific phobia (SP), or deter-mined by internal worry cues as happens in generalized anxiety disorder (GAD). These, together with obsessive-compulsive disorder, were the major diagnostic entities for the anxiety disorders in the Diagnostic and Statistical Manual of Mental Disorders (DSM-IV) [1]. In all disorders, anticipation and experience of feared events or situations cause negative affect often leading to avoidance. Anxiety problems are prevalent, costly and induce major suffering. Epidemiological studies [2, 3] demonstrate a lifetime prevalence of any anxiety disorder of around 30% with roughly twice as many affected women as men [2, 3]. In the DSM-5, obsessive-compulsive disorder is not included as an anxiety diagnosis but included within 'Obsessive Compulsive and Related Disorders' to be diagnosed separate from the anxiety syndromes. Also, PTSD is included within a separate category called 'Trauma and Stressor Related Disorders'. Anxiety disorders in DSM-5 then most likely will include: Separation Anxiety Disorder, Panic Disorder, Agoraphobia, Specific Phobia, Social Anxiety Disorder, (Social Phobia), Generalized Anxiety Disorder, Substance-Induced Anxiety Disorder, Anxiety Disorder Associated with a Known General Medical Condition, Other Specified Anxiety Disorder and Unspecified Anxiety Disorder. In this chapter we focused on anxiety disorders as they were diagnosed in the DSM-IV because all published studies reflect that nosology.

Etiology

Recent etiological theories of anxiety capitalize both on inborn and acquired mechanisms, but to a different extent. Anxiety disorders tend to run in families [4], most likely reflecting common genetic rather than environmental factors [5]. There are two independent genetic factors in anxiety disorders, the first associated predominantly with PD, GAD and agoraphobia, while a second mainly influences situationally elicited anxiety such as phobias [6]. Neurobiologically, it is not known what these two factors represent, but they may relate to neurochemical differences [7] or differences in anxiety sensitivity or conditionability. Genetic factors account for a moderate proportion of around 30–40% of the variance in anxiety disorders. Thus, environmental factors also contribute to fear and anxiety, particularly unique rather than commonly shared environmental factors that influence anxiety development, rendering gene-environmental interactions pivotal (see chapter on Genetic Factors in Anxiety Disorders, pp. 24–66).

Fear conditioning, a likely candidate mechanism both for the acquisition of anxiety and for mediating gene-environmental interactions, is moderately heritable, in the range of 35–45% [8]. In addition, there is tentative evidence that fear conditioning to stimuli like snakes and spiders, that often trigger fear, has a higher heritability than conditioning to neutral stimuli like circles and triangles [8]. Some candidate genes for fear conditioning have been identified in humans [9, 10], and certain moderately heritable personality traits may also act as vulnerability factors for the development of anxiety. To the extent that fear conditioning is an etiological mechanism, it could be predicted that patients with anxiety disorders should be characterized by better acquisition, slower extinction, retarded extinction retention and compromised disruption of reconsolidation [11].

Neuroimaging

An advantage with positron emission tomography (PET) and single-photon emission computed tomography (SPECT) is the virtually unlimited potential to use organic compounds like ^{18}F, ^{15}O, ^{13}N and ^{11}C serving as radioisotopes enabling the determination of brain perfusion, metabolism and neurochemistry. Magnetic resonance imaging (MRI) can be used to determine neural function and structure as well as to index metabolic compounds in the brain. Neuroimaging studies have been performed at rest and during symptomatic challenge using tracers that reflect both neural and neurochemical processes. We recently performed a systematic and comprehensive review of all neurochemical brain imaging studies in the anxiety disorders [7]. All but one were performed in the resting state. The only exception was a study from our lab where we induced anxiety and determined the uptake of a ligand (GR205171) that reflects neurokinin 1 (NK1) receptor availability. We observed that when persons with SP were challenged with visual presentations of their phobic object resulting in fear, an anxiety tracer uptake was reduced, indicating fewer available NK1 receptors in a fearful than a fearless state. This supports an endogenous release of substance P when anxious. The interpretation is further supported by the fact that NK1 receptor blockade reduces anxiety to a similar extent as does treatment with selective serotonin reuptake inhibitors (SSRIs) [12]. Both NK1 antagonists and SSRIs also reduce anxiety-induced amygdala reactivity to a similar extent [12, 13]. In patients with PD, the NK1 receptor system is downregulated in the resting state [14], suggestive of repeated anxiety-induced substance P release in the brain.

In the resting state, there exist around 30 published studies on brain neurochemistry in anxiety disorders using PET or SPECT [15–50]. If it is required that 2 independent studies demonstrate consistent alterations, then results show that patients with SAD display a reduced dopamine D_2 receptor binding potential. PTSD is associated with a compromised benzodiazepine binding site function, and in PD both benzodiazepine receptors and serotonergic (5-hydroxytryptamine 1A; 5-HT$_{1A}$) receptors are downregulated. Across the anxiety disorders then, there is downregulation of both benzodiazepine sites and 5-HT$_{1A}$ receptors. Reduction in benzodiazepine-binding site activity occur most frequently in limbic and frontal areas both for PD and PTSD, while monoaminergic alterations, both in serotonergic and dopaminergic neurotransmission were localized predominantly in the limbic system [7].

Spectroscopy has also been used to evaluate the anxious brain. One of the most well-replicated findings is that N-acetylaspartate is decreased in PTSD as compared to healthy controls suggesting compromised neural integrity and viability [51]. In PTSD for example dysfunctional tissue is found in the hippocampus and could contribute to PTSD symptomatology. There are studies in PD and SAD that also suggest reduced N-acetylaspartate [52–54]. Another well-replicated finding is that of increased lactate levels in patients with PD [55–57]. It has also been reported with some consistency that markers of GABA-ergic functions are reduced in PD but enhanced in SAD [58]. Brain imaging of SAD [59, 60], PTSD [61, 62], PD [55], cognitive behavioral therapy (CBT) [63] and phobia [64, 65] have recently been conceptually reviewed.

While initial brain imaging studies of mental disorders using tools like PET and SPECT focused on schizophrenia and depression, and were mainly performed in the resting state, the second wave of imaging studies included activation studies, where cognitive and emotional tasks are used to activate certain brain areas in order to isolate and localize the task-related processes. Symptom provocation studies were carried out in an attempt to define dysfunctional regions related to anxiety. Most of the second-wave studies utilized tracers like ^{18}F and ^{15}O to determine glucose metabolism and regional cerebral blood flow. The next wave of activation, provocation and perturbation studies were carried out using blood oxygen level-dependent (BOLD) signal changes determined by functional MRI (fMRI). In the anxiety disorders, a series of studies have been performed with these methods and different types of challenges to study brain networks underlying anxiety. In SAD, a number of studies have reported that the amygdala seem to be overactive in response to pictures displaying emotional faces. Stein et al. [66] for example demonstrated increased amygdala reactivity to angry and contemptuous faces in SAD patients. In PTSD, amygdala reactivity is enhanced in response to trauma reminders and the increased trauma-related reactivity also seems to generalize to other stimuli like fearful faces and may even be elicited outside awareness [67]. It is linked to aberrant prefrontal control of the amygdala as the anterior cingulate cortex (ACC) is underresponsive in PTSD patients as compared to healthy controls. In SP, there also exists a series of studies indicating altered fear network activity in the brain in response to symptomatic challenge. However, the generalized increased reactivity in the amygdala observed in PTSD for example is not observed in individuals with SP, where increased reactivity is observed to phobogenic but not to generally fear-inducing stimuli [68], suggesting a more circumscribed lesion than in PTSD.

In a number of studies investigating structural alterations in the anxiety disorders, it is striking that an altered volume or white matter integrity often is observed in the areas also linked to altered reactivity indicating a close relationship between structure and function [62, 69]. Some of the initial functional studies in the anxiety disorders were reviewed in a well-cited paper by Etkin and Wager [70]. They included between-group studies, where brain activity characteristic of a disordered group was compared to healthy control subjects. Their main conclusions were that emotion-generating areas such as the amygdala and the insula were hyperactive in patients with specific or social phobia as well as in PTSD, while activity in emotion-controlling areas in the dorsal and rostral ACC was compromised in PTSD patients only. The Etkin and Wager [70] paper was not restricted to symptomatic challenge but also included studies on emotional perception like reactivity to slides containing emotional content. The reactivity patterns may be different when observing emotional content and experiencing an emotion. It has been suggested that areas in the ACC and/or the ventromedial prefrontal cortex (vmPFC) modulate emotionally induced amygdala reactivity and that this relation is aberrant in anxiety disorders [71–73]. Therefore, we decided to evaluate the theoretically predicted functional connectivity between the ACC and the amygdala by performing a systematic review of symptom provocation studies in patients with phobia and PTSD because in these disorders it is possible to induce anxiety through visual, auditory and imaginary procedures.

The third wave of brain imaging studies using symptom provocation designs were performed using both fMRI and PET, but less often SPECT. We recently reviewed only PET and SPECT studies that had used symptom provocation [7]. The pattern resulting from symptom provocation supports the contention that activity in the brain's fear circuit is altered and characterized by increased reactivity in the amygdala, the midbrain and possibly also in the insular cortex, whereas activity in emotion-regulating areas in the PFC such as the subgenual ACC and the orbitofrontal cortex (OFC) seem compromised in the symptomatic state, predominantly in phobic disorders. We also noted that increased activity in nodes of the fear circuit was not only restricted to conditions of symptom provocation, but sometimes also occurs in response to nontraumatic but distressing cues in PTSD [74] and in the resting state in patients with PD [75, 76] and PTSD [77, 78], perhaps reflecting a disorder-related vulnerability factor or a 'scar' resulting from repeated anxiety activation. Because there are no longitudinal studies, it is not possible to determine this. Collectively, it can be concluded that parts of the fear circuit in patients with situationally elicited anxiety disorders are hyperactive. This may be a mechanism accounting for increased autonomic and endocrine drive present in anxiety-disordered patients [79], as well as in behavioral manifestations of anxiety [80]. However, a number of studies using fMRI were not included in our recent analysis, and we decided to perform a systematic review of studies that have evaluated brain blood flow in response to symptom provocation regardless of imaging modality.

A literature search was performed in PubMed and the Web of Science using the following key words: 'fMRI', 'PET', 'SPECT' and 'brain imaging' crossed one by one with the terms 'social anxiety disorder' or 'social phobia', 'specific phobia' and 'posttraumatic stress disorder' combined with 'symptom provocation' or 'challenge'. The reference lists of the retrieved articles were inspected for additional publications that fulfilled the inclusion criteria. All articles were scanned by reading abstracts to identify articles that reported original data fulfilling the criterion that the design included a symptom provocation study both with a resting and a provoked anxiety state reported in a way that it was possible to retrieve statistics (t test or z test) on a within-group basis. Thus, we analyzed studies that reported data for a diagnostic group separately but not studies that only reported a comparison between a diagnosed and a control group, where it was not possible to statistically estimate the change of only the disordered group. Only studies reporting voxels in three-dimensional Talairach and Tournoux [81] or Montreal Neurological Institute coordinates were included.

A sufficient number of studies in specific, social anxiety and PTSD resulted from the systematic search of the literature. In the anxiety disorders, a number of provocation studies have been published, both in SP and SAD [82–131]. There exist around 40 published studies from the early 1990 to 2012 that have used fMRI, PET or SPECT to determine activity in brain areas responsive to symptomatic challenge in the situationally elicited anxiety disorders SP, SAD and PTSD that also have described activations in the three-dimensional Montreal Neurological Institute or Talairach [81] space. Several additional studies use emotional probes other than symptom provocation such as aversive facial and affective pictures to elicit affective processes [for recent reviews see 132–134]. Also, other challenges like anticipation of anxiety induced by pentagastrin administration have been studied using PET [135]. There are additional studies that have used pharmacological and physiological perturbations to induce anxiety in healthy individuals and patients, like cholecystokinin tetrapeptide [136, 137] and carbon dioxide (CO_2) challenge [138]. We included none of these in the present meta-analysis because physiological perturbations besides their anxiety-inducing properties also have peripheral effects, and the CNS alterations in pharmacological studies are less straightforward to interpret when compared to studies that have used psychological procedures to induce anxiety.

Some studies have also imaged pharmacological and behavioral treatment effects [13, 88, 139–141]. We performed analyses also of studies that used exposure or cognitive behavioral treatment and reported within-group effects for brain activation to anxiety challenge before and after treatment [13, 89, 92, 95, 140, 142, 143]. There exist additional brain imaging studies that have used the [133]Xenon technique to demonstrate alterations in frontal brain activity as resulting from cognitive therapy for specific animal phobia [144] and studies using brain imaging to predict treatment response [13, 145].

Meta-Analysis of Anxiety Neuroimaging

Amygdala activity is central to anxiety and negative affect. The amygdala may code for arousal properties of stimuli, inherently related to anxiety or reflect stimulus ambiguity also integrated in anxious reactions [146]. Amygdala activity may not be specific to anxiety because also positive emotions activate the amygdala. The amygdala is a hub in the fear network of the brain [73]. It has been proposed that amygdala activity is regulated through activity in the vmPFC. Both the subgenual part of the ACC and the medial OFC (mOFC) have reciprocal connections with the amygdala [147] and have been suggested to guide or guard amygdala activity in response to environmental influences eliciting anxiety [148]. Early provocation studies in SP demonstrated profound reduction in prefrontal areas [87, 88], and more recent studies in patients with SPs have used network analyses to reveal that inhibitory ACC control of the amygdala present during nonanxious conditions is lost during conditions of anxiety

[82]. Recent theories on emotional regulation [73, 148] heavily emphasize the relation between prefrontally initiated control processes and amygdala activity. While reciprocal neural connections exist between the amygdala and subgenual ACC as well as the medial and lateral OFC, areas in the dorsolateral PFC do not reach amygdala directly but only through ACC and OFC couplings. However, no systematic review of fear-circuit connectivity between the amygdala and the anterior cingulate and orbitofrontal cortices during symptom provocation has been performed in anxiety disorders. Therefore, we focused our analysis on the amygdala, ACC and OFC. Thus, the primary aim of the present chapter was to perform a systematic review of symptom provocation studies in patients with situationally elicited anxiety disorders, that is specific and social phobia as well as PTSD, because symptoms can be elicited by thought, sight and sounds that remind patients of their feared situations or objects.

To evaluate areas in the amygdala, the ACC and the OFC that change in response to anxiety challenge, we averaged t or z scores from all individual studies reported for the amygdala on the one hand, and the ACC and OFC on the other hand, and analyzed these statistically. We then plotted brain coordinates associated with increased and decreased activity during the symptomatic state. Based on the extracted amygdala ACC and OFC coordinates, we then repeated the analyses specifically for the Brodmann's areas (BAs) in the ACC, BA25, BA32 and BA24 (subgenual, rostral and dorsal ACC) as well as BAs in the OFC (BA11 and BA47 or medial and lateral OFC). Finally, we estimated correlations between the z scores from individual studies reflecting neural activity in the amygdala on the one hand and the PFC on the other. Specifically, we evaluated ACC activity at large by averaging peaks from BA25, -32 and -24 reflecting the ACC. Then we performed the same set of analyses but for activity in the amygdala on the one hand and separate for the subgenual (BA25), ventromedial (BA32) and dorsal ACC (BA24) on the other. The same split was done for the OFC using the medial OFC (BA11 – roughly corresponding to the gyrus rectus) and lateral OFC (BA47) in order to evaluate the covariation between prefrontal areas and the amygdala.

Symptom Provocation and Fear Network Activity

Figure 1 (right panels in the top and middle rows) summarizes perfusion results from symptom provocation studies in specific and social phobia on the one hand and PTSD on the other. We grouped specific and social phobia together, because SAD studies were too few to be evaluated separately and no obvious or striking differences between the two phobia types were observed.

Both in phobias and PTSD, blood flow in the amygdala increased reliably across studies [$t(20) = 20.31$; $p < 0.0001$] with no difference between the two groups [$t(19) < 1$; n.s.]. In the phobic disorders, as a function of fear, activity in the ACC increased significantly [$t(16) = 20.51$; $p < 0.0001$] but decreased nonsignificantly [$t(8) = 1$; n.s.]

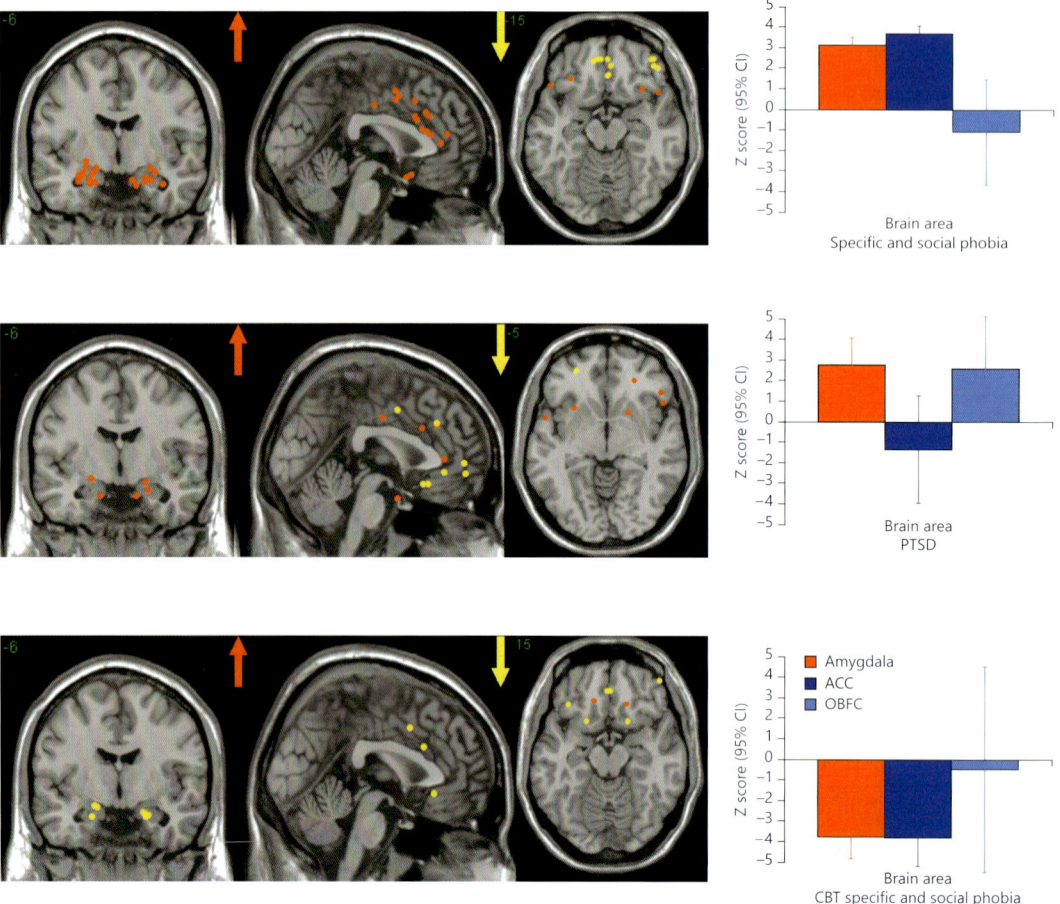

Fig. 1. Coronal, sagittal and transverse views of the amygdala, ACC and the orbitofrontal cortex (OFC), respectively, illustrating increased (red) and decreased (yellow) perfusion during symptom provocation in specific and social phobia (top row) and PTSD (middle row). The bottom row illustrates the effect of CBT. Note that in the sagittal views even though the hot spots (i.e. maximum peaks) are clearly not in the ACC, the extension of the original clusters comprise ACC regions. The right hand bar graph represents mean Z scores ± 95% confidence intervals based on blood flow estimates from the symptom provocation studies using PET, SPECT or fMRI illustrated in the brain plots.

in the OFC. In PTSD, average ACC activity was not significantly but only numerically reduced [t(7) = 1.18; n.s.] resulting in a significant difference between phobic patients and PTSD [t(18) = 5.32; p < 0.0001]. OFC activity tended to increase in PTSD [t(5) = 2.11; p < 0.09], resulting in a significant difference between PTSD and phobia [t(14) = 2.43; p < 0.05].

When evaluating more specifically where activity was altered in the ACC and the OFC, a clear pattern emerged (see fig. 2). In patients with phobia, activity increased in BA32 [t(6) = 23.02; p < 0.0001] and BA24 [t(6) = 10.64; p < 0.0001] but not BA25 [t(1) = 3.72; n.s.]. In PTSD patients, activity in the subgenual ACC (BA25) decreased

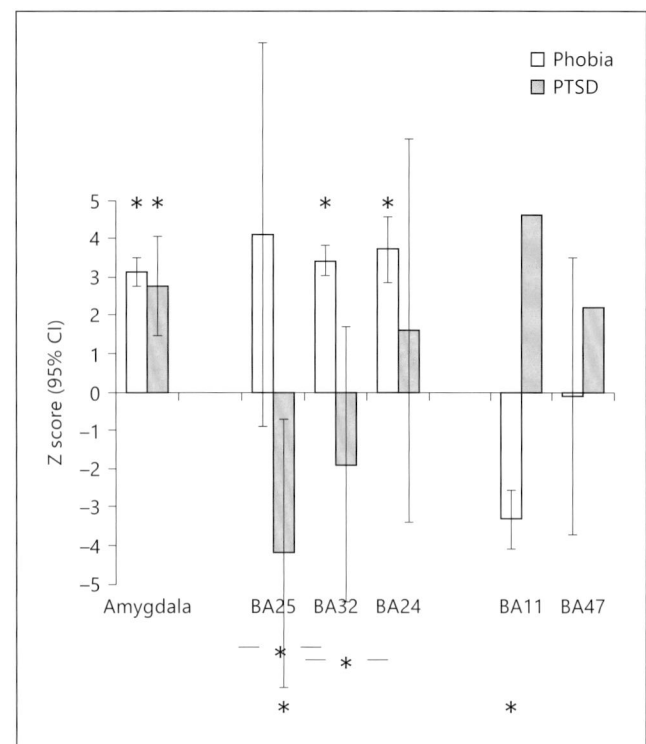

Fig. 2. Neural activity in the amygdala, subgenual ACC (BA25), ventromedial ACC (BA32) and dorsal ACC (BA24) as well as medial (BA11) and lateral OFC (BA47) in patients with phobic disorders or PTSD during symptom provocation. Single asterisks indicate significant differences from zero and asterisks within lines group differences.

during symptom provocation [t(1) = 15.12; p < 0.05] but was unaltered in BA24 [t(3) <1; n.s.] and BA32 [t(4) = 1.3; n.s.] resulting in significant differences between phobic and PTSD patients in the BA25 [t(2) = 7.30; p < 0.05], BA32 [t(10) = 4.35; p < 0.0015] but not BA24 [t(9) = 1.67; n.s.]. In the OFC, reactivity was attenuated in the mOFC (BA11) in phobic patients [t(4) = 12.03; p < 0.001] but not in PTSD. The data points in PTSD were too few to allow for a formal comparison in the BA11. Reactivity in BA47 was unaltered in patients with phobia [t(6) = <1; n.s.] or PTSD [t(4) = 1.54; n.s.] resulting in a nonsignificant difference between the two [t(10) = 1.06; n.s.].

Thus, the amygdala responds with increased reactivity to symptom provocation both in phobia and PTSD and is invariably positively correlated with measures of subjective fear and distress in individual studies [91, 92, 121, 122, 125, 142, 149]. Also, there are indications that reactivity in the vmPFC is compromised both in PTSD and phobia, albeit in different areas of the vmPFC. While reactivity in the subgenual cortex was attenuated in PTSD, it tended to be enhanced among phobic patients, while the reverse was true for mOFC, where activity decreased significantly across studies among patients with phobia but was increased in the only study that reported BA11 in PTSD patients. The fact that activity in the subgenual ACC is compromised speaks in favor of the hypothesis that the ACC, particularly BA25/-32 is involved in inhibitory emotional control in PTSD. Further supporting this, individual PTSD studies reporting correlations between activity in the ACC and subjective ratings more often report negative than positive correlations between the two [109, 111, 125, 149–152]. This may not be so in the phobic disorders because ACC activity is increased and is mainly positively correlated with symptom scores [99, 153], suggesting an appraising role for ACC activity in phobia. Activity in these ACC areas have sometimes [154, 155] but not always [156] been linked to generation and expression of fear reactions leading to conclusions that this area is involved in both evaluative and expressive aspects of emotions.

Studies that have evaluated connectivity within the PFC and the amygdala have demonstrated both negative and positive connectivity in SAD [157, 158], and negative in PTSD [125, 151]. It should be noted that for PTSD most of the areas being negatively correlated with subjective symptom reports indicate that inhibitory emotional control was located in the pregenual ACC [159]. Thus, the connectivity pattern in the two disorders seems more complex than just reflecting inhibitory areas regardless of symptomatology. For the amygdala, the interpretation is simpler. Reactivity is increased and invariably positively correlated with negative affect. Further supporting a role for the amygdala in generating fear, it should be noted that amygdala reactivity is reduced by therapy and also that the magnitude of reduction predicts long-term success [13, 89].

In the present meta-analysis, treatment with CBT resulted in reduced amygdala reactivity [$t(4) = 13.66$; $p < 0.0002$; see figure 1 bottom row]. Also, in patients with phobia the initially increased reactivity in the ACC was significantly reduced after therapy [$t(3) = 8.52$; $p < 0.005$]. The numbers of studies evaluating PTSD treatment were too few to allow for meaningful statistical analyses. However, it is of note that the initially increased ACC activity was significantly reduced by therapy in the phobic disorders while the initially decreased ACC activity in PTSD tended to be restored by increased activity after therapy [140]. This is an interesting observation forming the basis for a hypothesis of restorative processes activated by CBT.

A correlative approach including all studies in all groups that reported reactivity in the amygdala and areas of the ACC and OFC reveal that amygdala activity is positively correlated with ACC ($rxy = 0.80$; $p = 0.0005$), particularly BA24 ($rxy = 0.96$; $p = 0.0008$) but not OFC ($rxy = 0.19$; n.s.) activity. The correlation between amygdala reactivity and activity in the gyrus rectus (BA11) was strongly negative ($rxy = -0.99$; $p < 0.0001$), and in part reflects attenuating effects in the amygdala and enhancing effects in the mOFC in studies including CBT effects in SP.

Thus, supplemented with the correlations it might be argued that the dorsal ACC activates in concert with the amygdala and that the most parsimonious interpretation then is that activity in the dorsal ACC is related to fear evaluation or expression and not control. For the mOFC, data strongly suggest an inhibitory relation with the amygdala. Thus, we propose that the vmPFC is involved in inhibitory control of amygdala activity during anxiety provocation, but that the specific areas within the vmPFC differ depending on the type of anxiety. In adolescents with GAD, it was recently demonstrated that CBT increases activity in the PFC while viewing angry faces

[160], further supporting the view that successful CBT restores brain functionality. In patients with phobia, the mOFC may be pivotal for control, whereas in PTSD, the control function is most likely localized in the subgenual cortex. It is unclear if this pattern represents a risk factor present before the disorder onset, or a 'scar' resulting from the respective disorder. The treatment data for SP would suggest that dorsal ACC activity is critically involved in coding, generating or maintaining fear because treatment restores the initially enhanced ACC activity. The most robust finding evident across disorders though is reduced activity in the amygdala as a function of behavioral therapy. Also pharmacological interventions reduce medial temporal lobe activity including the amygdala in response to anxiety challenge [12, 13]. This is true for serotonergic reuptake inhibitors as well as NK1 receptor antagonists, suggesting that reduction in amygdala reactivity may be a final common pathway for efficient anxiety reduction. This notion is further supported by studies demonstrating that also responders but not nonresponders to placebo are characterized by reduced amygdala reactivity to symptom provocation [161, 162].

In patients with SAD, Phan et al. [163] recently presented evidence suggesting that SAD patients had significantly lower fractional anisotropy in the right uncinate fasciculus that connects the PFC with the temporal lobe. Thus, there might be structural underpinnings of the aberrant functional control of the amygdala eventually stemming from the mOFC. This may be a vulnerability factor for anxiety, because the brain structure seems to be under strong genetic control [164].

Multiple Mechanisms Mediating Anxiety

Altered neurotransmission could represent a vulnerability factor or a scar resulting from repeated anxiety experiences [7], and neurochemistry may be correlated with or modulate the activity of the fear network in the brain [73]. For example, Hariri and coworkers reported a negative correlation between $5\text{-}HT_{1A}$ receptor density and BOLD reactivity to emotional pictures in normal healthy volunteers. Fisher et al. [165] and Kienast et al. [166] demonstrated positive relations between serotonin and dopamine functions in the amygdala and BOLD reactivity to negative stimuli. This is in line with a modulating role for the monoaminergic system with respect to fear network activity, and suggests marked genetic influences because monoaminergic brain functions are strongly genetically determined [40]. Also data in patients with specific animal phobia suggest that the NK1-substance P system in the brain modulates activity in the amygdala. Ahs et al. [82] reported a positive correlation between amygdala regional cerebral blood flow and anxiety ratings and increased amygdala reactivity, while Michelgard et al. [167] observed a corresponding negative correlation between anxiety ratings and NK1 receptor activity associated with reduced receptor availability suggesting a potential coupling between neural activity in the fear circuit and neurotransmission. Neurochemical modulation of the central nervous system activity is further supported by imaging genetic studies linking functional serotonergic [168] and dopaminergic polymorphisms to emotionally determined amygdala reactivity [169] and by modulation of intrinsic couplings within the fear network [170]. One implication of the hypothesis that the monoaminergic as well as other neurotransmission systems modulate fear circuit activity is that treatments targeting specific neurochemical systems also should influence symptomatology through modulating fear network activity. A couple of studies from our and other laboratories are consistent with this notion, because reduction in anxiety achieved through administration of SSRI and a NK1 receptor antagonist attenuated amygdala reactivity in SAD [12, 13, 161]. In addition, in PTSD, initially reduced prefrontal activity was enhanced by SSRI treatment [171]. These findings were recently replicated in a larger cohort [172]. Thus, attenuation of amygdala reactivity may be a final common pathway for anxiety reduction irrespective of treatment modality and linked to prefrontal alterations.

Collectively, studies suggest that the fear network of the brain is altered in anxiety disorders with increased amygdala reactivity and decreased vmPFC activity in response to anxiety challenge coupled with neurochemical alterations. Activity in the fear network is restored by symptomatic treatment. A parsimonious working hypothesis is that both psychological and pharmacological interventions work through altering fear network activity either by bottom-up mechanisms reducing amygdala activity directly, or through prefrontal top-down control of fear-initiating areas. The hypothesis that neurotransmission is tightly coupled to fear network activity also implies that effective CBT is mediated by alterations in the neurochemistry of the brain. This was recently demonstrated for dopamine D_2 receptor binding [173] in an interesting first study on this topic. It will be a great challenge for the future to identify genes that affect brain connectivity in the anxiety disorders [174] and to evaluate the effect of treatment on the genetically determined connectome.

References

1 American Psychiatric Association: Diagnostic and Statistical Manual of Mental Disorders (DSM-IV), ed 4. Washington, American Psychiatric Press, 1994.
2 Kessler RC, McGonagle KA, Zhao S, Nelson CB, Hughes M, Eshleman S, Wittchen HU, Kendler KS: Lifetime and 12-month prevalence of DSM-III-R psychiatric disorders in the United States: results from the National Comorbidity Survey. Arch Gen Psychiatry 1994;51:8–19.
3 Kessler RC, Berglund P, Demler O, Jin R, Walters EE: Lifetime prevalence and age-of-onset distributions of DSM-IV disorders in the National Comorbidity Survey Replication. Arch Gen Psychiatry 2005;62:593–602.
4 Tillfors M, Furmark T, Ekselius L, Fredrikson M: Social phobia and avoidant personality disorder as related to parental history of social anxiety: a general population study. Behav Res Ther 2001;39:289–298.
5 Hettema JM, Neale MC, Kendler KS: A review and meta-analysis of the genetic epidemiology of anxiety disorders. Am J Psychiatry 2001;158:156–164.
6 Hettema JM, Prescott CA, Myers JM, Neale MC, Kendler KS: The structure of genetic and environmental risk factors for anxiety disorders in men and women. Arch Gen Psychiatry 2005;62:182–189.
7 Fredrikson M, Faria V, Furmark T: Neuroimaging of neurotransmission in anxiety disorders; in Dierckx RAJO, Otte A, Boer JA den, De Vries EFJ, Van Waarde A (eds): PET and SPECT in Psychiatry. Berlin, Springer, 2013, chapter 14, in press.

8 Hettema JM, Annas P, Neale MC, Kendler KS, Fredrikson M: A twin study of the genetics of fear conditioning. Arch Gen Psychiatry 2003;60:702–708.

9 Garpenstrand H, Annas P, Ekblom J, Oreland L, Fredrikson M: Human fear conditioning is related to dopaminergic and serotonergic biological markers. Behav Neurosci 2001;115:358–364.

10 Lonsdorf TB, Weike AI, Nikamo P, Schalling M, Hamm AO, Ohman A: Genetic gating of human fear learning and extinction: possible implications for gene-environment interaction in anxiety disorder. Psychol Sci 2009;20:198–206.

11 Agren T, Engman J, Frick A, Björkstrand J, Larsson E-M, Furmark T, Fredrikson M: Disruption of reconsolidation erases a memory trace in the human amygdala. Science 2012;337:1550–1552.

12 Furmark T, Appel L, Michelgard A, Wahlstedt K, Ahs F, Zancan S, Jacobsson E, Flyckt K, Grohp M, Bergström M, Pich EM, Nilsson LG, Bani M, Langström B, Fredrikson M: Cerebral blood flow changes after treatment of social phobia with the neurokinin-1 antagonist GR205171, citalopram, or placebo. Biol Psychiatry 2005;58:132–142.

13 Furmark T, Tillfors M, Marteinsdottir I, Fischer H, Pissiota A, Langström B, Fredrikson M: Common changes in cerebral blood flow in patients with social phobia treated with citalopram or cognitive-behavioral therapy. Arch Gen Psychiatry 2002;59:425–433.

14 Fujimura Y, Yasuno F, Farris A, Liow JS, Geraci M, Drevets W, Pine DS, Ghose S, Lerner A, Hargreaves R, Burns HD, Morse C, Pike VW, Innis RB: Decreased neurokinin-1 (substance P) receptor binding in patients with panic disorder: positron emission tomographic study with [18F]SPA-RQ. Biol Psychiatry 2009;66:94–97.

15 Bonne O, Gilboa A, Louzoun Y, Brandes D, Yona I, Lester H, Barkai G, Freedman N, Chisin R, Shalev AY: Resting regional cerebral perfusion in recent posttraumatic stress disorder. Biol Psychiatry 2003;54:1077–1086.

16 Bonne O, Bain E, Neumeister A, Nugent AC, Vythilingam M, Carson RE, Luckenbaugh DA, Eckelman W, Herscovitch P, Drevets WC, Charney DS: No change in serotonin type 1A receptor binding in patients with posttraumatic stress disorder. Am J Psychiatry 2005;162:383–385.

17 Brandt CA, Meller J, Keweloh L, Höschel K, Staedt J, Munz D, Stoppe G: Increased benzodiazepine receptor density in the prefrontal cortex in patients with panic disorder. J Neural Transm 1998;105:1325–1333.

18 Bremner JD, Innis RB, Southwick SM, Staib L, Zoghbi S, Charney DS: Decreased benzodiazepine receptor binding in prefrontal cortex in combat-related posttraumatic stress disorder. Am J Psychiatry 2000;157:1120–1126.

19 Bremner JD, Innis RB, White T, Fujita M, Silbersweig D, Goddard AW, Staib L, Stern E, Cappiello A, Woods S, Baldwin R, Charney DS: SPECT [I-123] iomazenil measurement of the benzodiazepine receptor in panic disorder. Biol Psychiatry 2000;47:96–106.

20 Cameron OG, Huang GC, Nichols T, Koeppe RA, Minoshima S, Rose D, Frey KA: Reduced gamma-aminobutyric acid(A)-benzodiazepine binding sites in insular cortex of individuals with panic disorder. Arch Gen Psychiatry 2007;64:793–800.

21 Czermak C, Staley JK, Kasserman S, Bois F, Young T, Henry S, Tamagnan GD, Seibyl JP, Krystal JH, Neumeister A: Beta2 nicotinic acetylcholine receptor availability in post-traumatic stress disorder. Int J Neuropsychopharmacol 2008;11:419–424.

22 Evans KC, Simon NM, Dougherty DD, Hoge EA, Worthington JJ, Chow C, Kaufman RE, Gold AL, Fischman AJ, Pollack MH, Rauch SL: A PET study of tiagabine treatment implicates ventral medial prefrontal cortex in generalized social anxiety disorder. Neuropsychopharmacology 2009;2:390–398.

23 Fujita M, Southwick SM, Denucci CC, Zoghbi SS, Dillon MS, Baldwin RM, Bozkurt A, Kugaya A, Verhoeff NP, Seibyl JP, Innis RB: Central type benzodiazepine receptors in Gulf War veterans with posttraumatic stress disorder. Biol Psychiatry 2004;56:95–100.

24 Geuze E, van Berckel BN, Lammertsma AA, Boellaard R, de Kloet CS, Vermetten E, Westenberg HG: Reduced GABAA benzodiazepine receptor binding in veterans with post-traumatic stress disorder. Mol Psychiatry 2008;13:74–83.

25 Hasler G, Nugent AC, Carlson PJ, Carson RE, Geraci M, Drevets WC: Altered cerebral gamma-aminobutyric acid type A-benzodiazepine receptor binding in panic disorder determined by [11C]flumazenil positron emission tomography. Arch Gen Psychiatry 2008;65:1166–1175.

26 Kaschka W, Feistel H, Ebert D: Reduced benzodiazepine receptor binding in panic disorders measured by iomazenil SPECT. J Psychiatr Res 1995;29:427–434.

27 Kent JM, Coplan JD, Lombardo I, Hwang DR, Huang Y, Mawlawi O, Van Heertum RL, Slifstein M, Abi-Dargham A, Gorman JM, Laruelle M: Occupancy of brain serotonin transporters during treatment with paroxetine in patients with social phobia: a positron emission tomography study with 11C McN 5652. Psychopharmacology (Berl) 2002;164:341–348.

28 Kuikka JT, Pitkänen A, Lepola U, Partanen K, Vainio P, Bergström KA, Wieler HJ, Kaiser KP, Mittelbach L, Koponen H, et al: Abnormal regional benzodiazepine receptor uptake in the prefrontal cortex in patients with panic disorder. Nucl Med Commun 1995;16:273–280.

29 Lanzenberger RR, Mitterhauser M, Spindelegger C, Wadsak W, Klein N, Mien LK, Holik A, Attarbaschi T, Mossaheb N, Sacher J, Geiss-Granadia T, Kletter K, Kasper S, Tauscher J: Reduced serotonin-1A receptor binding in social anxiety disorder. Biol Psychiatry 2007;61:1081–1089.

30 Liberzon I, Taylor SF, Phan KL, Britton JC, Fig LM, Bueller JA, Koeppe RA, Zubieta JK: Altered central micro-opioid receptor binding after psychological trauma. Biol Psychiatry 2007;61:1030–1038.

31 Malizia AL, Cunningham VJ, Bell CJ, Liddle PF, Jones T, Nutt DJ: Decreased brain GABA(A)-benzodiazepine receptor binding in panic disorder: preliminary results from a quantitative PET study. Arch Gen Psychiatry 1998;55:715–720.

32 Maron E, Kuikka JT, Shlik J, Vasar V, Vanninen E, Tiihonen J: Reduced brain serotonin transporter binding in patients with panic disorder. Psychiatry Res 2004;132:173–181.

33 Maron E, Kuikka JT, Ulst K, Tiihonen J, Vasar V, Shlik J: SPECT imaging of serotonin transporter binding in patients with generalized anxiety disorder. Eur Arch Psychiatry Clin Neurosci 2004;254:392–396.

34 Maron E, Nutt DJ, Kuikka J, Tiihonen J: Dopamine transporter binding in females with panic disorder may vary with clinical status. J Psychiatr Res 2010;44:56–59.

35 Maron E, Tõru I, Hirvonen J, Tuominen L, Lumme V, Vasar V, Shlik J, Nutt DJ, Helin S, NAgren K, Tiihonen J, Hietala J: Gender differences in brain serotonin transporter availability in panic disorder. J Psychopharmacol 2011;25:952–959.

36 Moriyama TS, Felicio AC, Chagas MH, Tardelli VS, Ferraz HB, Tumas V, Amaro-Junior E, Andrade LA, Crippa JA, Bressan RA: Increased dopamine transporter density in Parkinson's disease patients with Social Anxiety Disorder. J Neurol Sci 2011;15:53–57.

37 Murrough JW, Huang Y, Hu J, Henry S, Williams W, Gallezot JD, Bailey CR, Krystal JH, Carson RE, Neumeister A: Reduced amygdala serotonin transporter binding in posttraumatic stress disorder. Biol Psychiatry 2011;70:1033–1038.

38 Nash JR, Sargent PA, Rabiner EA, Hood SD, Argyropoulos SV, Potokar JP, Grasby PM, Nutt DJ: Serotonin 5-HT1A receptor binding in people with panic disorder: positron emission tomography study. Br J Psychiatry 2008;193:229–234.

39 Neumeister A, Bain E, Nugent AC, Carson RE, Bonne O, Luckenbaugh DA, Eckelman W, Herscovitch P, Charney DS, Drevets WC: Reduced serotonin type 1A receptor binding in panic disorder. J Neurosci 2004;24:589–591.

40 Pinborg LH, Arfan H, Haugbol S, Kyvik KO, Hjelmborg JV, Svarer C, Frokjaer VG, Paulson OB, Holm S, Knudsen GM: The 5-HT2A receptor binding pattern in the human brain is strongly genetically determined. Neuroimage 2008;40:1175–1180.

41 Schlegel S, Steinert H, Bockisch A, Hahn K, Schloesser R, Benkert O: Decreased benzodiazepine receptor binding in panic disorder measured by IOMAZENIL-SPECT. A preliminary report. Eur Arch Psychiatry Clin Neurosci 1994;244:49–51.

42 Schneier FR, Abi-Dargham A, Martinez D, Slifstein M, Hwang DR, Liebowitz MR, Laruelle M: Dopamine transporters, D2 receptors, and dopamine release in generalized social anxiety disorder. Depress Anxiety 2009;2:411–418.

43 Schneier FR, Liebowitz MR, Abi-Dargham A, Zea-Ponce Y, Lin SH, Laruelle M: Low dopamine D(2) receptor binding potential in social phobia. Am J Psychiatry 2000;157:457–459.

44 Schneier FR, Martinez D, Abi-Dargham A, Zea-Ponce Y, Simpson HB, Liebowitz MR, Laruelle M: Striatal dopamine D(2) receptor availability in OCD with and without comorbid social anxiety disorder: preliminary findings. Depress Anxiety 2008;25:1–7.

45 Spindelegger C, Lanzenberger R, Wadsak W, Mien LK, Stein P, Mitterhauser M, Moser U, Holik A, Pezawas L, Kletter K, Kasper S: Influence of escitalopram treatment on 5-HT 1A receptor binding in limbic regions in patients with anxiety disorders. Mol Psychiatry 2009;14:1040–1050.

46 Sullivan GM, Oquendo MA, Simpson N, Van Heertum RL, Mann JJ, Parsey RV: Brain serotonin1A receptor binding in major depression is related to psychic and somatic anxiety. Biol Psychiatry 2005;58:947–954.

47 Tiihonen J, Kuikka J, Bergström K, Lepola U, Koponen H, Leinonen E: Dopamine reuptake site densities in patients with social phobia. Am J Psychiatry 1997;154:239–242.

48 Tiihonen J, Kuikka J, Räsänen P, Lepola U, Koponen H, Liuska A, Lehmusvaara A, Vainio P, Könönen M, Bergström K, Yu M, Kinnunen I, Akerman K, Karhu J: Cerebral benzodiazepine receptor binding and distribution in generalized anxiety disorder: a fractal analysis. Mol Psychiatry 1997;2:463–471.

49 van der Wee NJ, van Veen JF, Stevens H, van Vliet IM, van Rijk PP, Westenberg HG: Increased serotonin and dopamine transporter binding in psychotropic medication-naive patients with generalized social anxiety disorder shown by 123I-beta-(4-iodophenyl)-tropane SPECT. J Nucl Med 2008;49:757–763.

50 Warwick JM, Carey PD, Cassimjee N, Lochner C, Hemmings S, Moolman-Smook H, Beetge E, Dupont P, Stein DJ: Dopamine transporter binding in social anxiety disorder: the effect of treatment with escitalopram. Metab Brain Dis 2012;27:151–158.

51 Karl A, Werner A: The use of proton magnetic resonance spectroscopy in PTSD research – meta-analyses of findings and methodological review. Neurosci Biobehav Rev 2010;34:7–22.

52 Trzesniak C, Uchida RR, Araújo D, Guimarães FS, Freitas-Ferrari MC, Filho AS, Santos AC, Busatto GF, Zuardi AW, Del-Ben CM, Graeff FG, Crippa JA: (1)H magnetic resonance spectroscopy imaging of the hippocampus in patients with panic disorder. Psychiatry Res 2010;182:261–265.

53 Davidson JR, Krishnan KR, Charles HC, Boyko O, Potts NL, Ford SM, Patterson L: Magnetic resonance spectroscopy in social phobia: preliminary findings. J Clin Psychiatry 1993;54:19–25.

54 Tupler LA, Davidson JR, Smith RD, Lazeyras F, Charles HC, Krishnan K: A repeat proton magnetic resonance spectroscopy study in social phobia. Biol Psychiatry 1997;42:419–424.

55 Kim JE, Dager SR, Lyoo IK: The role of the amygdala in the pathophysiology of panic disorder: evidence from neuroimaging studies. Biol Mood Anxiety Disord 2012;20:20.

56 Maddock RJ, Buonocore MH: MR spectroscopic studies of the brain in psychiatric disorders. Curr Top Behav Neurosci, E-pub ahead of print.

57 Corrigan NM, Richards TL, Friedman SD, Petropoulos H, Dager SR: Improving 1H MRSI measurement of cerebral lactate for clinical applications. Psychiatry Res 2010;182:40–47.

58 Maddock RJ, Buonocore MH, Copeland LE, Richards AL: Elevated brain lactate responses to neural activation in panic disorder: a dynamic 1H-MRS study. Mol Psychiatry 2009;14:537–545.

59 Freitas-Ferrari MC, Hallak JE, Trzesniak C, Filho AS, Machado-de-Sousa JP, Chagas MH, Nardi AE, Crippa JA: Neuroimaging in social anxiety disorder: a systematic review of the literature. Prog Neuropsychopharmacol Biol Psychiatry 2010;30:565–580.

60 Miskovic V, Schmidt LA: Social fearfulness in the human brain. Neurosci Biobehav Rev 2012;36:459–478.

61 Hughes KC, Shin LM: Functional neuroimaging studies of post-traumatic stress disorder. Expert Rev Neurother 2011;11:275–285.

62 Patel R, Spreng RN, Shin LM, Girard TA: Neurocircuitry models of posttraumatic stress disorder and beyond: a meta-analysis of functional neuroimaging studies. Neurosci Biobehav Rev 2012;36:2130–2142.

63 Porto PR, Oliveira L, Mari J, Volchan E, Figueira I, Ventura P: Does cognitive behavioral therapy change the brain? A systematic review of neuroimaging in anxiety disorders. J Neuropsychiatry Clin Neurosci 2009;21:114–125.

64 Del Casale A, Ferracuti S, Rapinesi C, Serata D, Piccirilli M, Savoja V, Kotzalidis GD, Manfredi G, Angeletti G, Tatarelli R, Girardi P: Functional neuroimaging in specific phobia. Psychiatry Res 2012;30: 181–197.

65 Linares IM, Trzesniak C, Chagas MH, Hallak JE, Nardi AE, Crippa JA: Neuroimaging in specific phobia disorder: a systematic review of the literature. Rev Bras Psiquiatr 2012;1:101–111.

66 Stein MB, Goldin PR, Sareen J, Zorrilla LT, Brown GG: Increased amygdala activation to angry and contemptuous faces in generalized social phobia. Biol Psychiatry 2000;47:769–776.

67 Rauch SL, Whalen PJ, Shin LM, McInerney SC, Macklin ML, Lasko NB, Orr SP, Pitman RK: Exaggerated amygdala response to masked facial stimuli in posttraumatic stress disorder: a functional MRI study. Biol Psychiatry 2000;47:769–776.

68 Wright CI, Martis B, McMullin K, Shin LM, Rauch SL: Amygdala and insular responses to emotionally valenced human faces in small animal specific phobia. Biol Psychiatry 2003;54:1067–1076.

69 Hayes JP, Hayes SM, Mikedis AM: Quantitative meta-analysis of neural activity in posttraumatic stress disorder. Biol Mood Anxiety Disord 2012;2:2–9.

70 Etkin A, Wager TD: Functional neuroimaging of anxiety: a meta-analysis of emotional processing in PTSD, social anxiety disorder, and specific phobia. Am J Psychiatry 2007;64:1476–1488.

71 Ray RD, Zald DH: Anatomical insights into the interaction of emotion and cognition in the prefrontal cortex. Neurosci Biobehav Rev 2012;36:479–501.

72 Rauch SL, Shin LM, Phelps EA: Neurocircuitry models of posttraumatic stress disorder and extinction: human neuroimaging research – past, present, and future. Biol Psychiatry 2006;60:376–382.

73 Shin LM, Liberzon I: The neurocircuitry of fear, stress, and anxiety disorders. Neuropsychopharmacology 2010;35:169–191.

74 Gold AL, Shin LM, Orr SP, Carson MA, Rauch SL, Macklin ML, Lasko NB, Metzger LJ, Dougherty DD, Alpert NM, Fischman AJ, Pitman RK: Decreased regional cerebral blood flow in medial prefrontal cortex during trauma-unrelated stressful imagery in Vietnam veterans with post-traumatic stress disorder. Psychol Med 2011;13:1–10.

75 Bisaga A, Katz JL, Antonini A, Wright CE, Margouleff CC, Gorman JM, Eidelberg D: Cerebral glucose metabolism in women with panic disorder. Am J Psychiatry 1998;166:1178–1183.

76 Sakai Y, Kumano H, Nishikawa M, Sakano Y, Kaiya H, Imabayashi E, Ohnishi T, Matsuda H, Yasuda A, Sato A, Diksic M, Kuboki T: Cerebral glucose metabolism associated with a fear network in panic disorder. Neuroreport 2005;16:927–931.

77 Mirzaei S, Knoll P, Keck A, Preitler B, Gutierrez E, Umek H, Köhn H, Pecherstorfer M: Regional cerebral blood flow in patients suffering from post-traumatic stress disorder. Neuropsychobiology 2001;43: 260–264.

78 Molina ME, Isoardi R, Prado MN, Bentolila S: Basal cerebral glucose distribution in long-term post-traumatic stress disorder. World J Biol Psychiatry 2010; 11:493–501.

79 Ahs F, Furmark T, Michelgard A, Langström B, Appel L, Wolf OT, Kirschbaum C, Fredrikson M: Hypothalamic blood flow correlates positively with stress-induced cortisol levels in subjects with social anxiety disorder. Psychosom Med 2006;68:859–862.

80 Laukka P, Ahs F, Furmark T, Fredrikson M: Neurofunctional correlates of expressed vocal affect in social phobia. Cogn Affect Behav Neurosci 2011;11: 413–425.

81 Talairach J, Tournoux P: Co-Planar Stereotactic Atlas of the Human Brain. Stuttgart, Germany, Thieme, 1988.

82 Ahs F, Pissiota A, Michelgard A, Frans O, Furmark T, Appel L, Fredrikson M: Disentangling the web of fear: amygdala reactivity and functional connectivity in spider and snake phobia. Psychiatry Res 2009;172: 103–108.

83 Alpers GW, Gerdes AB, Lagarie B, Tabbert K, Vaitl D, Stark R: Attention and amygdala activity: an fMRI study with spider pictures in spider phobia. J Neural Transm 2009;116:747–757.

84 Britton JC, Gold AL, Deckersbach T, Rauch SL: Functional MRI study of specific animal phobia using an event-related emotional counting stroop paradigm. Depress Anxiety 2009;26:796–805.

85 Carlsson K, Petersson KM, Lundqvist D, Karlsson A, Ingvar M, Ohman A: Fear and the amygdala: manipulation of awareness generates differential cerebral responses to phobic and fear-relevant (but non-feared) stimuli. Emotion 2004;4:340–353.

86 Dilger S, Straube T, Mentzel HJ, Fitzek C, Reichenbach JR, Hecht H, Krieschel S, Gutberlet I, Miltner WH: Brain activation to phobia-related pictures in spider phobic humans: an event-related functional magnetic resonance imaging study. Neurosci Lett 2003;348:29–32.

87 Fredrikson M, Wik G, Greitz T, Eriksson L, Stone-Elander S, Ericson K, Sedvall G: Regional cerebral blood flow during experimental phobic fear. Psychophysiology 1993;30:126–130.

88 Fredrikson M, Wik G, Annas P, Ericson K, Stone-Elander S: Functional neuroanatomy of visually elicited simple phobic fear: additional data and theoretical analysis. Psychophysiology 1995;32:43–48.

89 Hauner KK, Mineka S, Voss JL, Paller KA: Exposure therapy triggers lasting reorganization of neural fear processing. Proc Natl Acad Sci USA 2012;109:9203–9208.

90 Hermann A, Schäfer A, Walter B, Stark R, Vaitl D, Schienle A: Diminished medial prefrontal cortex activity in blood-injection-injury phobia. Biol Psychol 2007;75:124–130.

91 Hermann A, Schäfer A, Walter B, Stark R, Vaitl D, Schienle A: Emotion regulation in spider phobia: role of the medial prefrontal cortex. Soc Cogn Affect Neurosci 2009;4:257–267.

92 Paquette V, Lévesque J, Mensour B, Leroux JM, Beaudoin G, Bourgouin P, Beauregard M: Change the mind and you change the brain: effects of cognitive-behavioral therapy on the neural correlates of spider phobia. Neuroimage 2003;18:401–409.

93 Rauch SL, Savage CR, Alpert NM, Miguel EC, Baer L, Breiter HC, Fischman AJ, Manzo PA, Moretti C, Jenike MA: A positron emission tomographic study of simple phobic symptom provocation. Arch Gen Psychiatry 1995;52:20–28.

94 Rauch SL, van der Kolk BA, Fisler RE, Alpert NM, Orr SP, Savage CR, Fischman AJ, Jenike MA, Pitman RK: A symptom provocation study of post-traumatic stress disorder using positron emission tomography and script-driven imagery. Arch Gen Psychiatry 1996;53:380–387.

95 Schienle A, Schäfer A, Hermann A, Rohrmann S, Vaitl D: Symptom provocation and reduction in patients suffering from spider phobia: an fMRI study on exposure therapy. Eur Arch Psychiatry Clin Neurosci 2007;257:486–493.

96 Schienle A, Schäfer A, Walter B, Stark R, Vaitl D: Brain activation of spider phobics towards disorder-relevant, generally disgust- and fear-inducing pictures. Neurosci Lett 2005;388:1–6.

97 Straube T, Mentzel HJ, Glauer M, Miltner WH: Brain activation to phobia-related words in phobic subjects. Neurosci Lett 2004;372:204–208.

98 Straube T, Glauer M, Dilger S, Mentzel HJ, Miltner WH: Effects of cognitive-behavioral therapy on brain activation in specific phobia. Neuroimage 2006;29:125–135.

99 Straube T, Mentzel HJ, Miltner WH: Waiting for spiders: brain activation during anticipatory anxiety in spider phobics. Neuroimage 2007;37:1427–1436.

100 Tillfors M, Furmark T, Marteinsdottir I, Fischer H, Pissiota A, Langström B, Fredrikson M: Cerebral blood flow in subjects with social phobia during stressful speaking tasks: a PET study. Am J Psychiatry 2001;158:1220–1226.

101 Tillfors M, Furmark T, Marteinsdottir I, Fredrikson M: Cerebral blood flow during anticipation of public speaking in social phobia: a PET study. Biol Psychiatry 2002;52:1113–1119.

102 van Ameringen M, Mancini C, Szechtman H, Nahmias C, Oakman JM, Hall GB, Pipe B, Farvolden P: A PET provocation study of generalized social phobia. Psychiatry Res 2004;132:13–18.

103 Veltman DJ, Tuinebreijer WE, Winkelman D, Lammertsma AA, Witter MP, Dolan RJ, Emmelkamp PM: Neurophysiological correlates of habituation during exposure in spider phobia. Psychiatry Res 2004;132:149–158.

104 Wendt J, Lotze M, Weike AI, Hosten N, Hamm AO: Brain activation and defensive response mobilization during sustained exposure to phobia-related and other affective pictures in spider phobia. Psychophysiology 2008;45:205–215.

105 Wik G, Fredrikson M, Fischer H: Evidence of altered cerebral blood-flow relationships in acute phobia. Int J Neurosci 1997;91:253–263.

106 Wik G, Fredrikson M, Fischer H: Cerebral correlates of anticipated fear: a PET study of specific phobia. Int J Neurosci 1996;7:267–276.

107 Bremner JD, Narayan M, Staib LH, Southwick SM, McGlashan T, Charney DS: Neural correlates of memories of childhood sexual abuse in women with and without posttraumatic stress disorder. Am J Psychiatry 1999;156:1787–1795.

108 Bremner JD, Staib LH, Kaloupek D, Southwick SM, Soufer R, Charney DS: Neural correlates of exposure to traumatic pictures and sound in Vietnam combat veterans with and without posttraumatic stress disorder: a positron emission tomography study. Biol Psychiatry 1999;45:806–816.

109 Britton JC, Phan KL, Taylor SF, Fig LM, Liberzon I: Corticolimbic blood flow in posttraumatic stress disorder during script-driven imagery. Biol Psychiatry 2005;57:832–840.

110 Hendler T, Rotshtein P, Yeshurun Y, Weizmann T, Kahn I, Ben-Bashat D, Malach R, Bleich A: Sensing the invisible: differential sensitivity of visual cortex and amygdala to traumatic context. Neuroimage 2003;19:587–600.

111 Hopper JW, Frewen PA, van der Kolk BA, Lanius RA: Neural correlates of reexperiencing, avoidance, and dissociation in PTSD: symptom dimensions and emotion dysregulation in responses to script-driven trauma imagery. J Trauma Stress 2007;20: 713–725.

112 Hou C, Liu J, Wang K, Li L, Liang M, He Z, Liu Y, Zhang Y, Li W, Jiang T: Brain responses to symptom provocation and trauma-related short-term memory recall in coal mining accident survivors with acute severe PTSD. Brain Res 2007;4:165–174.

113 Lanius RA, Williamson PC, Densmore M, Boksman K, Gupta MA, Neufeld RW, Gati JS, Menon RS: Neural correlates of traumatic memories in posttraumatic stress disorder: a functional MRI investigation. Am J Psychiatry 2001;158:1920–1922.

114 Lanius RA, Williamson PC, Boksman K, Densmore M, Gupta M, Neufeld RW, Gati JS, Menon RS: Brain activation during script-driven imagery induced dissociative responses in PTSD: a functional magnetic resonance imaging investigation. Biol Psychiatry 2002;52:305–311.

115 Lanius RA, Williamson PC, Densmore M, Boksman K, Neufeld RW, Gati JS, Menon RS: The nature of traumatic memories: a 4-T FMRI functional connectivity analysis. Am J Psychiatry 2004;161:36–44.

116 Liberzon I, Taylor SF, Amdur R, Jung TD, Chamberlain KR, Minoshima S, Koeppe RA, Fig LM: Brain activation in PTSD in response to trauma-related stimuli. Biol Psychiatry 1999;45:817–826.

117 Lindauer RJ, Booij J, Habraken JB, Uylings HB, Olff M, Carlier IV, den Heeten GJ, van Eck-Smit BL, Gersons BP: Cerebral blood flow changes during script-driven imagery in police officers with posttraumatic stress disorder. Biol Psychiatry 2004;56:853–861.

118 Morey RA, Petty CM, Cooper DA, Labar KS, McCarthy G: Neural systems for executive and emotional processing are modulated by symptoms of posttraumatic stress disorder in Iraq War veterans. Psychiatry Res 2008;162:59–72.

119 Osuch EA, Willis MW, Bluhm R, CSTS Neuroimaging Study Group, Ursano RJ, Drevets WC: Neurophysiological responses to traumatic reminders in the acute aftermath of serious motor vehicle collisions using [15O]-H2O positron emission tomography. Biol Psychiatry 2008;64:327–335.

120 Osuch EA, Benson B, Geraci M, Podell D, Herscovitch P, McCann UD, Post RM: Regional cerebral blood flow correlated with flashback intensity in patients with posttraumatic stress disorder. Biol Psychiatry 2001;50:246–253.

121 Pissiota A, Frans O, Fernandez M, von Knorring L, Fischer H, Fredrikson M: Neurofunctional correlates of posttraumatic stress disorder: a PET symptom provocation study. Eur Arch Psychiatry Clin Neurosci 2002;252:68–75.

122 Protopopescu X, Pan H, Tuescher O, Cloitre M, Goldstein M, Engelien W, Epstein J, Yang Y, Gorman J, LeDoux J, Silbersweig D, Stern E: Differential time courses and specificity of amygdala activity in posttraumatic stress disorder subjects and normal control subjects. Biol Psychiatry 2005;57:464–473.

123 Semple WE, Goyer PF, McCormick R, Donovan B, Muzic RF Jr, Rugle L, McCutcheon K, Lewis C, Liebling D, Kowaliw S, Vapenik K, Semple MA, Flener CR, Schulz SC: Higher brain blood flow at amygdala and lower frontal cortex blood flow in PTSD patients with comorbid cocaine and alcohol abuse compared with normals. Psychiatry 2000;63: 65–74.

124 Semple WE, Goyer P, McCormick R, Morris E, Compton B, Muswick G, Nelson D, Donovan B, Leisure G, Berridge M, et al: Preliminary report: brain blood flow using PET in patients with posttraumatic stress disorder and substance-abuse histories. Biol Psychiatry 1993;3:115–118.

125 Shin LM, Orr SP, Carson MA, Rauch SL, Macklin ML, Lasko NB, Peters PM, Metzger LJ, Dougherty DD, Cannistraro PA, Alpert NM, Fischman AJ, Pitman RK: Regional cerebral blood flow in the amygdala and medial prefrontal cortex during traumatic imagery in male and female Vietnam veterans with PTSD. Arch Gen Psychiatry 2004;61:168–176.

126 Shin LM, Whalen PJ, Pitman RK, Bush G, Macklin ML, Lasko NB, Orr SP, McInerney SC, Rauch SL: An fMRI study of anterior cingulate function in posttraumatic stress disorder. Biol Psychiatry 2001; 50:932–942.

127 Shin LM, McNally RJ, Kosslyn SM, Thompson WL, Rauch SL, Alpert NM, Metzger LJ, Lasko NB, Orr SP, Pitman RK: Regional cerebral blood flow during script-driven imagery in childhood sexual abuse-related PTSD: a PET investigation. Am J Psychiatry 1999;156:575–584.

128 Shin LM, Kosslyn SM, McNally RJ, Alpert NM, Thompson WL, Rauch SL, Macklin ML, Pitman RK: Visual imagery and perception in posttraumatic stress disorder. Arch Gen Psychiatry 1997;54: 233–241.

129 Vermetten E, Schmahl C, Southwick SM, Bremner JD: Positron tomographic emission study of olfactory induced emotional recall in veterans with and without combat-related posttraumatic stress disorder. Psychopharmacol Bull 2007;40:8–30.

130 Yang P, Wu MT, Hsu CC, Ker JH: Evidence of early neurobiological alternations in adolescents with posttraumatic stress disorder: a functional MRI study. Neurosci Lett 2004;370:13–28.

131 Zubieta JK, Chinitz JA, Lombardi U, Fig LM, Cameron OG, Liberzon I: Medial frontal cortex involvement in PTSD symptoms: a SPECT study. J Psychiatr Res 1999;33:259–264.

132 Fusar-Poli P, Placentino A, Carletti F, Landi P, Allen P, Surguladze S, Benedetti F, Abbamonte M, Gasparotti R, Barale F, Perez J, McGuire P, Politi P: Functional atlas of emotional faces processing: a voxel-based meta-analysis of 105 functional magnetic resonance imaging studies. J Psychiatry Neurosci 2009;34:418–432.

133 Sergerie K, Chochol C, Armony JL: The role of the amygdala in emotional processing: a quantitative meta-analysis of functional neuroimaging studies. Neurosci Biobehav Rev 2008;32:811–830.

134 Sabatinelli D, Fortune EE, Li Q, Siddiqui A, Krafft C, Oliver WT, Beck S, Jeffries J: Emotional perception: meta-analyses of face and natural scene processing. Neuroimage 2011;54:2524–2533.

135 Boshuisen ML, Ter Horst GJ, Paans AM, Reinders AA, den Boer JA: rCBF differences between panic disorder patients and control subjects during anticipatory anxiety and rest. Biol Psychiatry 2002;52: 126–135.

136 Eser D, Leicht G, Lutz J, Wenninger S, Kirsch V, Schüle C, Karch S, Baghai T, Pogarell O, Born C, Rupprecht R, Mulert C: Functional neuroanatomy of CCK-4-induced panic attacks in healthy volunteers. Hum Brain Mapping 2009;30:511–522.

137 Schunck T, Erb G, Mathis A, Gilles C, Namer IJ, Hode Y, Demaziere A, Luthringer R, Macher JP: Functional magnetic resonance imaging characterization of CCK-4-induced panic attack and subsequent anticipatory anxiety. Neuroimage 2006;31: 1197–11208.

138 Ponto LL, Kathol RG, Kettelkamp R, Watkins GL, Richmond JC, Clark J, Hichwa RD: Global cerebral blood flow after CO_2 inhalation in normal subjects and patients with panic disorder determined with [15O]water and PET. J Anxiety Disord 2002;16: 247–258.

139 Lindauer RJ, Booij J, Habraken JB, van Meijel EP, Uylings HB, Olff M, Carlier IV, den Heeten GJ, van Eck-Smit BL, Gersons BP: Effects of psychotherapy on regional cerebral blood flow during trauma imagery in patients with post-traumatic stress disorder: a randomized clinical trial. Psychol Med 2008; 38:543–554.

140 Peres JF, Newberg AB, Mercante JP, Simão M, Albuquerque VE, Peres MJ, Nasello AG: Cerebral blood flow changes during retrieval of traumatic memories before and after psychotherapy: a SPECT study. Psychol Med 2007;37:1481–1491.

141 Sakai Y, Kumano H, Nishikawa M, Sakano Y, Kaiya H, Imabayashi E, Ohnishi T, Matsuda H, Yasuda A, Sato A, Diksic M, Kuboki T: Changes in cerebral glucose utilization in patients with panic disorder treated with cognitive-behavioral therapy. Neuroimage 2006;33:218–226.

142 Goossens L, Sunaert S, Peeters R, Griez EJ, Schruers KR: Amygdala hyperfunction in phobic fear normalizes after exposure. Biol Psychiatry 2007;62: 1119–1125.

143 Straube T, Mentzel HJ, Miltner WH: Neural mechanisms of automatic and direct processing of phobogenic stimuli in specific phobia. Biol Psychiatry 2006;59:162–170.

144 Johanson A, Gustafson L, Passant U, Risberg J, Smith G, Warkentin S, Tucker D: Brain function in spider phobia. Psychiatry Res 1998;84:101–111.

145 Doehrmann O, Ghosh SS, Polli FE, Reynolds GO, Horn F, Keshavan A, Triantafyllou C, Saygin ZM, Whitfield-Gabrieli S, Hofmann SG, Pollack M, Gabrieli JD: Predicting treatment response in social anxiety disorder from functional magnetic resonance imaging. JAMA Psychiatry 2013;70:87–97.

146 Davis M, Whalen PJ: The amygdala: vigilance and emotion. Mol Psychiatry 2001;1:13–34.

147 Barbas H, Zikopoulos B: Sequential and parallel circuits for emotional processing in primate orbitofrontal cortex; in Zald DH, Rauch SL: The Orbitofrontal Cortex. New York, Oxford University Press, 2006, pp 57–91.

148 Etkin A. Functional neuroanatomy of anxiety: a neural circuit perspective. Curr Top Behav Neurosci 2010;2:251–277.

149 Bryant RA, Felmingham K, Kemp A, Das P, Hughes G, Peduto A, Williams L: Amygdala and ventral anterior cingulate activation predicts treatment response to cognitive behaviour therapy for posttraumatic stress disorder. Psychol Med 2008;38: 555–561.

150 Kim SJ, Lyoo IK, Lee YS, Kim J, Sim ME, Bae SJ, Kim HJ, Lee JY, Jeong DU: Decreased cerebral blood flow of thalamus in PTSD patients as a strategy to reduce re-experience symptoms. Acta Psychiatr Scand 2007;116:145–153.

151 Shin LM, Wright CI, Cannistraro PA, Wedig MM, McMullin K, Martis B, Macklin ML, Lasko NB, Cavanagh SR, Krangel TS, Orr SP, Pitman RK, Whalen PJ, Rauch SL: A functional magnetic resonance imaging study of amygdala and medial prefrontal cortex responses to overtly presented fearful faces in posttraumatic stress disorder. Arch Gen Psychiatry 2005;62:273–281.

152 Williams LM, Kemp AH, Felmingham K, Barton M, Olivieri G, Peduto A, Gordon E, Bryant RA: Trauma modulates amygdala and medial prefrontal responses to consciously attended fear. Neuroimage 2006;29:347–357.

153 Caseras X, Giampietro V, Lamas A, Brammer M, Vilarroya O, Carmona S, Rovira M, Torrubia R, Mataix-Cols D: The functional neuroanatomy of blood-injection-injury phobia: a comparison with spider phobics and healthy controls. Psychol Med 2010;40:125–134.

154 Fredrikson M, Furmark T, Olsson MT, Fischer H, Andersson J, Långström B: Functional neuroanatomical correlates of electrodermal activity: a positron emission tomographic study. Psychophysiology 1998;35:179–185.

155 Critchley HD, Elliott R, Mathias CJ, Dolan RJ: Neural activity relating to generation and representation of galvanic skin conductance responses: a functional magnetic resonance imaging study. J Neurosci 2000;20:3033–3040.

156 Maier S, Szalkowski A, Kamphausen S, Perlov E, Feige B, Blechert J, Philipsen A, van Elst LT, Kalisch R, Tüscher O: Clarifying the role of the rostral dmPFC/dACC in fear/anxiety: learning, appraisal or expression? PLoS One 2012;7:e50120.

157 Blair K, Shaywitz J, Smith BW, Rhodes R, Geraci M, Jones M, McCaffrey D, Vythilingam M, Finger E, Mondillo K, Jacobs M, Charney DS, Blair RJ, Drevets WC, Pine DS: Response to emotional expressions in generalized social phobia and generalized anxiety disorder: evidence for separate disorders. Am J Psychiatry 2008;165:1193–1202.

158 Kilts CD, Kelsey JE, Knight B, Ely TD, Bowman FD, Gross RE, Selvig A, Gordon A, Newport DJ, Nemeroff CB: The neural correlates of social anxiety disorder and response to pharmacotherapy. Neuropsychopharmacology 2006;31:2243–2253.

159 Vogt BA: Pain and emotion interactions in subregions of the cingulate gyrus. Nat Rev Neurosci 2005;6:533–544.

160 Maslowsky J, Mogg K, Bradley BP, McClure-Tone E, Ernst M, Pine DS, Monk CS: A preliminary investigation of neural correlates of treatment in adolescents with generalized anxiety disorder. J Child Adolesc Psychopharmacol 2010;20:105–111.

161 Faria V, Appel L, Ahs F, Linnman C, Pissiota A, Frans O, Bani M, Bettica P, Pich EM, Jacobsson E, Wahlstedt K, Fredrikson M, Furmark T: Amygdala subregions tied to SSRI and placebo response in patients with social anxiety disorder. Neuropsychopharmacology 2012;37:2222–2232.

162 Furmark T, Appel L, Henningsson S, Ahs F, Faria V, Linnman C, Pissiota A, Frans O, Bani M, Bettica P, Pich EM, Jacobsson E, Wahlstedt K, Oreland L, Langström B, Eriksson E, Fredrikson M: A link between serotonin-related gene polymorphisms, amygdala activity, and placebo-induced relief from social anxiety. J Neurosci 2008;28:13066–13074.

163 Phan KL, Orlichenko A, Boyd E, Angstadt M, Coccaro EF, Liberzon I, Arfanakis K: Preliminary evidence of white matter abnormality in the uncinate fasciculus in generalized social anxiety disorder. Biol Psychiatry 2009;66:691–694.

164 Blokland GA, de Zubicaray GI, McMahon KL, Wright MJ: Genetic and environmental influences on neuroimaging phenotypes: a meta-analytical perspective on twin imaging studies. Twin Res Hum Genet 2012;15:351–371.

165 Fisher PM, Meltzer CC, Ziolko SK, Price JC, Moses-Kolko EL, Berga SL, Hariri AR: Capacity for 5-HT1A-mediated autoregulation predicts amygdala reactivity. Nat Neurosci 2006;9:1362–1363.

166 Kienast T, Hariri AR, Schlagenhauf F, Wrase J, Sterzer P, Buchholz HG, Smolka MN, Gründer G, Cumming P, Kumakura Y, Bartenstein P, Dolan RJ, Heinz A: Dopamine in amygdala gates limbic processing of aversive stimuli in humans. Nat Neurosci 2008;11:1381–1382.

167 Michelgard A, Appel L, Pissiota A, Frans O, Langström B, Bergström M, Fredrikson M: Symptom provocation in specific phobia affects the substance P neurokinin-1 receptor system. Biol Psychiatry 2007;61:1002–1006.

168 Munafò MR, Brown SM, Hariri AR: Serotonin transporter (5-HTTLPR) genotype and amygdala activation: a meta-analysis. Biol Psychiatry 2008; 63:852–857.

169 Domschke K, Dannlowski U: Imaging genetics of anxiety disorders. Neuroimage 2010;53:822–831.

170 Pezawas L, Meyer-Lindenberg A, Drabant EM, Verchinski BA, Munoz KE, Kolachana BS, Egan MF, Mattay VS, Hariri AR, Weinberger DR: 5-HTTLPR polymorphism impacts human cingulate-amygdala interactions: a genetic susceptibility mechanism for depression. Nat Neurosci 2005;8: 828–834.

171 Fernandez M, Pissiota A, Frans O, von Knorring L, Fischer H, Fredrikson M: Brain function in a patient with torture related post-traumatic stress disorder before and after fluoxetine treatment: a positron emission tomography provocation study. Neurosci Lett 2001;297:101–104.

172 Fani N, Ashraf A, Afzal N, Jawed F, Kitayama N, Reed L, Bremner JD: Increased neural response to trauma scripts in posttraumatic stress disorder following paroxetine treatment: a pilot study. Neurosci Lett 2011;491:196–201.

173 Cervenka S, Hedman E, Ikoma Y, Djurfeldt DR, Rück C, Halldin C, Lindefors N: Changes in dopamine D2-receptor binding are associated to symptom reduction after psychotherapy in social anxiety disorder. Transl Psychiatry 2012;2:e120.

174 Jahanshad N, Hibar DP, Ryles A, Toga AW, McMahon KL, de Zubicaray GI, Hansell NK, Montgomery GW, Martin NG, Wright MJ, Thompson PM: Discovery of genes that affect human brain connectivity: a genome-wide analysis of the connectome. Proc IEEE Int Symp Biomed Imaging 2012;542–545.

Mats Fredrikson
Department of Psychology, Uppsala University
Box 1225
SE–751 42 Uppsala (Sweden)
E-Mail Mats.Fredrikson@psyk.uu.se

Fredrikson · Faria

Baldwin DS, Leonard BE (eds): Anxiety Disorders.
Mod Trends Pharmacopsychiatry. Basel, Karger, 2013, vol 29, pp 67–84 (DOI: 10.1159/000351965)

Potential Neuroimmunological Targets in the Treatment of Anxiety Disorders

Ruihua Hou[a] · Zhen Tang[b] · David S. Baldwin[a, c]

[a]University Department of Psychiatry, Clinical and Experimental Sciences, Faculty of Medicine, University of Southampton, Southampton, UK; [b]Suzhou University Guangji Hospital, Suzhou, China; [c]Department of Psychiatry and Mental Health, University of Cape Town, Cape Town, South Africa

Abstract

In the translation of psychoneuroimmunology research into clinical practice, one critical step is to identify biomarkers for improved diagnosis and targeting of interventions. Inflammatory markers deserve special attention due to their crucial role linking various health conditions and disorders. In this chapter, we discuss the pivotal roles of cytokines in signalling to the brain and leading to behavioural changes. This is followed by a review of recent research findings into neuroimmunology of depression, and immunomodulating effects of antidepressants. The rest of the chapter focuses on neuroinflammatory hypothesis in anxiety disorders, and provides an overview of current research evidence on inflammatory responses in anxious state and anxiety disorders. Research suggestions are recommended, including study design, risk factors, medication effects, and measurement strategies. Clinical and pharmacotherapeutic implications and future research directions are also discussed in the final section.

Research into psychoneuroimmunology (PNI), the study of neural-endocrine-immune system interactions (see fig. 1), has led to substantial advances in the understanding of the reciprocal interactions between the central nervous system (CNS) and the immune system in neuropsychiatric disorders [1–4]. How the crosstalk of pathways and mechanisms enable immune systems to influence the brain and behaviour has become a question of immense significance. In the translation of PNI research developments into clinical practice to achieve better clinical outcomes, one critical step is to identify biomarkers for better diagnosis and interventions. Inflammatory markers deserve special attention due to their crucial role linking various health conditions and disorders [5]. In particular, experimental and clinical research reveals pivotal roles of cytokines in signalling to the brain to regulate important brain functions including neurotransmitter metabolism, neuroendocrine function and neurogenesis, ultimately leading to behavioural changes [6–10]. Further elucidation of inflammatory markers, cytokine networks, and immune-brain-behaviour interactions may reveal targets for

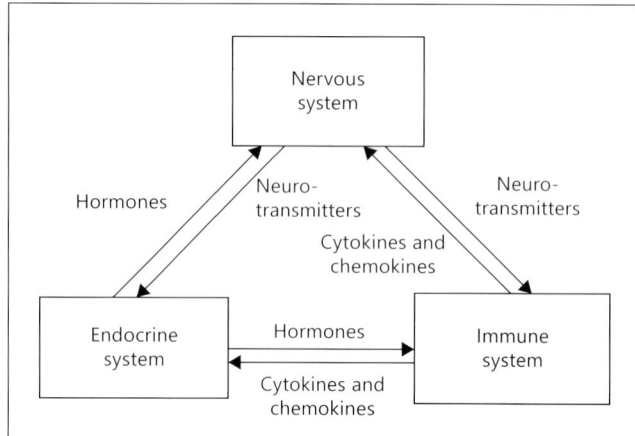

Fig. 1. PNI, study of the interactions between the nervous, immune and endocrine systems, illustrated based on the *Lancet* review by Ader et al. [1].

potential therapeutic development as well as strategies for the prevention of neuropsychiatric diseases in at risk populations. Greater understanding of the role of cytokines in bi-directional communications between the nervous and immune systems has inspired integrative, explanatory models for neuropsychiatric disorders. To date, the presence of inflammatory responses and the crucial role of cytokines in depression have received most attention, but greater awareness of the prevalence and burden of anxiety disorders is encouraging research into the role of cytokines in anxiety disorders.

The Pivotal Role of Cytokines

Just as the nervous and endocrine systems convey information to the immune system via neurotransmitters and hormones, the immune system conveys information to the nervous and endocrine systems via cytokines and chemokines [4]. Cytokines are soluble bioactive mediators released by various cell types both at the periphery (such as monocytes and macrophages) and in the brain (such as microglia, astrocytes, oligodendroglia and neurons), which operate within a complex network and act either synergistically or antagonistically. They are generally associated with inflammation, immune activation and cell differentiation or death, and include interleukins (ILs), tumour necrosis factors (TNFs), interferons (IFNs), chemokines and growth factors (such as brain-derived neurotrophic factor, BDNF) [11]. Based on the functional profile of an immune response, cytokine production is orchestrated by type 1 helper (Th1) cells which generally mediate a proinflammatory cellular immune response, and Th2 cells which enhance humoral immune reactions. Pro-inflammatory cytokines, such as IL-1, IL-6, INF-γ, and TNFα, enhance the immune response to help speed the elimination of pathogens and the resolution of the inflammatory challenge; by contrast, anti-inflammatory cytokines, such as IL-4, IL-10, and IL-13, serve to dampen the immune response via decreasing cell function and synthesis of pro-in-

Hou · Tang · Baldwin

flammatory cytokines [6]. The balance between Th1 and Th2 cells is an essential determinant in containing the inflammatory response [12], and a delicate balance of pro-inflammatory and anti-inflammatory cytokines is needed [8]. In addition to the Th1 and Th2 cytokines, Th3 cells exert their action primarily by secreting transforming growth factor-β_1 (TGF-β_1) which facilitates a balance between the Th1 and Th2 arms of cellular immunity [13].

Cytokines have been implicated in the modulation of neuronal activity in regions such as the amygdala, hippocampus, hypothalamus and cerebral cortex [14, 15]. Peripheral cytokine signals can reach the brain through humoral, neural and cellular pathways via five possible mechanisms: (1) passage of cytokines through 'leaky' regions of the blood-brain barrier; (2) active transport via saturable cytokine-specific transport molecules on brain endothelium; (3) activation of endothelial cells and inducing the release of second messengers such as prostaglandins and nitric oxide; (4) transmission via afferent nerve fibres such as the vagus nerve, and (5) entry into the brain parenchyma via peripherally activated monocytes (fig. 2) [9].

Physical or psychological stress, and infection or inflammation within the brain or the periphery can modulate cytokine expression in the CNS [16]. An acute immune challenge triggers an adaptive, temporary and controlled reaction of the CNS, but when immune challenge becomes chronic and/or dysregulated due to chronic medical illness, chronic stress, or cytokine treatments, the resultant chronic inflammatory response contributes to the development of maladaptive behavioural symptoms and neuropsychiatric disorders. Cytokines may lead to behavioural changes through their effects on: (1) neurotransmitter function – cytokines can alter the metabolism of serotonin, dopamine, and glutamate [17–19]; (2) neuroendocrine activity – cytokines can alter the function of the hypothalamic-pituitary-adrenal (HPA) axis via stimulant effects on the expression and release of corticotropin-releasing hormone (CRH), adrenocorticotropic hormone (ACTH), and cortisol [20, 21]; (3) neurogenesis – cytokines may affect neurogenesis via activation of NF-κB [22], and (4) neurocircuitry – the basal ganglia and subgenual and dorsal aspects of the anterior cingulate cortex (ACC) are target regions of cytokines [23, 24] (illustrated in fig. 3). Behavioural consequences of these effects include depression, anxiety, fatigue, psychomotor slowing, anorexia, cognitive dysfunction and sleep disturbance, all symptoms that overlap with those of a range of neuropsychiatric disorders [9]. Therefore, increased recognition of the role of cytokines in the CNS has opened important new areas for investigating the origin and treatment of neuropsychiatric disorders.

The Neuroimmunology of Depression

Since signs of immune disturbances in depression were first reported 20 years ago [25–28], the presence of inflammatory responses and the crucial role of cytokines in major depression have been addressed in numerous studies, and our understanding of depres-

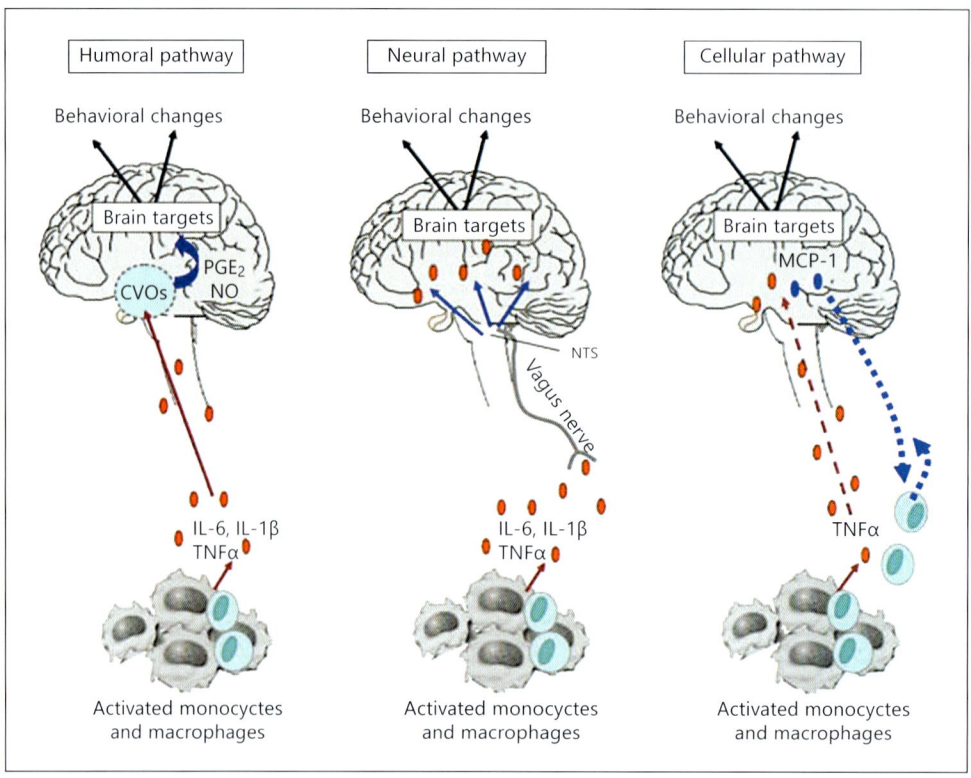

Fig. 2. Communication pathways from the periphery to the brain – different pathways by which cytokine signals access the brain, reproduced from Capuron and Miller [9]. CVOs = Circumventricular organs; PGE_2 = prostaglandins; NTS = nucleus of the tractus solitarius; MCP1 = monocyte chemoattractant protein-1.

sion has moved far beyond the 'monoamine hypothesis' or 'serotonin hypothesis' [29]. A recent meta-analysis of 24 studies reports significantly higher concentrations of the pro-inflammatory cytokines (such as TNFα and IL-6) in depressed subjects compared with control subjects, and stresses that depression is accompanied by activation of the immune system [30]. Specific depression-related symptoms, such as fatigue, insomnia and cognitive dysfunction, have been found to be related to inflammatory activation [31–33]. C-reactive protein (CRP) is an acute-phase protein in response to inflammation. Research has identified robust cross-sectional and longitudinal associations between CRP and depression [34–36]. Another recent meta-analysis also suggests strong positive associations between depression and CRP, IL-1, and IL-6 [37]. In addition, the immune dysregulation hypothesis of major depression, which considers an altered balance of Th1 pro-inflammatory cytokines and Th2 anti-inflammatory cytokines with Th1 pathway being predominant over Th2 pathway, has also been proposed [4, 38, 39].

Both external and internal stressors may trigger depression via acquired (e.g. T and B cell) and/or innate (e.g. macrophage) immune responses [40], while the HPA axis

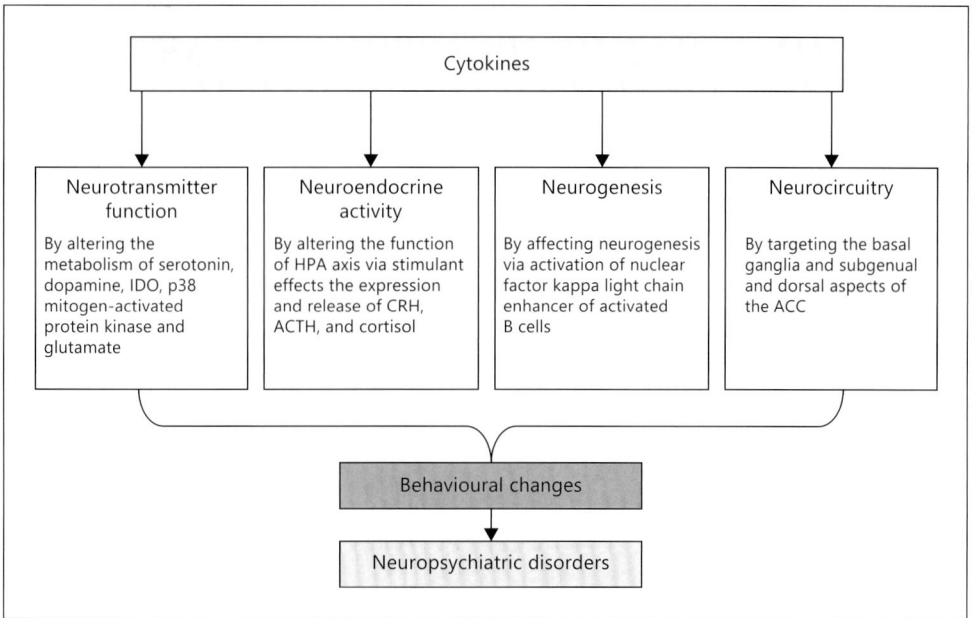

Fig. 3. Pathways through which cytokines lead to behavioural changes. Created based on the review by Capuron and Miller [9]. IDO = Indoleamine 2,3 dioxygenase.

and serotonin play pivotal roles in the connection between stress and depression [4]. Stress has been considered as a neuroinflammatory condition in the brain [41]. Depression is strongly associated with stress, especially in those individuals who have suffered childhood trauma [42]. There is also substantial evidence to suggest a relationship between psychological stress and increased levels of inflammatory markers in those who have experienced early life or recent stressors [2, 43]. It has been argued that childhood adversity can lead to long-term psychological and physical vulnerabilities, possibly mediated through inflammatory process [43–45]. Childhood trauma and recent stress were found to be significant risk factors for depression in cancer patients, and increased levels of inflammatory marks predict later depressive symptoms in colorectal cancer patients [46]. Based on epidemiological evidence [47, 48], it has been proposed that major depression may be a prelude to dementia in later life. It is not clear whether anxiety disorders also have this influencing role (fig. 4).

Immunomodulating Effects of Antidepressants

Antidepressants have marked effects on the production of cytokines [49–55]. Preclinical and clinical data demonstrate that antidepressant treatments, mainly selective serotonin reuptake inhibitors (SSRIs), are associated with decreases in inflammatory markers [2]. In contrast, recent results of two large clinical trials suggest that use of

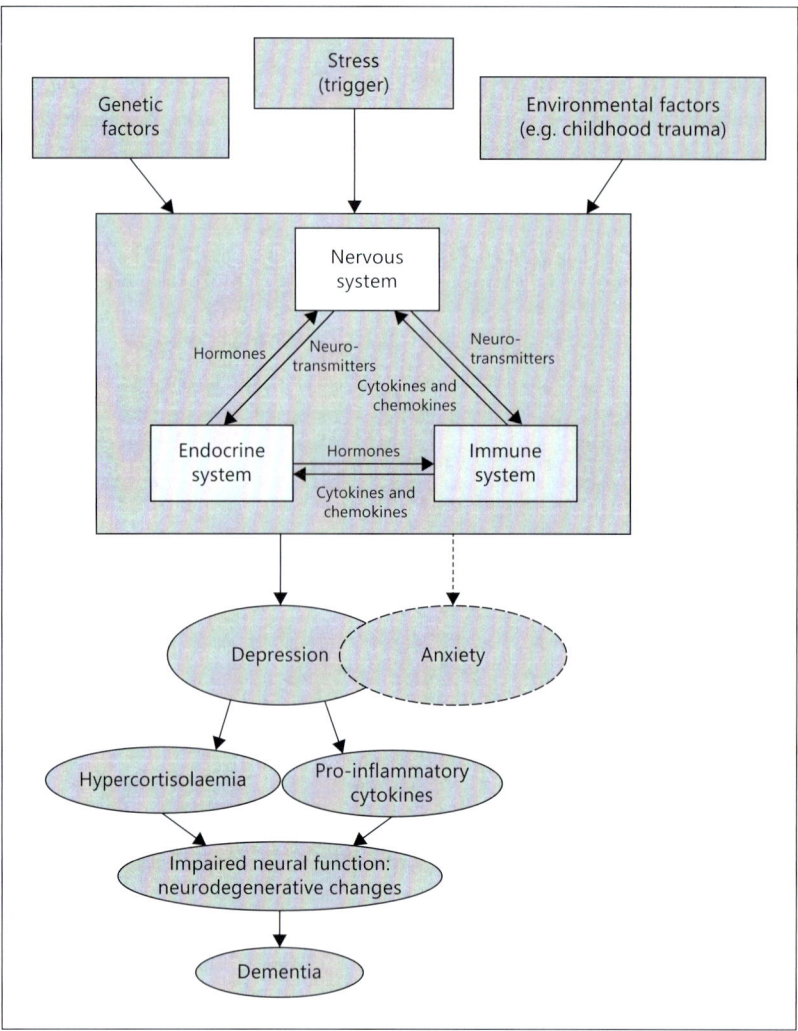

Fig. 4. Summary of links between stress, depression and dementia. Modified from Leonard and Myint [4].

antidepressants, mainly tricyclic antidepressants (TCAs), is associated with elevated inflammation levels [56].

Many antidepressants have shown specific anti-inflammatory effects [57, 58] and significant immunoregulatory activities, such as reducing the number of Th1 cells secreting IFN-γ, altering the production of IL-6 and IL-10, and inhibiting IFN-γ-induced microglial production of IL-6 and nitric oxide [8, 59]. A recent study demonstrates that inflammation was increased in men taking serotonin-norepinephrine reuptake inhibitors (SNRIs; CRP, IL-6) and in men and women taking tri- or tetracyclic antidepressants (CRP), but decreased among men using SSRIs (IL-6) [60]. While anti-inflammatory properties of SSRIs initially only related to work undertaken on cells of the peripheral immune system, Tynan et al. [61] recently examined anti-inflammatory effects of SSRIs on lipopolysaccharide (LPS)-stimulated microglia and demonstrated that the SSRIs (fluoxetine, sertraline, paroxetine, fluvoxamine and citalopram) and the SNRI venlafaxine suppressed microglial responses to an inflammatory stimulus, in particular SSRIs potently inhibited microglial TNFα and nitric oxide production. More importantly, clinical data also indicate that immune activation in patients with depression is associated with resistance to treatment with traditional antidepressants, and inflammatory biomarkers may hence provide an indicator of treatment response [62–64]. Antidepressants are often employed in the treatment of anxiety disorders, and immunological parameters have been found to predict or mediate the response to antidepressant drugs, although methodological inconsistencies have so far slowed progress along this path [65]. It is still difficult to identify certain patient subgroups which may respond preferentially to particular pharmacological interventions [66, 67].

A Neuroimmunology of Anxiety Disorders?

Similar treatment effects of antidepressants in anxiety disorders and depression suggest that similar neurobiological substrates may underlie both conditions. In addition, the pronounced response of central and peripheral cytokines to stress has prompted further interest in the role of cytokines in the pathogenesis of anxiety disorders. Experimental and clinical evidence shows that stress can produce an inflammatory reaction, indicated by a rise in circulating concentrations of pro-inflammatory cytokines; and chronic stress, by initiating changes in the HPA axis and the immune system, can therefore act as a trigger for anxiety and depression [4].

Inflammatory Responses and the Anxious State

Pre-clinical studies reveal that increased expression of cytokines in the periphery is associated with enhanced 'anxiety' in autoimmune mice [68–70], that mice over-expressing IL-6 or TNF reveal an anxious phenotype [71, 72], and that deletion of the gene encoding IFN-γ leads to heightened anxiety [72–74]. Human studies indicate that a chronic anxious state may have a deleterious impact on immune function [75–78], leading to damaged cellular and humoral immune responses [77, 79, 80] and increased incidence of viral and bacterial infections [81, 82]. Anxiety is also associated with an impaired immune response to several antiviral/bacterial vaccines, such as hepatitis B virus [83], pneumococcal bacteria [84], rubella virus [85], meningitis virus [86], and influenza virus [87–89].

The associations between inflammatory responses and anxious state have been evaluated in physically ill patients with known activation of inflammatory responses.

An early report showed an association between IFN-γ levels and anxiety in systemic lupus erythematosus [90], and both depressed and anxious states are associated with significantly lower ratios of IFN-γ (Th1 cells) versus IL-4 (Th2 cells) among ovarian cancer patients [91]. Patients receiving IFN-α for hepatitis C exhibit significantly greater activation in the dorsal ACC which is associated with increased anxiety and arousal compared with control subjects [92, 93].

While studies of subclinical psychoneuroimmunological variations in healthy populations demonstrate a positive correlation between anxious state and inflammation and coagulation markers, such as TNFα, IL-6, and CRP [79, 94, 95], a study by Zorrilla et al. [96] found that male subjects who were characteristically more anxious had significantly lower levels of circulating IL-1β compared to less anxious subjects, indicating a negative correlate. These inconsistent results may be due to small sample size and gender difference, indicating these results need to be confirmed in a larger sample exploring also gender differences. Normal volunteers injected with LPS, a well-known immune activator, have exhibited acute increases in symptoms of anxiety [97]. When compared with non-anxious participants, clinically anxious participants exhibited significantly higher levels of IL-6, independent of depressive symptoms, which indicates an anxiety-specific effect on inflammatory activity, and highlights a pathway by which anxiety may increase risk for inflammatory diseases [98].

Inflammatory Responses in Anxiety Disorders

Post-Traumatic Stress Disorder
Traumatic events can trigger peripheral cells to migrate, mediate inflammation, and decrease neurogenesis, potentially leading to CNS volume loss. Recent studies suggest that peripheral blood mononuclear cells could cause and/or exacerbate post-traumatic stress disorder (PTSD). The biological underpinnings for the role of the immune system in the pathogenesis of PTSD include crosstalk between the stress and immune systems, neurogenesis, and processes that underlie synaptic plasticity, such as learning and memory. Increased circulating levels of CRP, IL-6, TNFα, IL-1β and IL-8 have all been demonstrated in patients with PTSD, which may be due to an insufficient regulation of the immune function [99–103]. A recent review has suggested that cellular immunity is implicated in PTSD risk and resilience [104].

Panic Disorder
Alterations in circulating levels of IL-1 have previously been demonstrated [105]. Reductions in anxiety level by therapeutic interventions (CBT and the anxiolytic ethyl loflazepate) have been found to be associated with decreased cell-mediated immunity [80]. A prospective experimentally induced stress study demonstrates that 35% CO_2 inhalation induced significantly higher levels of anxiety in panic disorder (PD) patients as compared to the control subjects, but no differences in immune parameters

were found, either in basal conditions or after experimental panic induction [106]. Hoge et al. [107] found that patients with PD or PTSD had significantly elevated levels of IL-6, IL-1α, IL-1β, IL-8 and IFN-α compared with healthy controls.

Obsessive-Compulsive Disorder
Immunological findings from obsessive-compulsive disorder (OCD) studies are inconsistent. While several reports found no IL-6 differences in OCD, either in plasma or in cerebrospinal fluid (CSF) [108, 109], a decrease in production of TNFα and the low levels of LPS-stimulated IL-6 have been reported [110, 111], which is in contrast with the study by Konuk et al. [112], in which their findings demonstrated higher levels of TNFα and IL-6 in OCD patients, which may be due to high comorbidity with depression. Some research has suggested that the pathophysiology of OCD differs from that of other anxiety disorders, and the different cytokine profiles between OCD and other anxiety-related disorders inform the ongoing debate about the position of OCD within the group of anxiety disorders [113].

Generalized Anxiety Disorder
A recent prospective study demonstrates that generalized anxiety disorder (GAD) was associated with increased levels of CRP in bivariate cross-sectional analyses [36]. An evaluation of major depressive disorder and GAD in patients with stable coronary heart disease indicates a significant association between CRP levels and GAD [114]. Both studies imply that different inflammatory responses may occur in these two conditions. Recent studies conducted in 20 patients with GAD and 20 healthy controls demonstrated a T cell functional dysregulation in individuals with GAD via examining the T cell profile following in vitro activation in cultures: the cytokine profile in GAD revealed that Th1 and Th2 deficiencies were associated with dominant Th17 phenotype, which was enhanced by substance P [115, 116]. The profoundly altered composition of the peripheral T cell compartment might cause a state of compromised immune responsiveness, which may explain why some anxious patients show an increased susceptibility to infections, and inflammatory and autoimmune diseases.

The Limitations of Current Knowledge

Due to a reliance on cross-sectional study design, small sample sizes (an average of 20–40), the lack of standardized measurements, and high co-morbidity with depression, findings are not consistently observed across studies. There is a need for better understanding of both the heterogeneous role of specific cytokines in the control of anxious states and in different anxiety disorders, and of the immunomodulating effects of antidepressants on anxiety. Moreover, whether anxiety is associated with inflammatory activity either through a specific anxiety pathway, or through a more general negative emotionality pathway remains an interesting area to be explored.

Recommendations for Future Research

Longitudinal Study Design

Given well-known fluctuations in behavioural symptoms as well as immunologic status, research into neuroinflammation in anxiety should employ a longitudinal study design, in which repeated samples should be taken from the same subjects over a period ideally free of inflammatory clinical events. So far, most studies rely on cross-sectional design, with immune parameters measured by a single evaluation at a single time point.

Standardized Measures of Inflammatory Biomarkers

Inflammatory biomarkers should be standardized to allow comparison between studies:

a Assays based both on immunological detection of peptides (immunoassays) and biological responses (bioassays) are recommended to measure cytokine profile. Results with multiplex assays should be confirmed with standard ELISA assays. However, multiplex assays are considered to be ideal for assessing relevant inflammatory molecules in supernatants of stimulated cells in the context of hypothesis generation.

b Inflammation can fluctuate rapidly according to environmental and internal factors, such as circadian rhythm [117]. Thus, the timing of blood or tissue sampling may affect the cytokine profile. Ambulatory monitoring techniques, also known as the Experience Sampling Method and Ecological Momentary Assessment, are recommended for studying acute inflammatory fluctuations [118].

c Cytokine expression can vary depending on whether measurements are obtained from plasma, serum, CSF or stimulated peripheral blood samples; thus, the source of cytokines should be clearly defined.

d Proper sample handling and storage are important for reliable measurement of circulating cytokines. It has been suggested that serum and plasma should be separated immediately after sampling is taken and frozen at −80°C after blood draw. A delay of sample processing may cause degradation, absorption, or cellular production of cytokine, which leads to variable cytokine expression. Cytokines are stable for a period of 2 years of storage at −80°C [119].

e Given the delicate balance between pro-inflammatory and anti-inflammatory cytokines needed for normal regulation of neuropsychiatric functioning [8], it would be useful to test the pattern of immune dysregulation, such as whether an anxious state is characterized by a shift in the pro-/anti-inflammatory or Th1/Th2 cytokine ratio.

Standardized Behavioural Assessments and Record of Inflammatory Events

Clinical tools for assessing anxious state and recording inflammatory events should be standardized and made available for clinical research. Appropriate monitoring techniques should be developed for assessing short-term fluctuations in clinical symptoms.

Vulnerability Factors

A variety of vulnerability factors and demographic characteristics may potentially affect the direction and magnitude of cytokine changes in response to stress/anxious state including:

a   Body mass index (BMI). BMI has been shown to correlate with increased peripheral markers of inflammation, in part related to the capacity of adipose tissue to produce IL-6 and other cytokines [120, 121]. Obesity is associated with low-grade inflammatory processes, and with increased circulating levels of acute phase proteins (CRP in particular) and pro-inflammatory cytokines.

b   Ageing. Epidemiological studies indicate that anxiety disorders are more common among older age individuals [122]. Normal aging is characterized by chronic low-grade inflammatory factors, with an over-expression of periphery pro-inflammatory cytokines, and impaired pro- versus anti-inflammatory balance [9].

c   Medical conditions. The presence of medical conditions, in particular the presence of acute or chronic inflammatory challenge.

d   Childhood history. Adverse childhood experiences have been described as major environmental risk factors, the extent of prior stress exposure should be considered.

e   Exercise. Skeletal muscle has now been viewed as an immunogenic organ, which by contraction stimulates the production of cytokines, such as IL-6. Exercise affects circulating cytokine levels, and this impact has been a remarkably consistent research finding [123–125].

Effects of Medications

As described previously, anti-inflammatory effects of many antidepressant medications have been indicated in numerous studies [8, 57–59] controlling for the use of antidepressants and for any other medications known to affect inflammation, such as steroids, and should be considered when assessing the cytokine profile. In particular, the immunomodulatory effects may vary depending on different antidepressants used and the treatment duration.

Development of Novel Measurement Strategies

Novel approaches to measure inflammatory biomarkers are needed to improve the efficiency and ease of testing of relevant clinical populations. Such techniques would include development of blood spotting approaches, measurement of inflammatory markers in other body compartments, and the use of in vitro challenge strategies to reveal altered inflammatory response that might appear within normal limits without perturbation. In addition, application of computerized approaches to data collection and the use of multi-level statistical techniques for processing time series data are recommended. Sampling and biomarker characterization of other bodily compartments including CSF, joint spaces and amniotic fluid would be of relevance. As 'peripheral' cytokines can reach the brain, further development of strategies should include the measure of inflammatory biomarkers in the CSF.

Genetic Polymorphism of Cytokines

Genes encoding cytokines are highly polymorphic, single nucleotide polymorphisms being associated with increased or reduced cytokine production [126–129]. The presence of different pathogenetic polymorphism mechanisms has been indicated in the susceptibility to mood disorders [130], and polymorphisms in genes (e.g. IL-10) [131] and serotonergic proteins [128, 132] have been associated with an increased risk for major depressive disorder. A study of the association between genetic variant BDNF (Val66Met) polymorphism and anxiety-related behaviour found that variant BDNF may play a key role in genetic predispositions to anxiety disorders [133], indicating a new direction in therapeutic strategies to rescue anxiety symptoms in humans with this polymorphic allele. As significant cytokines are identified, research on genetic profiles encoding them would be warranted.

Clinical and Pharmacotherapeutic Implications

The availability of inflammatory biomarkers provides an opportunity to identify patients via specific pathophysiological processes and to monitor therapeutic responses within relevant pathways, which may represent an advance in the 'personalization' of treatment strategies. Therefore, further understanding of the mechanisms by which the immune system influences behaviour, in particular the role of specific cytokines in the control of anxious states, may provide novel intervention targets for potential therapeutic development as well as inform prevention strategies for neuropsychiatric disease in at-risk populations. Accumulating evidence has indicated modulatory effects of cytokines on neuronal communication and anxiety, but much is still to be understood about the nature of CNS inflammation before it can be successfully exploited for the development of clinical treatments. Research has not revealed consistent reproducible findings in anxiety disorders, and care is needed in their possible adoption as therapeutic targets for treating anxiety [134].

Future Research

To gain productive insights into interactions between the immune system and the CNS, and how these affect behaviour in anxiety disorders, with the goal of identifying new potential therapeutic targets, potentially fruitful investigations would include efforts to identify modifiable inflammatory processes or molecules in patients with anxiety disorders, assess the effects of conventional medications (such as antidepressants) on these processes or molecules, and based on experimental medicine paradigms, develop behavioural and/or psychopharmacological intervention approach to alter neuroimmune mechanisms with the aim of improving clinical outcomes.

References

1 Ader R, Cohen N, Felten D: Psychoneuroimmunology: interactions between the nervous system and the immune system. Lancet 1995;345:99–103.
2 Miller AH, Maletic V, Raison CL: Inflammation and its discontents: the role of cytokines in the pathophysiology of major depression. Biol Psychiatry 2009;65:732–741.
3 Raison CL, Capuron L, Miller AH: Cytokines sing the blues: inflammation and the pathogenesis of depression. Trends Immunol 2006;27:24–31.
4 Leonard BE, Myint A: The psychoneuroimmunology of depression. Hum Psychopharmacol 2009;24:165–175.
5 Yan Q: The role of psychoneuroimmunology in personalized and systems medicine. Methods Mol Biol (Clifton) 2012;934:3–19.
6 Kronfol Z, Remick DG: Cytokines and the brain: implications for clinical psychiatry. Am J Psychiatry 2000;157:683–694.
7 Maier SF: Bi-directional immune-brain communication: implications for understanding stress, pain, and cognition. Brain Behav Immun 2003;17:69–85.
8 Loftis JM, Huckans M, Morasco BJ: Neuroimmune mechanisms of cytokine-induced depression: current theories and novel treatment strategies. Neurobiol Dis 2010;37:519–533.
9 Capuron L, Miller AH: Immune system to brain signaling: neuropsychopharmacological implications. Pharmacol Ther 2011;130:226–238.
10 Dantzer R, O'Connor JC, Freund GG, Johnson RW, Kelley KW: From inflammation to sickness and depression: when the immune system subjugates the brain. Nat Rev 2008;9:46–56.
11 Allan SM, Rothwell NJ: Inflammation in central nervous system injury. Philos Trans R Soc Lond 2003;358:1669–1677.
12 Dantzer R, Capuron L, Irwin MR, Miller AH, Ollat H, Perry VH, Rousey S, Yirmiya R: Identification and treatment of symptoms associated with inflammation in medically ill patients. Psychoneuroendocrinology 2008;33:18–29.
13 Myint AM, Leonard BE, Steinbusch HW, Kim YK: Th1, Th2, and Th3 cytokine alterations in major depression. J Affect Dis 2005;88:167–173.
14 Besedovsky HO, del Rey A: Immune-neuro-endocrine interactions: facts and hypotheses. Endocr Rev 1996;17:64–102.
15 Elenkov IJ, Wilder RL, Chrousos GP, Vizi ES: The sympathetic nerve – an integrative interface between two supersystems: the brain and the immune system. Pharmacol Rev 2000;52:595–638.
16 Lucas SM, Rothwell NJ, Gibson RM: The role of inflammation in CNS injury and disease. Br J Pharmacol 2006;147(suppl 1):S232–S240.
17 Cai W, Khaoustov VI, Xie Q, Pan T, Le W, Yoffe B: Interferon-alpha-induced modulation of glucocorticoid and serotonin receptors as a mechanism of depression. J Hepatol 2005;42:880–887.

18 Moron JA, Zakharova I, Ferrer JV, Merrill GA, Hope B, Lafer EM, Lin ZC, Wang JB, Javitch JA, Galli A, Shippenberg TS: Mitogen-activated protein kinase regulates dopamine transporter surface expression and dopamine transport capacity. J Neurosci 2003; 23:8480–8488.

19 Ida T, Hara M, Nakamura Y, Kozaki S, Tsunoda S, Ihara H: Cytokine-induced enhancement of calcium-dependent glutamate release from astrocytes mediated by nitric oxide. Neurosci Lett 2008;432: 232–236.

20 Raison CL, Borisov AS, Woolwine BJ, Massung B, Vogt G, Miller AH: Interferon-alpha effects on diurnal hypothalamic-pituitary-adrenal axis activity: relationship with proinflammatory cytokines and behavior. Mol Psychiatry 2010;15:535–547.

21 Pariante CM, Miller AH: Glucocorticoid receptors in major depression: relevance to pathophysiology and treatment. Biol Psychiatry 2001;49:391–404.

22 Ben Menachem-Zidon O, Goshen I, Kreisel T, Ben Menahem Y, Reinhartz E, Ben Hur T, Yirmiya R: Intrahippocampal transplantation of transgenic neural precursor cells overexpressing interleukin-1 receptor antagonist blocks chronic isolation-induced impairment in memory and neurogenesis. Neuropsychopharmacol 2008;33:2251–2262.

23 Brydon L, Harrison NA, Walker C, Steptoe A, Critchley HD: Peripheral inflammation is associated with altered substantia nigra activity and psychomotor slowing in humans. Biol Psychiatry 2008;63: 1022–1029.

24 Miller AH: Norman Cousins Lecture. Mechanisms of cytokine-induced behavioral changes: psychoneuroimmunology at the translational interface. Brain Bev Immun 2009;23:149–158.

25 Maes M, Bosmans E, Suy E, Vandervorst C, De Jonckheere C, Raus J: Immune disturbances during major depression: upregulated expression of interleukin-2 receptors. Neuropsychobiology 1990;24: 115–120.

26 Maes M, Bosmans E, Suy E, Vandervorst C, DeJonckheere C, Raus J: Depression-related disturbances in mitogen-induced lymphocyte responses and interleukin-1 beta and soluble interleukin-2 receptor production. Acta Psychiatr Scand 1991;84: 379–386.

27 Maes M, Scharpe S, Bosmans E, Vandewoude M, Suy E, Uyttenbroeck W, Cooreman W, Vandervorst C, Raus J: Disturbances in acute phase plasma proteins during melancholia: additional evidence for the presence of an inflammatory process during that illness. Prog Neuropsychopharmacol Biol Psychiatry 1992;16:501–515.

28 Maes M, Van der Planken M, Stevens WJ, Peeters D, DeClerck LS, Bridts CH, Schotte C, Cosyns P: Leukocytosis, monocytosis and neutrophilia: hallmarks of severe depression. J Psychiatr Res 1992;26:125–134.

29 Gardner A, Boles RG: Beyond the serotonin hypothesis: mitochondria, inflammation and neurodegeneration in major depression and affective spectrum disorders. Prog Neuropsychopharmacol Biol Psychiatry 2011;35:730–743.

30 Dowlati Y, Herrmann N, Swardfager W, Liu H, Sham L, Reim EK, Lanctot KL: A meta-analysis of cytokines in major depression. Biol Psychiatry 2010; 67:446–457.

31 Irwin M, Rinetti G, Redwine L, Motivala S, Dang J, Ehlers C: Nocturnal proinflammatory cytokine-associated sleep disturbances in abstinent African American alcoholics. Brain Behav Immun 2004;18: 349–360.

32 Meyers CA, Albitar M, Estey E: Cognitive impairment, fatigue, and cytokine levels in patients with acute myelogenous leukemia or myelodysplastic syndrome. Cancer 2005;104:788–793.

33 Van Der Ven A, Van Diest R, Hamulyak K, Maes M, Bruggeman C, Appels A: Herpes viruses, cytokines, and altered hemostasis in vital exhaustion. Psychosom Med 2003;65:194–200.

34 Danner M, Kasl SV, Abramson JL, Vaccarino V: Association between depression and elevated C-reactive protein. Psychosom Med 2003;65:347–356.

35 Crnkovic D, Buljan D, Karlovic D, Krmek M: Connection between inflammatory markers, antidepressants and depression. Acta Clin Croat 2012;51:25–33.

36 Copeland WE, Shanahan L, Worthman C, Angold A, Costello EJ: Generalized anxiety and C-reactive protein levels: a prospective, longitudinal analysis. Psychol Med 2012;42:2641–2650.

37 Howren MB, Lamkin DM, Suls J: Associations of depression with C-reactive protein, IL-1, and IL-6: a meta-analysis. Psychosom Med 2009;71:171–186.

38 Gabbay V, Klein RG, Guttman LE, Babb JS, Alonso CM, Nishawala M, Katz Y, Gaite MR, Gonzalez CJ: A preliminary study of cytokines in suicidal and nonsuicidal adolescents with major depression. J Child Adolesc Psychopharmacol 2009;19:423–430.

39 Brietzke E, Stertz L, Fernandes BS, Kauer-Sant'anna M, Mascarenhas M, Escosteguy Vargas A, Chies JA, Kapczinski F: Comparison of cytokine levels in depressed, manic and euthymic patients with bipolar disorder. J Affect Dis 2009;116:214–217.

40 Mossner R, Mikova O, Koutsilieri E, Saoud M, Ehlis AC, Muller N, Fallgatter AJ, Riederer P: Consensus paper of the WFSBP Task Force on Biological Markers: biological markers in depression. World J Biol Psychiatry 2007;8:141–174.

41 Garcia-Bueno B, Caso JR, Leza JC: Stress as a neuroinflammatory condition in brain: damaging and protective mechanisms. Neurosci Biobehav Rev 2008; 32:1136–1151.

42 Kendler KS, Gardner CO, Prescott CA: Toward a comprehensive developmental model for major depression in women. Am J Psychiatry 2002;159:1133–1145.

43 Kiecolt-Glaser JK, Gouin J-P, Weng NP, Malarkey WB, Beversdorf DQ, Glaser R: Childhood adversity heightens the impact of later-life caregiving stress on telomere length and inflammation. Psychosom Med 2011;73:16–22.

44 Danese A, Moffitt TE, Harrington H, Milne BJ, Polanczyk G, Pariante CM, Poulton R, Caspi A: Adverse childhood experiences and adult risk factors for age-related disease depression, inflammation, and clustering of metabolic risk markers. Arch Pediatr Adolesc Med 2009;163:1135–1143.

45 Danese A, Pariante CM, Caspi A, Taylor A, Poulton R: Childhood maltreatment predicts adult inflammation in a life-course study. Proc Natl Acad Sci USA 2007;104:1319–1324.

46 Archer JA, Hutchison IL, Dorudi S, Stansfeld SA, Korszun A: Interrelationship of depression, stress and inflammation in cancer patients: a preliminary study. J Affect Dis 2012;143:39–46.

47 Steffens DC, Payne ME, Greenberg DL, Byrum CE, Welsh-Bohmer KA, Wagner HR, MacFall JR: Hippocampal volume and incident dementia in geriatric depression. Am J Geriatr Psychiatry 2002;10: 62–71.

48 Green RC, Cupples LA, Kurz A, Auerbach S, Go R, Sadovnick D, Duara R, Kukull WA, Chui H, Edeki T, Griffith PA, Friedland RP, Bachman D, Farrer L: Depression as a risk factor for Alzheimer disease – The MIRAGE study. Arch Neurol 2003;60:753–759.

49 Kenis G, Maes M: Effects of antidepressants on the production of cytokines. Int J Neuropsychopharmacol 2002;5:401–412.

50 Kubera M, Kenis G, Bosmans E, Jaworska-Feil L, Lason W, Scharpe S, Maes M: Suppressive effect of TRH and imipramine on human interferon-gamma and interleukin-10 production in vitro. Pol J Pharmacol 2000;52:481–486.

51 Kubera M, Kenis G, Bosmans E, Kajta M, Basta-Kaim A, Scharpe S, Budziszewska B, Maes M: Stimulatory effect of antidepressants on the production of IL-6. Int Immunopharmacol 2004;4:185–192.

52 Kubera M, Kenis G, Bosmans E, Scharpe S, Maes M: Effects of serotonin and serotonergic agonists and antagonists on the production of interferon-gamma and interleukin-10. Neuropsychopharmacol 2000; 23:89–98.

53 Kubera M, Lin AH, Kenis G, Bosmans E, van Bockstaele D, Maes M: Anti-Inflammatory effects of antidepressants through suppression of the interferon-gamma/interleukin-10 production ratio. J Clin Psychopharmacol 2001;21:199–206.

54 Kubera M, Maes M, Kenis G, Kim YK, Lason W: Effects of serotonin and serotonergic agonists and antagonists on the production of tumor necrosis factor alpha and interleukin-6. Psychiatry Res 2005;134: 251–258.

55 Maes M, Song C, Lin AH, Bonaccorso S, Kenis G, De Jongh R, Bosmans E, Scharpe S: Negative immuno-regulatory effects of antidepressants: inhibition of interferon-gamma and stimulation of interleukin-10 secretion. Neuropsychopharmacology 1999;20:370–379.

56 Hamer M, Batty GD, Marmot MG, Singh-Manoux A, Kivimaeki M: Anti-depressant medication use and C-reactive protein: results from two population-based studies. Brain Behav Immun 2011;25: 168–173.

57 Lim CM, Kim SW, Park JY, Kim C, Yoon SH, Lee JK: Fluoxetine affords robust neuroprotection in the postischemic brain via its anti-inflammatory effect. J Neurosci Res 2009;87:1037–1045.

58 Carvalho LA, Pariante CM: In vitro modulation of the glucocorticoid receptor by antidepressants. Stress (Amsterdam) 2008;11:411–424.

59 Hashioka S, Klegeris A, Monji A, Kato T, Sawada M, McGeer PL, Kanba S: Antidepressants inhibit interferon-gamma-induced microglial production of IL-6 and nitric oxide. Exp Neurol 2007;206:33–42.

60 Vogelzangs N, Duivis HE, Beekman ATF, Kluft C, Neuteboom J, Hoogendijk W, Smit JH, de Jonge P, Penninx BWJH: Association of depressive disorders, depression characteristics and antidepressant medication with inflammation. Transl Psychiatry 2012; 2:e71.

61 Tynan RJ, Weidenhofer J, Hinwood M, Cairns MJ, Day TA, Walker FR: A comparative examination of the anti-inflammatory effects of SSRI and SNRI antidepressants on LPS stimulated microglia. Brain Behav Immun 2012;26:469–479.

62 O'Brien SM, Scully P, Fitzgerald P, Scott LV, Dinan TG: Plasma cytokine profiles in depressed patients who fail to respond to selective serotonin reuptake inhibitor therapy. J Psychiatr Res 2007;41:326–331.

63 Eller T, Vasar V, Shlik J, Maron E: Pro-inflammatory cytokines and treatment response to escitalopram in major depressive disorder. Prog Neuropsychopharmacol Biol Psychiatry 2008;32:445–450.

64 Eller T, Vasar V, Shlik J, Maron E: Effects of bupropion augmentation on pro-inflammatory cytokines in escitalopram-resistant patients with major depressive disorder. J Psychopharmacol (Oxford) 2009;23:854–858.

65 Hou R, Baldwin DS: A neuroimmunological perspective on anxiety disorders. Hum Psychopharmacol 2012;27:6–14.

66 Baldwin DS, Waldman S, Allgulander C: Evidence-based pharmacological treatment of generalized anxiety disorder. Int J Neuropsychopharmacol 2011; 14:697–710.

67 Baldwin DS, Bolognesi F: On predicting the response to antidepressant treatment. Hum Psychopharmacol 2012;27:343–344.

68 Schrott LM, Crnic LS: Increased anxiety behaviors in autoimmune mice. Behav Neurosci 1996;110:492–502.

69 Sakic B, Szechtman H, Talangbayan H, Denburg SD, Carbotte RM, Denburg JA: Disturbed emotionality in autoimmune MRL-lpr mice. Physiol Behav 1994;56:609–617.

70 Bluthe RM, Dantzer R, Kelley KW: Effects of interleukin-1 receptor antagonist on the behavioral effects of lipopolysaccharide in rat. Brain Res 1992;573:318–320.

71 Connor TJ, Leonard BE: Depression, stress and immunological activation: the role of cytokines in depressive disorders. Life Sci 1998;62:583–606.

72 Fiore M, Alleva E, Probert L, Kollias G, Angelucci F, Aloe L: Exploratory and displacement behavior in transgenic mice expressing high levels of brain TNF-alpha. Physiol Behav 1998;63:571–576.

73 Kustova Y, Sei Y, Morse HC Jr, Basile AS: The influence of a targeted deletion of the IFNgamma gene on emotional behaviors. Brain Behav Immun 1998;12:308–324.

74 Lesch KP: Mouse anxiety: the power of knockout. Pharmacogenomics J 2001;1:187–192.

75 Boscarino JA: Posttraumatic stress disorder and physical illness: results from clinical and epidemiologic studies. Ann N Y Acad Sci 2004;1032:141–153.

76 Schneiderman N, Ironson G, Siegel SD: Stress and health: psychological, behavioral, and biological determinants. Ann Rev Clin Psychol 2005;1:607–628.

77 Zhou FL, Zhang WG, Wei YC, Xu KL, Hui LY, Wang XS, Li MZ: Impact of comorbid anxiety and depression on quality of life and cellular immunity changes in patients with digestive tract cancers. World J Gastroenterol 2005;11:2313–2318.

78 Godbout JP, Glaser R: Stress-induced immune dysregulation: implications for wound healing, infectious disease and cancer. J Neuroimmune Pharmacol 2006;1:421–427.

79 Arranz L, Guayerbas N, De la Fuente M: Impairment of several immune functions in anxious women. J Psychosom Res 2007;62:1–8.

80 Koh KB, Lee Y: Reduced anxiety level by therapeutic interventions and cell-mediated immunity in panic disorder patients. Psychother Psychosom 2004;73:286–292.

81 Takkouche B, Regueira C, Gestal-Otero JJ: A cohort study of stress and the common cold. Epidemiology 2001;12:345–349.

82 Aviles H, Johnson MT, Monroy FP: Effects of cold stress on spleen cell proliferation and cytokine production during chronic *Toxoplasma gondii* infection. Neuroimmunomodulation 2004;11:93–102.

83 Jabaaij L, van Hattum J, Vingerhoets JJ, Oostveen FG, Duivenvoorden HJ, Ballieux RE: Modulation of immune response to rDNA hepatitis B vaccination by psychological stress. J Psychosom Res 1996;41:129–137.

84 Glaser R, Sheridan J, Malarkey WB, MacCallum RC, Kiecolt-Glaser JK: Chronic stress modulates the immune response to a pneumococcal pneumonia vaccine. Psychosom Med 2000;62:804–807.

85 Morag M, Morag A, Reichenberg A, Lerer B, Yirmiya R: Psychological variables as predictors of rubella antibody titers and fatigue – a prospective, double blind study. J Psychiatry Res 1999;33:389–395.

86 Burns VE, Drayson M, Ring C, Carroll D: Perceived stress and psychological well-being are associated with antibody status after meningitis C conjugate vaccination. Psychosom Med 2002;64:963–970.

87 Miller GE, Cohen S, Pressman S, Barkin A, Rabin BS, Treanor JJ: Psychological stress and antibody response to influenza vaccination: when is the critical period for stress, and how does it get inside the body? Psychosom Med 2004;66:215–223.

88 Vedhara K, Cox NK, Wilcock GK, Perks P, Hunt M, Anderson S, Lightman SL, Shanks NM: Chronic stress in elderly carers of dementia patients and antibody response to influenza vaccination. Lancet 1999;353:627–631.

89 Vedhara K, McDermott MP, Evans TG, Treanor JJ, Plummer S, Tallon D, Cruttenden KA, Schifitto G: Chronic stress in nonelderly caregivers: psychological, endocrine and immune implications. J Psychosom Res 2002;53:1153–1161.

90 Figueiredo-Braga M, Mota-Garcia F, O'Connor JE, Garcia JR, Mota-Cardoso R, Cardoso CS, de Sousa M: Cytokines and anxiety in systemic lupus erythematosus (SLE) patients not receiving antidepressant medication: a little-explored frontier and some of its brief history. Ann N Y Acad Sci 2009;1173:286–291.

91 Lutgendorf SK, Lamkin DM, DeGeest K, Anderson B, Dao M, McGinn S, Zimmerman B, Maiseri H, Sood AK, Lubaroff DM: Depressed and anxious mood and T-cell cytokine expressing populations in ovarian cancer patients. Brain Behav Immun 2008;22:890–900.

92 Capuron L, Pagnoni G, Demetrashvili M, Woolwine BJ, Nemeroff CB, Berns GS, Miller AH: Anterior cingulate activation and error processing during interferon-alpha treatment. Biol Psychiatry 2005;58:190–196.

93 Harrison NA, Brydon L, Walker C, Gray MA, Steptoe A, Dolan RJ, Critchley HD: Neural origins of human sickness in interoceptive responses to inflammation. Biol Psychiatry 2009;66:415–422.

94 Pitsavos C, Panagiotakos DB, Papageorgiou C, Tsetsekou E, Soldatos C, Stefanadis C: Anxiety in relation to inflammation and coagulation markers, among healthy adults: the ATTICA study. Atherosclerosis 2006;185:320–326.

95 Maes M, Song C, Lin A, De Jongh R, Van Gastel A, Kenis G, Bosmans E, De Meester I, Benoy I, Neels H, Demedts P, Janca A, Scharpe S, Smith RS: The effects of psychological stress on humans: increased production of pro-inflammatory cytokines and a Th1-like response in stress-induced anxiety. Cytokine 1998;10:313–318.

96 Zorrilla EP, Redei E, DeRubeis RJ: Reduced cytokine levels and T-cell function in healthy males: relation to individual differences in subclinical anxiety. Brain Behav Immun 1994;8:293–312.

97 Reichenberg A, Yirmiya R, Schuld A, Kraus T, Haack M, Morag A, Pollmacher T: Cytokine-associated emotional and cognitive disturbances in humans. Arch Gen Psychiatry 2001;58:445–452.

98 O'Donovan A, Hughes BM, Slavich GM, Lynch L, Cronin MT, O'Farrelly C, Malone KM: Clinical anxiety, cortisol and interleukin-6: evidence for specificity in emotion-biology relationships. Brain Behav Immun 2010;24:1074–1077.

99 Gill J, Vythilingam M, Page GG: Low cortisol, high DHEA, and high levels of stimulated TNF-alpha, and IL-6 in women with PTSD. J Trauma Stress 2008;21:530–539.

100 Rohleder N, Joksimovic L, Wolf JM, Kirschbaum C: Hypocortisolism and increased glucocorticoid sensitivity of pro-Inflammatory cytokine production in Bosnian war refugees with posttraumatic stress disorder. Biol Psychiatry 2004;55:745–751.

101 Pace TW, Heim CM: A short review on the psychoneuroimmunology of posttraumatic stress disorder: from risk factors to medical comorbidities. Brain Behav Immun 2011;25:6–13.

102 von Kanel R, Begre S, Abbas CC, Saner H, Gander ML, Schmid JP: Inflammatory biomarkers in patients with posttraumatic stress disorder caused by myocardial infarction and the role of depressive symptoms. Neuroimmunomodulation 2010;17:39–46.

103 Gill JM, Saligan L, Woods S, Page G: PTSD is associated with an excess of inflammatory immune activities. Perspect Psychiatr Care 2009;45:262–277.

104 Baker DG, Nievergelt CM, O'Connor DT: Biomarkers of PTSD: neuropeptides and immune signaling. Neuropharmacology 2012;62:663–673.

105 Brambilla F, Bellodi L, Perna G, Bertani A, Panerai A, Sacerdote P: Plasma interleukin-1 beta concentrations in panic disorder. Psychiatry Res 1994;54: 135–142.

106 van Duinen MA, Schruers KR, Kenis GR, Wauters A, Delanghe J, Griez EJ, Maes MH: Effects of experimental panic on neuroimmunological functioning. J Psychosom Res 2008;64:305–310.

107 Hoge EA, Brandstetter K, Moshier S, Pollack MH, Wong KK, Simon NM: Broad spectrum of cytokine abnormalities in panic disorder and posttraumatic stress disorder. Depress Anxiety 2009;26:447–455.

108 Carpenter LL, Heninger GR, McDougle CJ, Tyrka AR, Epperson CN, Price LH: Cerebrospinal fluid interleukin-6 in obsessive-compulsive disorder and trichotillomania. Psychiatry Res 2002;112:257–262.

109 Monteleone P, Catapano F, Fabrazzo M, Tortorella A, Maj M: Decreased blood levels of tumor necrosis factor-alpha in patients with obsessive-compulsive disorder. Neuropsychobiology 1998;37:182–185.

110 Fluitman S, Denys D, Vulink N, Schutters S, Heijnen C, Westenberg H: Lipopolysaccharide-induced cytokine production in obsessive-compulsive disorder and generalized social anxiety disorder. Psychiatry Res 2010;178:313–316.

111 Denys D, Fluitman S, Kavelaars A, Heijnen C, Westenberg H: Decreased TNF-alpha and NK activity in obsessive-compulsive disorder. Psychoneuroendocrinology 2004;29:945–952.

112 Konuk N, Tekin IO, Ozturk U, Atik L, Atasoy N, Bektas S, Erdogan A: Plasma levels of tumor necrosis factor-alpha and interleukin-6 in obsessive compulsive disorder. Mediators Inflamm 2007;2007: 65704–65704.

113 Bartz JA, Hollander E: Is obsessive-compulsive disorder an anxiety disorder? Prog Neuropsychopharmacol Biol Psychiatry 2006;30:338–352.

114 Bankier B, Barajas J, Martinez-Rumayor A, Januzzi JL: Association between C-reactive protein and generalized anxiety disorder in stable coronary heart disease patients. Eur Heart J 2008;29:2212–2217.

115 Barros PO, Ferreira TB, Vieira MM, Almeida CR, Araujo-Lima CF, Silva-Filho RG, Hygino J, Andrade RM, Andrade AF, Bento CA: Substance P enhances Th17 phenotype in individuals with generalized anxiety disorder: an event resistant to glucocorticoid inhibition. J Clin Immun 2011;31: 51–59.

116 Vieira MM, Ferreira TB, Pacheco PA, Barros PO, Almeida CR, Araujo-Lima CF, Silva-Filho RG, Hygino J, Andrade RM, Linhares UC, Andrade AF, Bento CA: Enhanced Th17 phenotype in individuals with generalized anxiety disorder. J Neuroimmunol 2010;229:212–218.

117 Coogan AN, Wyse CA: Neuroimmunology of the circadian clock. Brain Res 2008;1232:104–112.

118 Tournier M, Sorbara F, Gindre C, Swendsen JD, Verdoux H: Cannabis use and anxiety in daily life: a naturalistic investigation in a non-clinical population. Psychiatry Res 2003;118:1–8.

119 de Jager W, Bourcier K, Rijkers GT, Prakken BJ, Seyfert-Margolis V: Prerequisites for cytokine measurements in clinical trials with multiplex immunoassays. BMC Immun 2009;10:52.

120 Kern PA, Ranganathan S, Li C, Wood L, Ranganathan G: Adipose tissue tumor necrosis factor and interleukin-6 expression in human obesity and insulin resistance. Am J Physiol 2001;280:E745–E751.

121 Vgontzas AN, Papanicolaou DA, Bixler EO, Hopper K, Lotsikas A, Lin HM, Kales A, Chrousos GP: Sleep apnea and daytime sleepiness and fatigue: relation to visceral obesity, insulin resistance, and hypercytokinemia. J Clin Endocrinol Metab 2000;85: 1151–1158.

122 Wolitzky-Taylor KB, Castriotta N, Lenze EJ, Stanley MA, Craske MG: Anxiety disorders in older adults: a comprehensive review. Depress Anxiety 2010;27:190–211.

123 Pedersen BK, Febbraio MA: Muscle as an endocrine organ: focus on muscle-derived interleukin-6. Physiol Rev 2008;88:1379–1406.

124 Woods JA, Vieira VJ, Keylock KT: Exercise, inflammation, and innate immunity. Neurol Clin 2006;24: 585–599.

125 Suzuki K, Nakaji S, Yamada M, Totsuka M, Sato K, Sugawara K: Systemic inflammatory response to exhaustive exercise. Cytokine kinetics. Exerc Immunol Rev 2002;8:6–48.

126 Yu YWY, Chen T-J, Hong C-J, Chen H-M, Tsai S-J: Association study of the interleukin-1beta (C-511T) genetic polymorphism with major depressive disorder, associated symptomatology, and antidepressant response. Neuropsychopharmacology 2003;28:1182–1185.

127 Hwang J, Tsai S, Hong C, Yang C, Hsu C, Liou Y: Interleukin-1 beta -511C/T genetic polymorphism is associated with age of onset of geriatric depression. Neuromolecular Med 2009;11:322–327.

128 Lotrich FE, Ferrell RE, Rabinovitz M, Pollock BG: Risk for depression during interferon-alpha treatment is affected by the serotonin transporter polymorphism. Biol Psychiatry 2009;65:344–348.

129 Maletic V, Raison CL: Neurobiology of depression, fibromyalgia and neuropathic pain. Front Biosci 2009;14:5291–5338.

130 Clerici M, Arosio B, Mundo E, Cattaneo E, Pozzoli S, Dell'Osso B, Vergani C, Trabattoni D, Altamura AC: Cytokine polymorphisms in the pathophysiology of mood disorders. CNS Spectr 2009;14:419–425.

131 Traks T, Koido K, Eller T, Maron E, Kingo K, Vasar V, Vasar E, Koks S: Polymorphisms in the interleukin-10 gene cluster are possibly involved in the increased risk for major depressive disorder. BMC Med Genet 2008;9:111.

132 Kraus MR, Al-Taie O, Schaefer A, Pfersdorff M, Lesch K-P, Scheurlen M: Serotonin-1A receptor gene HTR1A variation predicts interferon-induced depression in chronic hepatitis C. Gastroenterology 2007;132:1279–1286.

133 Chen Z-Y, Jing D, Bath KG, Ieraci A, Khan T, Siao C-J, Herrera DG, Toth M, Yang C, McEwen BS, Hempstead BL, Lee FS: Genetic variant BDNF (Val66Met) polymorphism alters anxiety-related behavior. Science 2006;314:140–143.

134 Millan MJ: The neurobiology and control of anxious states. Prog Neurobiol 2003;70:83–244.

Ruihua Hou
University Department of Psychiatry, Academic Centre, College Keep
4–12 Terminus Terrace
Southampton SO14 3DT (UK)
E-Mail R.Hou@soton.ac.uk

Baldwin DS, Leonard BE (eds): Anxiety Disorders.
Mod Trends Pharmacopsychiatry. Basel, Karger, 2013, vol 29, pp 85–97 (DOI: 10.1159/000351945)

Anxiety and Cardiovascular Disease

Simon J.C. Davies[a, b] · Christer Allgulander[c]

[a]Geriatric Psychiatry Division, Centre for Addiction and Mental Health, Department of Psychiatry, University of Toronto, Toronto, Ont., Canada; [b]Academic Unit of Psychiatry, University of Bristol, Bristol, UK; [c]Section of Psychiatry, Department of Clinical Neuroscience, Karolinska Institutet, Stockholm, Sweden

Abstract

This chapter examines the association of anxiety disorders and anxiety symptoms with cardiovascular disease, focussing on hypertension (an independent risk factor for myocardial infarction and stroke) and coronary heart disease. In both cases, epidemiological data linking the cardiovascular disorder with specific anxiety disorders and anxiety symptoms are examined first, and evidence relating to putative mechanisms that may underlie these associations is explored. For hypertension, an association with panic attacks and panic disorder has been reported most consistently, but the literature relating to other forms of anxiety is inconsistent, especially as some studies have reported an association of anxiety with low blood pressure. Recent work which has attempted to elucidate this confusing situation is presented. Mechanisms which may be responsible for the link between hypertension and panic include autonomic nervous system dysfunction (which may be under serotonergic control), respiratory mechanisms, cytokines, platelet dysfunction and behavioural factors. While an association of depression with coronary heart disease has been studied extensively, the association with anxiety disorders has been slower to emerge. Studies contributing to this evidence base are examined, and as for hypertension putative mechanisms are discussed.

Copyright © 2013 S. Karger AG, Basel

In this chapter, the associations of anxiety and anxiety disorders with cardiovascular disease will be examined. As the bulk of the evidence relates to hypertension and coronary heart disease (CHD), the focus of this paper will be on these common cardiovascular problems.

Anxiety and Hypertension

Hypertension is a common disorder with increasing prevalence through the lifespan. It is a prognostic factor for myocardial infarction, heart failure and stroke [1], but this risk is modifiable by antihypertensive drugs. The term 'essential hypertension' has traditionally been applied to high blood pressure (BP) of unknown aetiology as it was thought that hypertension was commonly a compensatory mechanism to ensure that adequate perfusion was maintained when arteries became sclerosed [2]. However, hypertension previously considered 'essential' can often now be linked to pathologies including insulin resistance, salt sensitivity, sleep apnoea and dysfunction of the sympathetic nervous system [3, 4].

Association of Anxiety Disorders with Hypertension

Clinical observation suggests that panic attacks are associated with transient increases in BP [5]. Controlled studies have reported higher rates of panic attacks or panic disorder with hypertension [6, 7] but had methodological limitations, such as failure to adjust for confounders other than age and sex.

Meanwhile, rather different conclusions have been drawn about the association between hypertension and generalized anxiety disorder (GAD) or non-specific measures of anxiety. In studies employing hypertension as a dichotomous end point, all kinds of relationships have been reported. For instance, hypertension as a category was associated with both panic disorder and GAD in a recent study from South Africa [8], and with anxiety disorders distinct from panic in further studies [9, 10], but in others no association with anxiety [11, 12] was found. In contrast, large population-based studies, using continuous BP measures rather than a hypertension diagnosis, have reported associations between *low* BP and general psychological morbidity and related symptoms [13, 14]. These latter findings are in line with clinical practice in some countries where a syndrome of low BP, tiredness and (generalized) anxiety is well recognized [15].

To summarise, measures of anxiety have been associated both with low and high BP; and among all the anxiety symptoms and disorders, panic attacks/panic disorder have most consistently been associated with hypertension. To reconcile these diverse findings, we have employed data from the population-based HUNT study where all 92,936 individuals aged 20 or more residing in one Norwegian county were invited to participate and just under 65,000 had BP recorded. We examined the hypothesis that there is a non-linear relationship between systolic BP and panic and an association of low BP with generalized anxiety [16]. Both unadjusted (n = 61,408) and adjusted analyses provided evidence for a non-linear relationship between panic and systolic BP, represented by a 'U'-shaped curve with a minimum prevalence of panic around 140 mm Hg (fig. 1). The relationship was strengthened after adjustment for multiple confounders with the quadratic term significantly associated with panic (p = 0.03). Generalized anxiety symptoms were associated only with low systolic BP (fig. 1). The 'U'-shaped relation between systolic BP and panic provides a unifying explanation for the separate strands of published literature in this area, as high BP appears to be associated only with panic symptoms, while several forms of anxiety including panic and generalized anxiety may be associated with low BP.

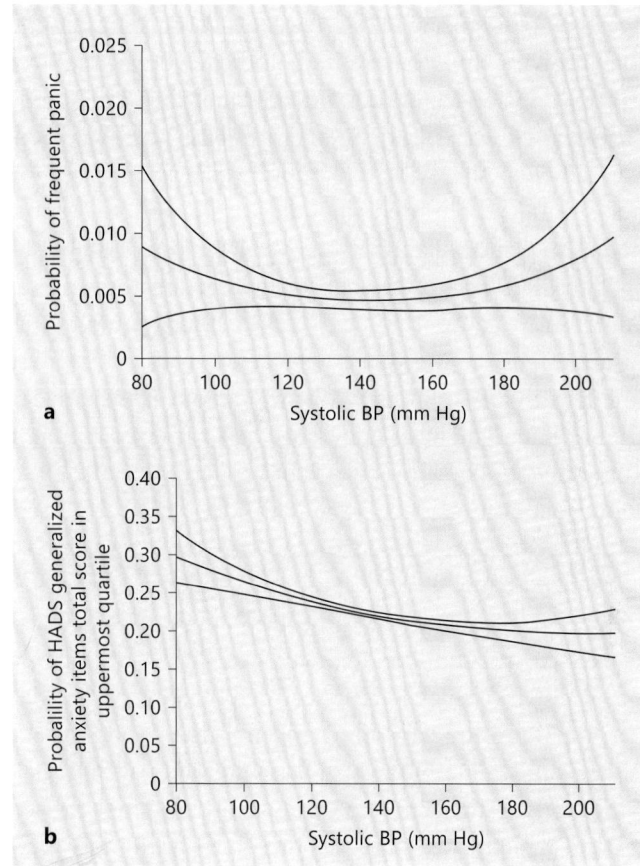

Fig. 1. a Probability of frequent panic by systolic BP after adjustment for potential confounding variables (n = 43,974). **b** Probability of Hospital Anxiety and Depression Scale-derived generalized anxiety symptoms (score in uppermost quartile of sample) by systolic BP after adjustment for potential confounding variables (n = 39,755). Dotted lines indicate 95% confidence limits. Reproduced from Davies et al. [16].

Mechanisms in the Association of Hypertension and Panic Attacks/Panic Disorder

What mechanisms might explain why panic attacks and panic disorder, but not other anxiety disorders, are associated with high BP? A prime candidate is the autonomic nervous system. A study examining panic attack symptoms [17] illustrated that only the typical autonomic symptoms of sweating and flushes are significantly more common in attacks reported by hypertensive patients compared with normotensives, and on factor analysis only the autonomic dominated factor (comprising sweating, flushing, shaking and the non-specific symptom of nausea) was associated significantly with hypertension.

At the neurochemical level, central or peripheral catecholamine dysfunction has been described in both panic disorder and hypertension. Despite the majority of cases of hypertension being classified as 'essential hypertension', there has been an acknowledgement that in many cases a dysfunction of the autonomic nervous system may be the underlying pathology [18]. Evidence from the studies by Esler et al. [19] of clinical microneurography and direct measurement of noradrenaline spillover from cardiac nerve terminals suggests sympathetic dysfunction in hypertensives. 'Spillover' is the overflow of a substance to an organ's venous drainage. Catheterisation, in this case of the coronary sinus, is required, and catecholamine overflow is measured through an isotope dilution technique with constant infusion of radiolabelled noradrenaline. Similarly, excess adrenaline spillover from the heart has been reported during panic attacks [20]. There is also evidence of abnormal central catecholamine function in both disorders. Nutt [21] reported altered central α_2-adrenoceptor sensitivity in panic disorder, and excess catecholamine spillover from the brain has been seen in hypertension [22].

There has been interest as to whether serotonin systems and their dysfunction may contribute to autonomic nervous system dysfunction and thereby to the association of hypertension and panic disorder. Serotonin-promoting antidepressants are first-line treatments in anxiety disorders, and transient depletion of serotonin by acute tryptophan depletion renders treated patients with a history of panic disorder more vulnerable to panic on stress challenge [23]. Polyak has reported that selective serotonin reuptake inhibitor (SSRI) antidepressants can assist BP control in hypertensive patients with co-morbid panic [24]. After 3–6 months' drug treatment, patients with co-morbid panic disorder and mild hypertension experienced more pronounced BP reduction if on treatment with the SSRI fluoxetine than those treated with the antihypertensive moxonidine. Reduced heart rate variability has been reported in panic disorder [25, 26] which can be rectified by SSRIs [27].

Thus, lowering serotonin concentrations using the acute tryptophan depletion technique should alter both cardiovascular and psychological parameters relevant to these conditions. In patients with treated panic disorder or social anxiety disorder, acute tryptophan depletion left participants vulnerable to significantly greater BP and psychological responses to stress challenges than that seen under nondepleted conditions [28]. Serotonin may have an anti-stress role in both psychological and cardiovascular domains.

We have previously constructed a model to illustrate possible neuroanatomical pathways that may be involved in the association of panic and hypertension through common autonomic dysfunction, illustrating the possibility that failure of serotonin-modulated control mechanisms may play a role [29]. The model (fig. 2) highlights serotonin-dependent pathways in the ventrolateral periaqueductal gray (VLPAG) and raphe pallidum which may exert control over the C1 cells of the rostral ventrolateral medulla. The C1 cells are in turn responsible for sympathetic activation. Serotonergic control of the VLPAG may impinge also on behavioural symptoms of panic, mediated through the dorsal periaqueductal gray.

Other Putative Mechanisms

Although some evidence of cytokine disturbance in panic disorder exists (involving reports of increased interleukin-1β [30] and IL-2 plasma concentrations [31] in panic disorder compared with controls), overall the evidence is as yet insufficient to underpin an association with hypertension.

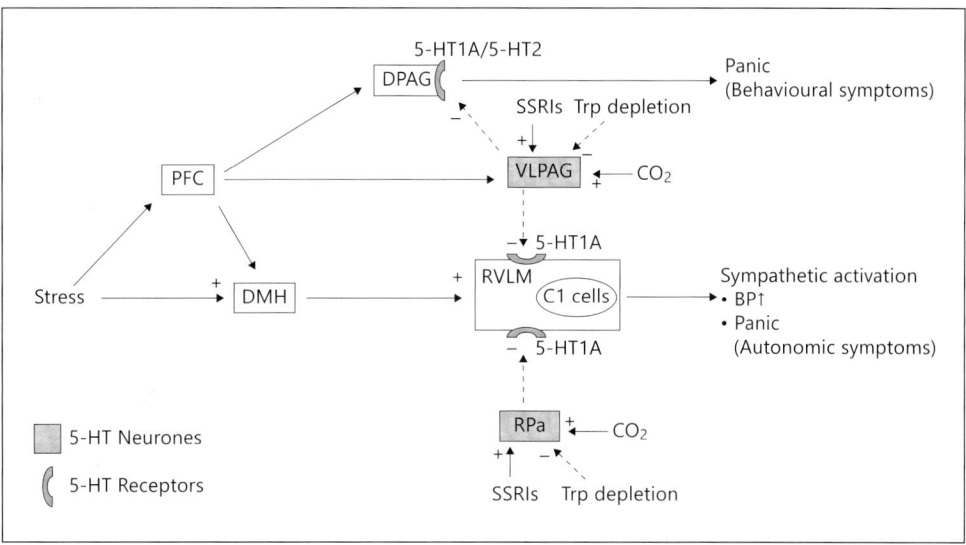

Fig. 2. Hypothetical model of neural systems underlying the association between hypertension and panic disorder. According to the model, deficiencies in inhibitory control, either local GABAergic inhibitory mechanisms within the dorsomedial hypothalamus (DMH), or serotonergic inhibitory mechanisms, acting within the dorsal periaqueductal gray (DPAG; 5-HT_{1A}/5-HT_2 receptors) or rostral ventrolateral medulla (RVLM; 5-HT_{1A} receptors), would result in vulnerability to both hypertension and panic disorder. Serotonergic neurons in both the ventrolateral part of the dorsal raphe nucleus (DRVL)/VLPAG region and the medullary raphe pallidum (RPa) are directly excited by the panicogenic agent CO_2 or decreases in extracellular pH. Normally, this mechanism would serve as a negative feedback system, with increasing concentrations of CO_2 or decreasing pH-activating serotonergic neuronal firing rates, preventing an overactivation of both the behavioural and autonomic symptoms of panic. If these serotonergic neurons are compromised, either by changes in their intrinsic properties or changes in the neural input regulating their activity (e.g. changes in executive function in the prefrontal cortex, PFC), behavioural and autonomic responses would continue unchecked. Chronic, reduced activity of serotonergic neurons in the DRVL/VLPAG region would be expected to lead to vulnerability to both hypertension and the behavioural and autonomic symptoms of panic. Chronic, reduced activity of serotonergic neurons in the RPa region would be expected to lead to vulnerability to both hypertension and the autonomic, but not behavioural, symptoms of panic. Indeed tryptophan depletion can exacerbate panic symptoms. In contrast, SSRIs, possibly by increasing serotonergic neurotransmission in these systems, can alleviate panic symptoms. C1 = C1-adrenergic cell group. Reproduced from Davies et al. [29].

Among other biological mechanisms postulated to underlie the association of hypertension and panic disorder, respiratory mechanisms have attracted interest. Hyperventilation is a prominent component of panic attacks, and acutely has a significant but short-lived pressor effect, averaging 9/8 mm Hg in normotensive subjects [32]. Klein [33] divided panic attacks into two subtypes, the first due to 'false suffocation alarms' and characterized by panic with a predominance of respiratory symptoms and the second group attributable to sympathetic nervous system or hypothalamo-pituitary-adrenal axis deficits. However, in the factor analysis of panic attack symptoms in hypertensive and normotensive patients described earlier [17], the factor significantly associated with hypertension was that comprising symptoms typical of sympathetic nervous system dysfunction, whereas respiratory panic symptoms were no more common in hypertensives than normotensives, and the factor dominated by respiratory symptoms had no association with hypertension.

It remains possible that the association of hypertension with panic attacks and panic disorder is due to illness behaviour, so-called 'white coat responses' or labelling effects. Psychological symptoms may impair the ability of patients both to tolerate or adhere to medication regimes and to follow interventions that reduce cardiovascular risk after myocardial infarction. Panic attacks, anxiety and depression are associated with episodes of intolerance to antihypertensive agents [34] provided the intolerances reported are not typical of the drugs implicated (non-specific intolerance). The number of episodes of non-specific intolerance was significantly associated with poor outcome in BP control [34].

It has been suggested that reported associations of hypertension and panic disorder may be that patients with panic disorder appear artefactually to have higher BPs due to a greater 'white coat response' (i.e. medical setting anxiety-induced hypertension) response compared with patients without panic disorder. Patients who are prone to panic attacks may perceive a primary care facility or hospital clinic as threatening, and could have a pressor effect as a conditioned response to these situations [35]. However in an earlier clinical study, we found no excess 'white coat effect' in patients with panic disorder and panic attacks making this explanation unlikely [36].

Finally, it is conceivable that the association of panic disorder and hypertension might be due at least in part to a 'labelling effect'. Patients' awareness of a diagnosis of hypertension may lead to subsequent adverse effects on psychological well-being [37] and to vulnerability to the development of panic disorder. Indeed, in the one study which examined the temporal relationship of the onset of panic attacks and hypertension [7], the diagnosis of hypertension preceded panic attacks significantly more often than vice versa (p < 0.01).

Anxiety and Coronary Heart Disease

CHD includes ischaemic heart disease, angina and cardiac events such as myocardial infarction. Depression has been recognized as an independent risk factor for CHD in numerous prospective studies and several meta-analyses [38, 39]. Some studies have questioned the strength of the relation. A recent systematic review of 48 studies concluded that while the majority of individual studies did report an association and that there was an association overall, attention was drawn to methodological issues in many papers, especially in that 85% of studies had not controlled for any measure of anxiety despite the high rates of co-morbidity between anxiety and depression [40]. This left most studies open to the possibility of residual confounding through the presence of anxiety symptoms assuming that the association of anxiety and CHD is itself important.

The evidence for an association of CHD with anxiety disorders has been slower to emerge. The abundance of literature relating to depression compared with that relating to anxiety disorders in this area might be seen as indicating that depression is indeed more strongly associated with CHD than are anxiety disorders. However, there are alternative explanations for this focus on depression. Research collaborations designing prospective studies with complex medical outcomes may have been more immediately familiar with depression than anxiety disorders (and therefore included measures of depression in preference to those of anxiety) or considered anxiety as insufficiently distinct from depression to merit investigation. The multiplicity of anxiety symptoms, existence of several different anxiety disorders, and diagnoses which have changed markedly in their criteria over time may be further disincentives to study anxiety in addition to depression as a cardiovascular risk factor.

A meta-analysis [41] has brought together prospective studies examining the link between anxiety or anxiety disorders and subtypes of CHD. Roest et al. [41] identified 20 studies with varying types of anxiety or anxiety disorder as baseline risk factors and end points related to CHD as the outcome. Illustrating the heterogeneous nature of these studies with regard to the type of anxiety considered, one study examined the impact of panic attacks, one post-traumatic symptoms and a further 2 GAD or its core symptoms of excess worry. A further 4 employed the 'phobic anxiety' subscale of the Crown-Crisp Experiential Index, the remaining 12 employed end points described as 'general' measures of anxiety (as opposed to GAD) using scales which were not designed to differentiate between specific types of anxiety or anxiety disorder. Many of these 'general' scales contain items which predominantly describe symptoms of generalized anxiety, with questions on episodic panic attacks and the autonomic activation symptoms typically experienced in panic underrepresented. Overall, anxious persons were at a significantly higher risk of incident CHD independent of demographic variables, biological risk factors and health behaviours (hazard ratio 1.21; 95% CI: 1.15–1.38, p < 0.0001) in a sample of around 250,000 people with a mean follow-up of 11.2 years.

What cannot be established from the existing evidence base of prospective studies is whether there is a differential risk of CHD between different types of anxiety. Notably, the single study which had panic attacks as the exposure [42] produced the largest hazard ratio of 4.20 (95% CI: 1.76–10.00). This study was undertaken in a population of 3,369 post-menopausal women for an outcome of cardiac events (fatal and nonfatal myocardial infarction and stroke) over a 5.3-year follow-up period. Other studies not included in the meta-analysis of Roest et al. [41] may shed further light on the potential importance of panic and panic disorder. Using a managed care database of 78,000 patients, a 2-fold increased risk for CHD was reported in patients with panic disorder (based on the ICD-9 diagnostic system), independent of the presence of major depressive disorder [43]. A large cohort study based on the British General

Practice Research database reported that panic attacks/panic disorder conferred a significantly increased risk of myocardial infarction if panic onset was before age 50 years, and elevated risk of CHD at all ages [44], while a Taiwanese longitudinal study reported an increased risk of myocardial infarction in panic disorder of around 1.75-fold which was independent of hypertension [45]. Most recently, a prospective study using data from a well-known cohort of young Swedish men examined for military service, which included a baseline assessment for 'anxiety neurosis' has been published [46]. This diagnostic forerunner of panic disorder and GAD containing some aspects of both modern-day diagnoses appeared in ICD-8 which was the predominant diagnostic system at the time the cohort was established. Over an impressive follow-up period of 37 years for almost 50,000 participants, anxiety neurosis conferred a hazard ratio of 2.17 (95% CI: 1.28–3.67) for CHD. Finally, strong associations of panic or anxiety neurosis with CHD and cardiovascular mortality are supported by cross-sectional data in smaller studies [47, 48] and data derived from the Epidemiological Catchment Area study [6]. A significant excess of cardiovascular conditions including history of 'heart attack' which had an odds ratio of 4.54 in panic disorder compared to subjects with no psychiatric illness was reported.

Roest cited four studies which examined the association of CHD with 'phobic anxiety' symptoms by a subscale of the Crown Crisp Experiential Index. This questionnaire [49] dates from the mid-1960s and incorporates eight items, four of which refer to the concept of agoraphobia, two to specific phobias (claustrophobia and height phobia) and two to worries about family members and about health which might now be considered to refer to generalized anxiety symptoms or hypochondriasis. In one study, phobic anxiety scores of 5 or more had relative risk of 3.77 for fatal CHD (95% CI: 1.64–8.64) compared to those scoring 0 or 1 on the subscale in white males followed up for an average of 6.7 years [50]. In similar studies [51, 52] of men free of CHD at baseline, phobic anxiety was associated with excess CHD mortality, which was entirely due to excess sudden deaths. A further study by the same authors [53] showed an association between baseline phobic anxiety, and increased risk of sudden cardiac death over 32 years of follow-up. In another prospective study, Watkins et al. [54] reported associations of phobic anxiety and depressive symptomatology with ventricular arrhythmias. Fleet and Beitman's review [55] concluded that panic and phobic anxiety taken together, which he termed 'panic-like anxiety' appeared to be an independent risk factor for cardiovascular death. However, the heterogeneous nature of the Crown Crisp Experiential Index phobic anxiety subscale – with half of the measure being made up of items approximating to agoraphobia, which is known to be closely linked to panic disorder – leaves questions to be answered as to whether the anxiety associated with phobias carries a similarly elevated risk of CHD and its consequences as described above with panic disorder.

In contrast, a number of studies have examined the association of cardiovascular disease with measures of anxiety more closely related to GAD. A meta-analysis of anxiety as a risk factor for cardiovascular disease in studies up to 2003 concluded that the evidence for generalized anxiety as a cardiovascular risk factor was relatively sparse [56], with several studies finding no association. In total, Roest et al. [41] cited 14 studies in which the anxiety measure at baseline was either GAD, its core symptom, worry, or a 'general' measure of anxiety made up predominantly of GAD symptoms (e.g. HADS-A, Spielberger Trait Inventrory, EDS Anxiety Subscale). Around half of these studies, including 6 of the 9 published since 2006 reported a significant association of the GAD-related measure with incident CHD. Although Roest's group did not pool these studies for comparison with the effect size of the single panic study, there is some suggestion that generalized anxiety symptoms and disorder may be a weaker risk factor for CHD than panic, mirroring the situation described earlier with panic disorder. However, only a larger prospective study with robust ascertainment of panic disorder diagnoses at baseline will allow this to be ascertained with a greater degree of certainty.

Finally, a recent study [57] highlights an interesting paradox relating to the impact of GAD on cardiovascular outcome. In a sample of patients with acute coronary syndrome followed over 5 years, GAD at baseline was associated with significantly better cardiovascular outcomes after adjustment for depression and medical comorbidity. The authors suggested that GAD may increase the likelihood of seeking treatment and of adhering to cardiac rehabilitation, and described this phenomenon as 'constructive worrying'.

Mechanisms in the Association of Coronary Heart Disease and Anxiety

Just as the epidemiological evidence for the association with anxiety and CHD has lagged behind that for depression, elucidation of the biological causes of an association is not yet well developed. Mechanisms which have been put forward to explain why depression may be an independent risk factor for CHD include autonomic nervous system dysfunction, inflammatory mediators, platelet dysfunction and atherosclerosis. Some of these ideas have been applied to the arena of anxiety and CHD.

We have discussed mechanisms relating to autonomic dysfunction in examining the association of panic and hypertension. Many of the same concepts have been invoked to explain an association of CHD primarily with panic disorder. Of course, this association may merely be based on hypertension being on the causal pathway as an important risk factor for CHD, but some markers of autonomic dysfunction are abnormal in the presence of CHD irrespective of hypertension, for example reduced heart rate variability [58]. As with hypertension, serotonin may have a role in moderating autonomic nervous system dysfunction in ischaemic heart disease. The SADHART study [59] reported a trend towards SSRI treatment reducing further ischaemic heart disease-related morbidity in people who had experienced myocardial infarction or unstable angina, while in depressed patients who had experienced stroke cardiovascular outcomes were significantly better in patients randomized to an SSRI [60]. It is possible that the association could act through anxiety disorders causing cardiac arrhythmias, and increased serotonin availability is known to reduce vulnerability to ventricular fibrillation in the cat [61].

There is evidence of changes in concentrations of inflammatory markers such as IL-1, IL-2, IL-6, TNFα and CRP in cardiovascular disease [62], and indeed in depression [62; see also chapter by Hou et al., pp. 67–84]. Increased anxiety symptoms have also been correlated with raised CRP, IL-6 and TNFα levels in one large study of 853 people free of cardiovascular disease [63]. In more controlled conditions, the Trier social stress test, which is an acute psychological stressor designed as a laboratory probe of social anxiety symptoms, has been consistently reported to produce a transient increase in plasma IL-6 [64] and IL-1β [65]. As noted earlier, some evidence exists for elevated IL-6 and IL-2 in panic disorder [30, 31]. However, although the possibility that cytokines may be responsible for the association of anxiety disorders with ischemic heart disease is still to be fully investigated, there have been some recent intriguing reports which suggest that immune functioning may link risk factors for cardiovascular disease and anxiety (or at least psychological stress). For example, an increased body mass index confers an excessively large proinflammatory cytokine response to experimentally induced anxiety [66], and the combination of immune stimulus and experimental anxiety challenge produces a synergistic increase in proinflammatory cytokine production, negative mood and BP [67].

Recent studies examining potential platelet dysfunction in panic disorder have addressed 'second messenger' systems. Initial studies reported decreased serotonin receptor coupling [68], decreased platelet cyclic adenosine monophosphate (cAMP) concentrations [69] and altered subunit ratios of protein kinase A [70] in panic disorder patients. As elevated platelet cAMP concentrations are known to inhibit platelet activation [71], it is possible that platelets are more aggregable in panic disorder. However, some previous studies have shown that platelets show less aggregation in response to serotonin challenge in panic disorder patients than controls [72]. Overall, it remains unclear as to the degree of involvement platelets have in mediating the link between panic disorder and cardiovascular disease. A further study used an anxiety measure more closely linked to GAD than to panic (the anxiety subscale of the Hospital Anxiety and Depression Scale). Anxiety was associated with excess platelet aggregation in response to serotonin and ephedrine combinations in people with CHD [73] and was a better predictor of this abnormal response than was depression.

One study [74] has reported an association of subclinical atherosclerosis with anxiety disorders, and it has been postulated that the impact of anxiety on CHD risk may act through this pathway. The authors suggested several ways in which subclinical atherosclerosis could be linked to anxiety disorders; these include (a) activation of immune system pathways, (b) hypothalamic pituitary adrenal axis dysfunction, (c) pro-atherogenic metabolic abnormalities, such as abdominal obesity and dyslipidemia, and (d) sympathetic nervous overactivity in anxious persons.

Acknowledgement

The authors would like to thank Dr. David M. Christmas for his assistance especially in the area of cytokines/inflammatory markers.

References

1 Lewington S, Clarke R, Qizilbash N, Peto R, Collins R: Age-specific relevance of usual blood pressure to vascular mortality: a meta-analysis of individual data for one million adults in 61 prospective studies. Lancet 2002;360:1903–1913.

2 White GW: The New Hampshire Academy of Science. Science 1931;74:98.

3 Mancia G, Grassi G, Parati G, Zanchetti A: The sympathetic nervous system in human hypertension. Acta Physiol Scand Suppl 1997;640:117–121.

4 Esler M: The sympathetic system and hypertension. Am J Hypertens 2000;13:99S-105S.

5 White WB, Baker LH: Episodic hypertension secondary to panic disorder. Arch Int Med 1986;146: 1129–1130.

6 Weissman MM, Markowitz JS, Ouellette R, Greenwald S, Kahn JP: Panic disorder and cardiovascular/cerebrovascular problems: results from a community survey. Am J Psychiatry 1990;147:1504–1508.

7 Davies SJC, Ghahramani P, Jackson PR, Noble TW, Hardy P, Hippisley-Cox J, Yeo WW, Ramsay LE: Association of panic disorder and panic attacks with hypertension. Am J Med 1999;107:310–316.

8 Grimsrud A, Stein DJ, Seedat S, Williams D, Myer L: The association between hypertension and depression and anxiety disorders: results from a nationally-representative sample of South African adults. PLoS One 2009;4:e5552.

9 Jonas BS, Franks P, Ingram DD: Are symptoms of anxiety and depression risk factors for hypertension? Longitudinal evidence from the National Health and Nutrition Examination Survey I Epidemiologic Follow-up Study. Arch Fam Med 1997;6:43–49.

10 Paterniti S, Alperovitch A, Ducimetiere P, Dealberto MJ, Lepine JP, Bisserbe JC: Anxiety but not depression is associated with elevated blood pressure in a community group of French elderly. Psychosom Med 1999;61:77–83.

11 Shinn EH, Poston WS, Kimball KT, St Jeor ST, Foreyt JP: Blood pressure and symptoms of depression and anxiety a prospective study. Am J Hypertens 2001;14:660–664.

12 Sparrow D, Garvey AJ, Rosner B, Thomas HE Jr: Factors in predicting blood pressure change. Circulation 1982;65:789–794.

13 Pilgrim JA, Stansfeld S, Marmot M: Low blood pressure, low mood? BMJ 1992;304:75–78.

14 Hildrum B, Mykletun A, Stordal E, Bjelland I, Dahl AA, Holmen J: Association of low blood pressure with anxiety and depression: the Nord-Trondelag Health Study. J Epidemiol Community Health 2007; 61:53–58.

15 Pemberton J: Does constitutional hypotension exist? BMJ 1989;298:660–662.

16 Davies SJC, Bjerkeset O, Nutt DJ, Lewis G: A U-shaped relationship between systolic blood pressure and panic symptoms: the HUNT study. Psychol Med 2012;17:1–8.

17 Davies SJC, Jackson PR, Lewis G, Hood SD, Nutt DJ, Potokar JP: Is the association of hypertension and panic disorder explained by the clustering of autonomic panic symptoms in hypertensive patients? J Affect Disord 2008;111:344–350.

18 Mann SJ: Neurogenic essential hypertension revisited: the case for increased clinical and research attention. Am J Hypertens 2003;16:881–888.

19 Esler M, Rumantir M, Kaye D, Jennings G, Hastings J, Socratous F, et al: Sympathetic nerve biology in essential hypertension. Clin Exp Pharmacol Physiol 2001;28:986–989.

20 Wilkinson DJ, Thompson JM, Lambert GW, Jennings GL, Schwarz RG, Jefferys D, et al: Sympathetic activity in patients with panic disorder at rest, under laboratory mental stress, and during panic attacks. Arch Gen Psychiatry 1998;55:511–520.

21 Nutt DJ: Altered central alpha 2-adrenoceptor sensitivity in panic disorder. Arch Gen Psychiatry 1989; 46:165–169.

22 Ferrier C, Cox H, Esler M: Elevated total body noradrenaline spillover in normotensive members of hypertensive families. Clin Sci (Lond) 1993;84:225–230.

23 Bell C, Forshall S, Adrover M, Nash J, Hood S, Argyropoulos S, et al: Does 5-HT restrain panic? A tryptophan depletion study in panic disorder patients recovered on paroxetine. J Psychopharmacol (Oxf) 2002;16:5–14.

24 Polyák J: How should we manage cardiovascular panic disorder accompanied by hypertension? J Hypertens 2001;19:S64.

25 Yeragani VK, Sobolewski E, Igel G, Johnson C, Jampala VC, Kay J, et al: Decreased heart-period variability in patients with panic disorder: a study of Holter ECG records. Psychiatry Res 1998;20;78:89–99.

26 Friedman BH, Thayer JF: Autonomic balance revisited: panic anxiety and heart rate variability. J Psychosom Res 1998;44:133–151.

27 Yeragani VK, Jampala VC, Sobelewski E, Kay J, Igel G: Effects of paroxetine on heart period variability in patients with panic disorder: a study of holter ECG records. Neuropsychobiology 1999;40:124–128.

28 Davies SJ, Hood SD, Argyropoulos SV, Morris K, Bell C, Witchel HJ, et al: Depleting serotonin enhances both cardiovascular and psychological stress reactivity in recovered patients with anxiety disorders. J Clin Psychopharmacol 2006;26:414–418.

29 Davies SJ, Lowry CA, Nutt DJ: Panic and hypertension: brothers in arms through 5-HT? J Psychopharmacol 2007;21:563–566.

30 Weizman R, Laor N, Wiener Z, Wolmer L, Bessler H: Cytokine production in panic disorder patients. Clin Neuropharmacol 1999;22:107–109.

31 Norman TR, Judd FK, Gregory M, James RH, Kimber NM, McIntyre IM, et al: Platelet serotonin uptake in panic disorder. J Affect Disord 1986;11:69–72.

32 Kaplan NM: Anxiety-induced hyperventilation: a common cause of symptoms in patients with hypertension. Arch Intern Med 1997;157:945–948.

33 Klein DF: False suffocation alarms, spontaneous panics, and related conditions. Arch Gen Psychiatry 1993,50:306–317.

34 Davies SJC, Jackson PR, Ramsay LE, Ghahramani P: Drug intolerance due to non-specific side effects related to psychiatric morbidity in hypertensive patients. Arch Intern Med 2003;163:592–600.

35 Pickering TG, Devereux RB, Gerin W, James GD, Pieper C, Schlussel YR, et al: The role of behavioral factors in white coat and sustained hypertension. J Hypertens Suppl 1990;8:S141–S147.

36 Davies SJ, Jackson PR, Ramsay LE, Ghahramani P, Palmer RL, Hippisley-Cox J: No evidence that panic attacks are associated with the white coat effect in hypertension. J Clin Hypertens (Greenwich) 2003;5:145–152.

37 Macdonald LA, Sackett DL, Haynes RB, Taylor DW: Labelling in hypertension: a review of the behavioural and psychological consequences. J Chronic Dis 1984;37:933–942.

38 Van der Kooy K, van Hout H, Marwijk H, Marten H, Stehouwer C, Beekman A: Depression and the risk for cardiovascular diseases: systematic review and meta-analysis. Int J Geriatr Psychiatry 2007;22:613–626.

39 Frasure-Smith N, Lespérance F: Recent evidence linking coronary heart disease and depression. Can J Psychiatry 2006;51:730–737.

40 Stamfer HG, Hince DA, Dimmett SB: Depression as a risk factor for coronary heart disease – How strong is the evidence? Open J Psychiatry 2012;2:284–291.

41 Roest AM, Martens EJ, de Jone P, et al: Anxiety and risk of incident coronary heart disease: A meta-analysis. J Am Coll Cardiol 2010;56:38–46.

42 Smoller JW, Pollack MH, Wassertheil-Smoller S, Jackson RD, Oberman A, Wong ND, et al: Panic attacks and risk of incident cardiovascular events among postmenopausal women in the Women's Health Initiative Observational Study. Arch Gen Psychiatry 2007;64:1153–1160.

43 Gomez-Caminero A, Blumentals WA, Russo LJ, Brown RR, Castilla-Puentes R: Does panic disorder increase the risk of coronary heart disease? A cohort study of a national managed care database. Psychosom Med 2005;67:688–691.

44 Chen YH, Tsai SY, Lee HC, Lin HC: Increased risk of acute myocardial infarction for patients with panic disorder: a nationwide population-based study. Psychosom Med 2009;71:798–804.

45 Walters K, Rait G, Petersen I, Williams R, Nazareth I: Panic disorder and risk of new onset coronary heart disease, acute myocardial infarction, and cardiac mortality: cohort study using the general practice research database. Eur Heart J 2008;29:2981–2988.

46 Janszky I, Ahnve S, Lundberg I, et al: Early-onset depression, anxiety and risk of subsequent coronary heart disease. 37-year follow-up of 49,321 young Swedish men. J Am Coll Cardiol 2010;56:31–37.

47 Coryell W, Noyes R, Clancy J: Excess mortality in panic disorder: a comparison with primary unipolar depression. Arch Gen Psychiatry 1982;39:701–703.

48 Coryell W, Noyes R Jr, House JD: Mortality among outpatients with anxiety disorders. Am J Psychiatry 1986;143:508–510.

49 Crown S, Crisp AH: A short clinical diagnostic self-rating scale for psychoneurotic patients. The Middlesex Hospital Questionnaire (M.H.Q.). Br J Psychiatry 1966;112:917–923.

50 Haines AP, Imeson JD, Meade TW: Phobic anxiety and ischaemic heart disease. BMJ (Clin Res Ed) 1987; 295:297–299.

51 Kawachi I, Sparrow D, Vokonas PS, Weiss ST: Symptoms of anxiety and risk of coronary heart disease: the Normative Aging Study. Circulation 1994; 90:2225–2229.

52 Albert CM, Chae CU, Rexrode KM, Manson JE, Kawachi I: Phobic anxiety and risk of coronary heart disease and sudden cardiac death among women. Circulation 2005;111:480–487.

53 Kawachi I, Colditz GA, Ascherio A, Rimm EB, Giovannucci E, Stampfer MJ, et al: Prospective study of phobic anxiety and risk of coronary heart disease in men. Circulation 1994;89:1992–1997.

54 Watkins LL, Blumenthal JA, Davidson JR, Babyak MA, McCants CB Jr, Sketch MH Jr: Phobic anxiety, depression, and risk of ventricular arrhythmias in patients with coronary heart disease. Psychosom Med 2006;68:651–656.

55 Fleet RP, Beitman BD: Cardiovascular death from panic disorder and panic-like anxiety: a critical review of the literature. J Psychosom Res 1998;44:71–80.

56 Suls J, Bunde J: Anger, anxiety, and depression as risk factors for cardiovascular disease: the problems and implications of overlapping affective dispositions. Psychol Bull 2005;131:260–300.

57 Parker G, Hyett M, Hadzi-Pavlovic D, Brotchie H, Walsh W: GAD is good? Generalized anxiety disorder predicts a superior five-year outcome following an acute coronary syndrome. Psychiatry Res 2011; 188:383–389.

58 Kleiger RE, Miller JP, Bigger JT Jr, et al: Decreased heart rate variability and its association with increased mortality after acute myocardial infarction. Am J Cardiol 1987;59:256–262.

59 Glassman AH, O'Connor CM, Califf RM, Swedberg K, Schwartz P, Bigger JT Jr, et al: Sertraline treatment of major depression in patients with acute MI or unstable angina. JAMA 2002;288:701–709.

60 Rasmussen A, Lunde M, Poulsen DL, Sørensen K, Qvitzau S, Bech P: A double-blind, placebo-controlled study of sertraline in the prevention of depression in stroke patients. Psychosomatics 2003;44:216–221.

61 Lehnert H, Lombardi F, Raeder EA, Lorenzo AV, Verrier RL, Lown B, et al: Increased release of brain serotonin reduces vulnerability to ventricular fibrillation in the cat. J Cardiovasc Pharmacol 1987;10:389–397.

62 Miller GE, Stetler CA, Carney RM, Freedland KE, Banks WA: Clinical depression and inflammatory risk markers for coronary heart disease. Am J Cardiol 2002;90:1279–1283.

63 Pitsavos C, Panagiotakos DB, Papageorgiou C, Tsetsekou E, Soldatos C, Stefanadis C: Anxiety in relation to inflammation and coagulation markers, among healthy adults: the ATTICA study. Atherosclerosis 2006;185:320–326.

64 von Känel R, Kudielka BM, Metzenthin P, Helfricht S, Preckel D, Haeberli A, Stutz M, Fischer JE: Aspirin, but not propranolol, attenuates the acute stress-induced increase in circulating levels of interleukin-6: a randomized, double-blind, placebo-controlled study. Brain Behav Immun 2008;22:150–157.

65 Yamakawa K, Matsunaga M, Isowa T, Kimura K, Kasugai K, Yoneda M, Kaneko H, Ohira H: Transient responses of inflammatory cytokines in acute stress. Biol Psychol 2009;82:25–32.

66 Wirtz PH, Ehlert U, Emini L, Suter T: Higher body mass index (BMI) is associated with reduced glucocorticoid inhibition of inflammatory cytokine production following acute psychosocial stress in men. Psychoneuroendocrinology 2008;33:1102–1110.

67 Brydon L, Walker C, Wawrzyniak A, Whitehead D, Okamura H, Yajima J, Tsuda A, Steptoe A: Synergistic effects of psychological and immune stressors on inflammatory cytokine and sickness responses in humans. Brain Behav Immun 2009;23:217–224.

68 Dell'Osso L, Carmassi C, Palego L, Trincavelli ML, Tuscano D, Montali M, et al: Serotonin-mediated cyclic AMP inhibitory pathway in platelets of patients affected by panic disorder. Neuropsychobiology 2004;50:28–36.

69 Marcourakis T, Gorenstein C, Brandao de Almeida PE, Ramos RT, Glezer I, Bernardes CS, et al: Panic disorder patients have reduced cyclic AMP in platelets. J Psychiatr Res 2002;36:105–110.

70 Tardito D, Zanardi R, Racagni G, Manzoni T, Perez J: The protein kinase A in platelets from patients with panic disorder. Eur Neuropsychopharmacol 2002;12:483–487.

71 Schwartz UR, Walter U, Eigenthaler M: Taming platelets with cyclic nucleotides. Biochem Pharmacol 2001;62:1153–1161.

72 Butler J, O'Halloran A, Leonard BE: The Galway Study of Panic Disorder. II: Changes in some peripheral markers of noradrenergic and serotonergic function in DSM III-R panic disorder. J Affect Disord 1992;26:89–99.

73 Zafar MU, Paz-Yepes M, Shimbo D, Vilahur G, Burg MM, Chaplin W, Fuster V, Davidson KW, Badimon JJ: Anxiety is a better predictor of platelet reactivity in coronary artery disease patients than depression. Eur Heart J 2010;31:1573–1582.

74 Seldenrijk A, Vogelzangs N, van Hout HP, van Marwijk HW, Diamant M, Penninx BW: Depressive and anxiety disorders and risk of subclinical atherosclerosis. Findings from the Netherlands Study of Depression and Anxiety (NESDA). J Psychosom Res 2010;69:203–210.

Simon J.C. Davies
Geriatric Psychiatry Division, Centre for Addiction and Mental Health
Department of Psychiatry, University of Toronto
Toronto, ON M6J 1H4 (Canada)
E-Mail simon_davies@camh.net

Baldwin DS, Leonard BE (eds): Anxiety Disorders.
Mod Trends Pharmacopsychiatry. Basel, Karger, 2013, vol 29, pp 98–110 (DOI: 10.1159/000351931)

The Early Phases of Anxiety Disorders: From Prevention to Treatment

Javier Vázquez-Bourgon · Andres Herrán · José Luis Vázquez-Barquero

Department of Psychiatry, Psychiatric Research Unit of Cantabria, University Hospital Marqués de Valdecilla, IFIMAV, CIBERSAM, Santander, Spain

Abstract

The 'early intervention' model has been applied with good results to the care of a range of serious medical conditions. The key rationale for this model is to guarantee early identification and treatment for the illness, thus preventing its progression to a more advanced and severe stage. It would also provide a framework for optimal treatment according to the stage of the disorders. Although in the field of psychiatry this model has mainly been implemented in nonaffective psychosis, research evidence supports its application in other mental disorders. To promote this initiative, the chapter explores the available evidence demonstrating the feasibility of adopting the key elements of the model in the care of the whole spectrum of anxiety disorders. In addition, the chapter describes the different stages that are possible to identify in the process of developing an illness, and also the phase-specific interventions that could be applied. Finally, the service repercussions of implementing an early intervention model in anxiety disorders are discussed.

The advantages of prevention and the benefits of early diagnosis and treatment have been assumed for a long time as a major standard of medical practice. So much so that in modern health care systems this model has been successfully applied to malignant medical conditions. This has not been the case, however, in the area of mental health where psychiatric knowledge and practice have been derived from patients with well-established, often chronic, disorders. In these circumstances, the nature of the illness tends to be confounded with variables related to long-term treatment and clinical course. This has conditioned the understanding of key elements of mental disorders in general and particularly of the entire spectrum of anxiety disorders. Although the application of the early intervention model has proved to be useful in advanced medical care, it has only recently been extended to mental health, focusing mainly on psychosis [1]. As a result of this, there has been a significant emergence of early intervention services for psychosis worldwide. Despite this, there have been only limited initiatives to extend the clinical staging model to other mental disorders.

In anxiety disorders, the onset of the illness is difficult to distinguish from transient and benign psychopathological changes. The situation is even more critical when we consider their differentiation from unspecific emotional dysfunctions and from normal anxiety states. This means that the application of an early intervention model to anxiety disorders is dependent both on the differentiation of the boundaries between normal and preclinical psychological experiences, and on a more precise characterization of the different stages of the illness process. The focus of this chapter is on describing the different stages that it is possible to identify in anxiety disorders, and reviewing their early clinical manifestations. In addition, the foundations of the application of the early intervention model to these disorders are discussed.

Application of the Early Intervention Model to Anxiety Disorders

The application of the early intervention model is based on the idea that the course of a disease is likely to progress from an 'at-risk' to a prodromal state and finally to a fully developed diagnostic entity. It also implies that the disease progresses through different stages that are characterized by phase-specific clinical manifestations and treatment susceptibility. From a clinical perspective, it also assumes that the earlier stages have better prognosis, require less intensive treatments, and tend to respond better to interventions. A series of concepts are incorporated into this model, the most relevant of which are reviewed in this chapter.

New Concepts for Health Prevention

In modern health care, the focus of prevention has been extended to noninfectious and chronic diseases, including mental illness and emotional disturbances. For this, the traditional classification system for prevention, differentiating the three levels of primary, secondary and tertiary prevention has been regarded as unsatisfactory. In the early 1990s the Committee on Prevention of Mental Disorders of the Institute of Medicine (IOM) proposed a new model of preventive intervention describing the three levels of universal, selective and indicated prevention. At the universal level, prevention is focused on the general public or on a whole population group that has not been identified on the basis of individual risk. At the selective level, interventions are directed at asymptomatic populations, with a higher risk of a particular disorder. Finally, at the indicated level, preventive interventions are targeted at high-risk individuals who are identified as having minimal, but detectable, signs or symptoms foreshadowing a particular mental disorder, but who do not meet the diagnostic criteria for the disease. In these populations, defined for example by the occurrence of attenuated and/or subthreshold 'illness-specific' clinical symptoms, or by the presence of a decline in functioning and a positive family history, phase-specific interventions could be implemented to prevent or postpone the onset of a 'full-blown' disorder. The relevance of this model of prevention is due to the fact that it allows the integration into a comprehensive construct of the clinical manifestations of different stages of a particular psychiatric condition, with interventions directed at promoting mental health and preventing the illness. As exemplified in its application to anxiety disorders by Lau and Rapee [2], the new concept of indicated prevention set the basis for implementing preventive strategies in the early phases of the disease.

Predictors of Anxiety Disorders

The relative contribution of genetic and environmental factors for the development of anxiety disorders has been extensively explored. In this respect, clinical genetic studies propose a genetic contribution to the pathogenesis of anxiety disorders with a heritability of about 20–50%, suggesting that a significant degree of variance is explained by environmental factors and gene-environment interactions [3]. These findings emphasize the important role that discrete environmental factors play in the liability for anxiety psychopathology, and the relevance of interactions of candidate genes and stressful life events.

A key issue related to the inherited spectrum of factors is to determine how much personality traits and personality disorders, may contribute to the development of anxiety disorders. Bienvenue et al. [4] have shown that avoidant and dependent personality traits are predisposing factors, or at least markers of risk, for panic disorders and agoraphobia. Similarly, the presence of higher scores on neuroticism was, in combination with stressful life events, associated with an increased risk of developing a panic attack [5], an association which has been replicated in the Cantabria First Episode Study of Panic Disorders [6]. It is clear, therefore, that certain personality traits, in combination with specific environment factors, appear to contribute to the development of anxiety disorders. An additional predisposing factor for these disorders is the presence of prenatal exposure to biological and psychological maternal stress [7]. This raises the possibility that preventing or reducing the presence of maternal distress during the prenatal period may have long-term beneficial effects through diminishing the risk for developing anxiety problems in the next generation.

In addition to genetic components, considerable attention has been given to the impact that adverse experiences in early life have on the development of anxiety disorders later in life, and on the way in which these factors interact with any genetic predisposition. Evidence mainly from preclinical studies suggests that stress early in life results in persistent central corticotropin-releasing factor hyperactivity and increased stress reactivity in adulthood [8]. Thus, genetic disposition combined with early stress in critical phases of development may result in a phenotype that is neurobiologically vulnerable to stress and consequently reduces the threshold for developing an anxiety disorder under the exposure during adulthood to stress. Given this, research findings have increasingly supported the notion that certain adverse life events may be more substantive to their etiological explanations. Among these events, physical/sexual abuse and loss/separation experiences during childhood have received much research attention: the presence of childhood physical and sexual abuse constitutes an important predisposing factor for the development of anxiety disorders [9], as does the presence of loss/separation experiences in childhood [10].

Duration of Untreated Illness in Anxiety Disorders

There is increasing evidence indicating that, even in countries with sophisticated health care systems, when a person develops a particular mental disease there is usually a long period of time before it is correctly identified and receives appropriate treatment [11]. This was initially demonstrated in psychosis, where the duration of the untreated illness ranged from several weeks to many years [12]. It is now assumed that this long period of untreated illness also appears in other mental disorders, including anxiety disorders, in which although the onset of the illness usually occurs during the first three decades of life, effective treatment is typically not initiated until a number of years later [13, 14] (see chapter on Duration of Untreated Illness and Duration of Illness in Anxiety Disorders, pp. 111–118). In accordance with this, findings from research in anxiety and obsessive compulsive disorders demonstrate that the duration of untreated illness (DUI) extends for at least one year. The Cantabria First Episode of Panic Disorders Study demonstrated that for these disorders the DUI reached one year [15]. Similarly, others have demonstrated that the DUI for panic disorders reached nearly 45 months, the one for generalized anxiety disorders 87 months, and for obsessive compulsive disorders 90.6 months [16]. The relevance of this long period of untreated mental illness is based on its presumed association with a poorer outcome and treatment response, as demonstrated for psychosis and other major mental disorders [12, 17–19]. Similarly, research evidence is accumulating to support the idea that also in anxiety and obsessive compulsive disorders the presence of a long DUI is associated with a poorer outcome and reduced treatment response [15, 20, 21].

It has been postulated that in psychosis and other major mental disorders this association is due to a possible neuro-psycho-socio-toxic effect of untreated illness. Regarding anxiety disorders, despite this hypothesis being coherent with impressions derived from clinical practice, we still lack sufficient research evidence to believe unequivocally that the existence of a long delay in initiating appropriate treatment may promote the progression of an illness-related neuro-psycho-socio-toxic effect. A complementary explanation for the association between long DUI and poor outcome is derived from the 'critical period hypothesis'. This was originally formulated for psychosis, and proposes that the early phase of the illness constitutes a 'critical period' during which symptomatic and psychosocial deterioration progresses rapidly [22]. It also contends that subsequent progression of morbidity slows or stops and the level of the recovery attained, by the end of the critical period, persists into the long-term. There is increasing evidence supporting the notion that existence of a similar critical period could be postulated in major mental disorders [17, 18]. The relevance of this concept relies on the fact that it provides evidence for postulating an optimal period for neuroprotective interventions, in either the prodromal phase or early stages of the illness. Thus, it appears that there are grounds for arguing that effective early intervention procedures should be applied during this stage of maximum susceptibility to the damaging effects of illness and the neuro-psycho-socio protective effects of interventions. Whether this postulation is applicable to anxiety disorders is a pressing issue for future studies.

The Early Stages of Anxiety Disorders

A key element of the early intervention model is the operationalization of the sequence of the prediagnostic and diagnostic stages of the illness (table 1). As the different anxiety disorders do not as yet have biological markers to define these different stages, the characterization should be mainly identified by symptoms and signs. The stages may in turn correlate with prognosis and treatment, and potentially with a specific pathophysiology from which can be derived reliable and phase-specific biological markers. To guide clinicians in identifying the stages at which an individual is at a particular time, different concepts have been proposed. Although originally developed for psychosis, in recent years they have been applied, with certain adaptations, to other mental disorders, including anxiety disorders.

The 'at Risk Asymptomatic'

The first stage in the model (stage 0) is defined as a 'at risk asymptomatic' where a range of risk factors may be operating in asymptomatic persons. In the case of psychosis, several risk factors have been identified. Such is the case of family history of mental illness, substance abuse and premorbid personality traits [17]. Similarly, in patients who develop anxiety and obsessive compulsive disorders long before the illness appears, it is possible to identify a series of predisposing conditions: among them being prenatal and environmental factors and factors related to personality traits. In addition, the presence in young children of 'behavioral inhibition' (a conduct characterized by reactions of withdrawal, shyness and avoidance in novel, unfamiliar situations) and the subsequent development of anxiety disorders is well established [23]. It has also been demonstrated that children who have anxious parents or overinvolved mothers tend to develop anxiety disorders later in life [24]. The relevance of this is the fact that it can be used to identify potential candidates for early prevention and for establishing appropriate intervention targets.

Vázquez-Bourgon · Herrán · Vázquez-Barquero

Table 1. Application of the early intervention model to anxiety disorders

Stage	Clinical definition	Target population	Potential interventions
0	Increased risk of disorder No symptoms currently	Young age first-degree relatives of probands	Psychoeducation for young persons and family Promotion of health life styles Resilience training
1	Mild or nonspecific subthreshold symptoms of the disorder Could include the presence of 'ultra-high risk' syndrome (moderate but subthreshold symptoms) Mild functional (psychosocial) change or decline Mild/moderate neurocognitive deficits (GAF <70)	Screening of a risk young population Referred from: school, primary care; social welfare, and so on	Identification of early signs, and risk factors, for the illness Prevention of risk factors for transition Psychoeducation for young persons and family Promotion of health lifestyles Simple CBT skill training Problem solving
2	First episode Full threshold disorder Moderate to severe typical symptoms Functional decline (GAF: 30–50) Possible cognitive deficits	Referrals from: primary care; specialist care agencies; emergency department; welfare agencies	Pharmacological treatment Psychological treatment (CBT) Psychoeducation including: promotion of treatment adherence; relapse prevention; identification of early relapse signs
3	Incomplete remission from first episode Recurrence of relapse of the disorder Residual symptoms and/or psychosocial decline (GAF, cognition functioning, and so on) below the best level of improvement at remission from first episode	Referrals from: primary care; specialist care agencies	As in stage 2 Emphasizing on long-term pharmacological treatment Promotion and maintenance of social integration Rehabilitation of deficits
4	Failure to respond to treatment or/and severe, persistent symptoms Marked psychosocial deficits as indicated in GAF, neurocognition, functioning, and so on	Referrals from: primary care; specialist care agencies	Emphasis on long-term pharmacological treatment Maintenance of social integration Rehabilitation of deficits

Adapted from McGorry et al. [40]. GAF = Global assessment of functioning.

The Prodrome

In the process of illness development, individuals may start to exhibit a range of mild, nonspecific, subthreshold symptoms (stage 1). They have been traditionally defined as a 'prodrome' or 'precursor' of a full threshold disorder. The clinical relevance of this symptomatic, yet preclinical, stage is derived from the fact that it constitutes the earliest point at which 'indicated' preventive interventions could be implemented in order to avoid, or reduce, the transition to a full-blown disorder. This justifies the efforts that are made in applying this concept to clinical practice.

The idea that prodromal manifestations started to appear long before the onset of a disorder, or before a relapse, is in common use in medicine and has been applied to psychosis since the 1930s. Since then, its clinical use in psychosis has grown significantly in parallel with the development of early intervention services [1]. Based on the success of its application in psychosis, in recent years the extension of this concept to other psychiatric disorders, including anxiety and obsessive compulsive disorders, has been tentatively shown [15, 18, 19, 25].

However, the application of the concept of the prodrome to routine clinical practice still has its limitations. The most relevant lies in the fact that this clinical entity is mainly composed of nonspecific features, which tend to overlap from one disorder to another. For example, the data from the ABC study indicate that depression and schizophrenia shared 8 of the 11 most frequent prodromal symptoms [17], and the same may apply for the overlap of prodromal features across anxiety disorders. So much so that it may be that the prodrome should be regarded as a nonspecific precursor for the development of mental disturbances in general. In a recent conceptual paper McGorry [26] proposed the possibility that in phenotypically similar disorders there may be a 'pluri-potential prodrome' characterized by common features which at later stage may develop into one of a range of disorders, which may include psychotic disorders, bipolar disorder, unipolar depression and anxiety disorders.

The second limitation is related to the fact that the concept of prodrome can only be applied retrospectively once the person has developed an illness. This is due to the practical difficulties in detecting this clinical entity prospectively. This is a situation which is more manifest in disorders in which the criteria of 'caseness' is difficult to establish, as in anxiety disorders. In these illnesses, it would be necessary to define the boundary between the prodromal clinical stage and normal human experiences, and to distinguish this status from premorbid manifestations. It would also be essential to identify, in a reliable way, the point at which the preclinical manifestations start to meet the diagnostic criteria. In an attempt to resolve these limitations in the case of psychosis, the concept of 'ultra-high risk' was developed, incorporating a more specific operational definition. Unfortunately, even for psychosis the validity of this concept has not been fully demonstrated. Thus, although the application of the 'ultra-high-risk' concept to anxiety disorders shows promise from a clinical perspective, its clinical formulation is still at an early stage [15].

Although great advances have been made, currently recognized risk indicators for the development of the different mental diseases are not sufficiently predictive to identify persons at risk who later will develop the illness. Further progress is needed to improve the predictability of the risk criteria for mental disorders, including anxiety and obsessive-compulsive disorders. As Klosterkötter et al. [27] have suggested, we should strive to improve the risk criteria to be used by applying the strategy of: (a) risk enrichment with the inclusion of biological risk factors, and (b) stronger individualization of the risk estimation by stratification. Among the risk enrichment strategy we could, for example, expect that incorporation of brain morphological changes, genetic markers, and specific cognitive impairments may play – as Kapczinski et al. [28] have proposed for bipolar disorder – a significant role in the future. The applicability of this strategy to anxiety disorders, although at a preliminary stage, is becoming feasible in parallel to the progressive accumulation of research findings. Regarding the risk stratification approach, we could argue that in psychiatry as in other medical disciplines (such as oncology), it would be desirable to establish risk modeling strategies to define population subgroups with progressive prognostic indices of the transition to a clear diagnosis. This approach was tentatively introduced in the EPOS study in which a multivariate prognostic index, with four risk levels, was constructed for the stratification of the risk of transition to psychosis from a prodromal stage [29]. Further research is needed to explore whether such risk-enriched models could be constructed in the case of the different anxiety disorders and whether their application could result in early identification of individuals who would later develop the disorder.

The First Episode

The next stage involves a clinical focus on the period following the onset of a first episode of the disorder. It includes early detection and treatment, and the goal is to minimize the duration of the untreated mental illness. For this, specialized early intervention services and clinical programs have extensively been developed for psychosis, bipolar disorders or depression. In the case of anxiety disorders, the First Episode Panic Disorder Program developed in the University Hospital Marques de Valdecilla has demonstrated the feasibility and utility of implementing this sort of intervention program [30].

Incomplete Recovery, Relapse and Treatment Resistance after the First Episode

Stage 3 includes the first few years following the onset of the disorder. It is generally assumed that during this period the parameters for the long-term course of the disorder are established. It has also been suggested that during this phase, which tends to last between 3 and 5 years, the patient and family insight into the nature and consequences of the illness is acquired, the development of comorbidity emerges, suicide is prevented, and adherence to treatment is established. Thus, in contrast to the previous phases in which the emphasis is more on early identification and treatment, in this stage the focus is on symptom resolution, prevention of relapse, comorbidity and disability, and on potentiating social integration and treatment adherence.

Finally, stage 4 is defined as a failure to respond to treatment and the presence of severe persistent symptoms and marked psychosocial deficits. Regarding anxiety disorders, the presence of nonremitting symptoms and psychosocial deficits is due to the fact that the degree of response to current pharmacological and psychological treatment is often disappointing. As Baldwin et al. [31] have shown, the evidence for further management of patients who have not responded to initial pharmacological or psychological treatment is limited. Taking this into consideration, the consensus statement formulated by the Anxiety Disorders Research Network established as one of its main research priorities to undertake research in 'treatment-resistant' anxiety disorders [14]. The objective of this effort would be to find the most effective combinations of intensive pharmacological and psychosocial interventions. In addition, strategies directed to reduce disability and enhance social integration should also be incorporated.

Objectives of Early Intervention in Anxiety Disorders

The objectives of early intervention extend to clinical management, research and health service provision. Clinical objectives include: early detection of patients at risk, or at the initial outbreak of the illness; effective prevention of the illness in patients at risk, and optimal early treatment for those who have already presented a first episode. In addition, the prevention of relapse, comorbidities and disabilities constitutes an important clinical task. Implementation of early intervention services and programs constitutes an important complementary objective [26].

The early intervention model also provides a useful framework for research. The aims here will be directed to: (a) acquire precise information on the origin and course of illness; (b) clarify the psychosocial and biological bases of the disorders; (c) identify the predictors of transition from one stage to the other, and (d) to develop and test effective interventions for reducing the symptoms and associated disabilities of the illness, and for controlling the progression of the disease from one stage to the next. To accomplish all these objectives, the implementation of early intervention programs and services for anxiety disorders, such as the one developed in the Autonomous Community of Cantabria, has proved most useful [30].

Prevention and Intervention in the Early Stages of Anxiety Disorders

The early intervention paradigm provides a useful framework for developing, in mental health, phase-specific intervention and prevention strategies. However, in conducting intervention strategies for the early stages of anxiety disorders, a prerequisite is that individuals at risk should establish contact with mental health services. As the general population, and especially young people, tend to be reluctant to seek help for mental disorders, it is necessary to develop actions to encourage individuals at risk to access mental health services, making possible the process of early identification and treatment. For this, specific educational and help-seeking facilitative actions, at the level of general population and primary care services, need to be developed.

During the 'at risk' stage (stage 0), promotion of healthy lifestyles, resilience training and psychoeducation, for the general population, and more so for young persons, have proven to be beneficial for optimizing mental health and quality of life. The universal prevention project conducted by Dadds and Roth [32] examined the effects of a brief anxiety prevention program, based on resilience training, for preschool children: although the results were encouraging, the dropout rates were high in the intervention groups, resulting in a self-selection of families into the program. This is a common difficulty faced when conducting a universal prevention program, in which participants with no or low interference from the disorder show low levels of motivation and engagement [2]. A systematic review on the effectiveness of school-based prevention and intervention strategies for anxiety disorders conducted by Neil and Christensen [33] indicated that while universal prevention programs to date have produced mixed results, the findings of universal intervention studies were far more positive. Future developments and methodological refinements should result in an improvement of the efficacy and cost-effectiveness of the prevention and intervention strategies that could be applied in anxiety disorders.

At the prodromal stage (stage 1), the emphasis is on psychological interventions directed mainly to prevent the transition to a full threshold disorder. Great emphasis should be placed on psychoeducation for persons at risk and families, promotion of heath lifestyles and cognitive behavior therapy (CBT) skill training. More specific psychosocial interventions have also been extensively used at this stage with positive effects in anxiety disorders. Gardenswartz and Craske [34] conducted with satisfactory results an indicated prevention program for panic disorders in young students, combining psychoeducation, cognitive and behavioral interventions and exposure techniques to prevent the transition to full panic disorder. Similar positive results have been shown in other indicated prevention programs for young children at risk of developing anxiety disorders [35].

At the onset of a first episode of the disorder (stage 2), in addition to appropriate pharmacological treatment, psychological interventions in the form of psychoeducation and CBT, are usually required. Meulenbeek et al. [36] have shown that simple group interventions based on cognitive-behavioral principles were effective in the early phases of panic disorders. In addition, there is increasing evidence demonstrating that the combination of pharmacologic treatments with specific psychological interventions such as psychoeducation, self-help, or health-exercise therapies increases the treatment effectiveness in the early stages of the disorder [19, 37, 38]. In prescribing pharmacological treatments at this stage, we should be using a dosage with maximal effectiveness but minimal side effects. Finally, when combining different therapeutic strategies, we should be aiming not only at resolution of symptoms but also at the promotion of social integration and prevention of comorbidity and relapse.

Following the first episode (stages 3 and 4), the therapeutic emphasis should be on long-term pharmacological and psychosocial interventions. The objectives should focus on resolving any remaining symptoms and deficits, preventing relapses and promoting treatment adherence. For this, according to existing studies, a combination of pharmacological and psychological interventions has proved to have greater efficacy in anxiety disorders [38].

Service Repercussions of Applying the Early Intervention Model to Anxiety and Obsessive Compulsive Disorders

The application of the early intervention model in mental health should impact both the theory and practice of psychiatry. At present, neither diagnostic and evaluation systems, nor available intervention programs and health care services, are well adapted to the early phases of mental disorders. From a theoretical perspective, an early intervention model will allow investigation of the origin and nature of mental disorder without the effects of illness chronicity and secondary effects of long-term treatment. This will promote a more precise clarification of the mechanisms underlying the origin and course of the disorder. The possibility to differentiate the key biological and psychological processes underlying the origin and course of the disorder from epiphenomena, and clinical sequel, should allow a more precise understanding of the intrinsic nature of mental illness. Recent studies conducted in different mental disorders show that clinical staging might be a useful approach to achieve early diagnosis and to facilitate research into the natural course of the disorder in subjects at risk [26]. The information obtained on the way in which social and biological factors may condition the transition of the illness from one stage to another should also facilitate the development of more precise preventive interventions.

Furthermore, the new paradigm should also allow refining the present psychiatric diagnostic systems. The traditional diagnostic system is derived from a categorical delimitation of illness based on the combination of well-established psychopathological manifestations organized through syndromes and symptom dimensions. However, this conceals the nature of the different stages and 'flow' of the illness, and pays insufficient attention to the dimensions of time, sequence, severity, and repercussion which characterize the illness process. In establishing the diagnosis of a particular disease, consideration should be given to the symptom dimensions at different points of presentation, and also to the severity, persistence, and recurrence of symptomatology. A new conceptualization is needed to integrate the clinical features of the early phases of mental illness. Staging has been promoted by different authors as a course specifier for future mental illness classificatory systems, which should allow establishing a more precise classificatory system for the whole spectrum of anxiety disorders. By incorporating the new information on the classificatory system, it should be possible to develop more precise and phase-specific evaluation procedures.

From the perspective of clinical practice, this new model would also provide a framework for optimal treatment according to the stages of the disorders not only for psychosis and other major mental disorders, but also for the whole spectrum of anxiety disorders [18, 19, 25, 37]. A direct consequence of this will be to obtain more accurate information regarding the influence of risk and protective factors acting on the transition from one stage to another and the ways to intervene in this process. Delimiting discrete stages according to the natural history of the illness would facilitate the development of a prevention-orientated framework for the treatment of patients.

Finally, from a mental health service planning perspective, the early intervention model would set the theoretical basis for the reform of mental health services and for the delivery of new and more efficient phase-specific services [39]. As we have seen in the Cantabria First Episode Panic Disorder Study [30], these new services will maximize the chances of treatment engagement, continuity of care, family and social support, vocational recovery and ultimately the disappearance of stigma attached to mental illness and its treatment.

References

1 McGorry PD, Edwards J, Mihlopoulos C, Harrigan SM, Jackson HJ: EPPIC: an evolving system of early detection and optimal management. Schizoph Bull 1996;22:305–326.

2 Lau EX, Rapee RM: Prevention of anxiety disorders. Curr Psychiatry Rep 2011;13:258–266.

3 Eley TC: Bases Geneticas de los Trastornos de Ansiedad; in Vázquez-Barquero JL, Herran Gomez A (eds): Las Fases Iniciales de las Enfermedades Mentales: Trastornos de Ansiedad. Barcelona, Elsevier-Masson, 2007, chapter 8, pp 53–62.

4 Bienvenue OJ, Stein MB, Samuels JF, Onyike ChU, Eaton WW, Nestadt G: Personality disorder traits as predictors of subsequent first-onset panic disorder or agoraphobia. Compr Psychiatry 2009;50:209–214.

5 Watanabe A, Nakao K, Tokuyama M, Takeda M: Prediction of first episode of panic attack among white-collar workers. Psychiatry Clin Neurosci 2005;59:119–126.

6 Carrera-Arce M, Herran A, Ramirez ML, Ayestaran A, Sierra-Biddle D, Hoyuela-Zaton F, Rodriguez Cabo B, Vázquez-Barquero JL: Personality traits in early phase of panic disorders: implications on the presence of agorofobia, clinical severity and short-term outcome. Acta Psychiatr Scand 2006;114:417–425.

7 Davis EP, Sandman CA: Prenatal psychobiological predictors of anxiety risk in preadolescent children. Psychoneuroendocrinology 2012;37:1224–1233.

8 Heim C, Nemeroff CB: The impact of early adverse experiences on brain system involved in pathophysiology of anxiety and affective disorders. Biol Psychiatry 1999;46:1509–1522.

9 Coougle JR, Timpano KR, Sachs-Ericsson N, Keough ME, Riccardi CJ: Examining the unique relationship between anxiety disorder and childhood physical and sexual abuse in the National Comorbidity Survey-Replication. Psychiatry Res 2010;177:150–155.

10 Klauke B, Deckert J, Reif A, Pauli P, Domschke K: Life events in panic disorder an update of candidate stressors. Depress Anxiety 2010;27:716–730.

11 Kohn R, Saxena S, Levav I, Saraceno B: The treatment gap in mental health care. Bull World Health Organ 2004;11:858–866.

12 Marshall M, Harrigan S, Lewis S: Duration of untreated psychosis: definition, measurement and association with outcome; in Jackson J, McGorry, PD (eds): The Recognition and Management of Early Psychosis: A preventive Approach. Cambridge, Cambridge University Press, 2009, chapter 8, pp 125–145.

13 McGorry PD, Purcell R, Goldstone S, Amminger GP: Age of onset and timing of treatment for mental and substance use disorders: implication for preventive intervention strategies and models of care. Curr Opin Psychiatry 2011;24:301–306.

14 Baldwin DS, Allgulander CH, Altamura AC, Angst J, Bandelow B, den Boer J, Boyer P, Davies S, Dell'osso B, Eriksson E, Fineberg N, Fredrikson M, Herran A, Maron E, Metspalu A, Nutt D, van der Wee N, Vázquez-Barquero JL, Zohar J: Manifesto for a European Anxiety Disorders Research Network. Eur Neuropsychopharmacol 2010;20:426–432.

15 Vázquez-Barquero JL, Herran Gómez A: Feasibility of applying the early phase paradigm to the early phases of anxiety disorders; in Vázquez-Barquero JL, Herran Gomez A (eds): Las Fases Iniciales de las Enfermedades Mentales: Trastornos de Ansiedad. Barcelona, Elsevier-Masson, 2007, chapter 1, pp 1–7.

16 Altamura AC, Buolli M, Albano A, Dell'Osso B: Age at onset and latency to treatment (duration of untreated illness) in patients with mood and anxiety disorders: a naturalistic study. Int Clin Psychopharmacol 2010;25:172–179.

17 Häfner H, Maurer K: Podromal symptoms and early detection of schizophrenia; in Maj M, Lopez-Ibor JJ, Sartorius N, Sato M, Okasha A (eds): Early Detection and Management of Mental Disorders. Chichester, Wiley, 2005, chapter 1, pp 1–50.

18 Vieta E, Reinares M, Rosa AR: Staging bipolar disorder. Neurotox Res 2011;19:279–285.

19 Hetrick SE, Parker AG, Hickie IB, Purcell R, Yung AR, McGorry PD: Early identification and intervention in depressive disorder: towards a clinical staging model. Psychother Psychosom 2008;77:263–270.

20 Dell'Osso B, Buolli M, Hollander E, Altamura AC: Duration of untreated illness as a predictor of treatment response and remission in obsessive-compulsive disorder. World J Biol Psychiatry 2010;11:59–65.

21 Altamura AC, Dell'Osso B, DÜrso N, Russo M, Fumagalli S, Mundo E: Duration of untreated illness as a predictor of treatment response and clinical course in general anxiety disorder. CNS Spectr 2008;13:415–422.

22 Birchwood M, Fowler D, Jackson C: Early intervention in psychosis. The critical period hypothesis. Br J Psychiatry Suppl 1998;172:53–59.

23 Chronis-Tuscano A, Degnan KA, Pine DS, Perez-Edagard K, Henderson HA: Stable early maternal report of behavioral inhibition predicts lifetime social anxiety disorders in adolescence. J Am Acad Child Psychiatry 2009;48:928–935.

24 McLeod BD, Wood JJ, Weisz JR: Examining the association between parenting and childhood anxiety: a meta-analysis. Clin Psychol Rev 2007;27:155–172.

25 Kapczinski F, Vasco D, Kauer-Sant'Anna M, Frey BN, Grassi-Oliveira R, Colom B, Berk M: Clinical implications of a staging model for bipolar disorders. Expert Rev Neurother 2009a;9:957–966.

26 McGorry PD: Staging in neuropsychiatry: a heuristic model for understanding, prevention and treatment. Neurotox Res 2010;18:244–255.

27 Klosterkötter J, Schultze-Lutter F, Bechdolf A, Ruhrmann S: Prediction and prevention of schizophrenia: what has been achieved and where go next. World Psychiatry 2011;10:165–174.

28 Kapczinski F, Dias VV, Kauer-Sant'Anna M, Frey BN, Grassi-Oliveira R, Colom B, Berk M: The potential use of biomarkers as an adjunctive tool for staging bipolar disorders. Prog Neuropsychopharmacol 2009;33:1366–1371.

29 Ruhrmann S, Schultze-Lutter F, Salokangas RK, et al: Prediction of psychosis in adolescents and young adults at high risk: results from the prospective European Prediction of Psychosis Study (EPOS). Arch Gen Psychiatry 2010;67:241–251.

30 Herran-Gomez A, Ramirez ML, Ayestaran A, Hoyuela F, Carrera-Arce M, Sierra-Bidle D, Vázquez-Barquero JL: El programa de fases tempranas del trastorno de angustia del Hospital Universitario Marques de Valdecilla; in Vázquez-Barquero JL, Herran Gomez A (eds): Las Fases Iniciales de las Enfermedades Mentales: Trastornos de Ansiedad. Barcelona, Elsevier-Masson, 2007, chapter 21, pp 181–187.

31 Baldwin DS, Anderson IM, Nutt DJ, Bandelow B, Bond A, Davidson JR, den Boer JA, Fineberg NA, Knapp M, Scott J, Wittchen HU, British Association for Psychopharmacology: Evidence-based guidelines for the pharmacological treatment of anxiety disorders: recommendations from the British Association for Psychopharmacology. J Psychopharmacol 2005;19:567–596.

32 Dadds M, Roth J: Prevention of anxiety disorders: results of a universal trial with young children. J Child Fam Stud 2008;17:320–335.

33 Neil AL, Christensen H: Efficacy and effectiveness of school-based prevention and intervention programs for anxiety. Clin Psychol Rev 2009;29:208–215.

34 Gardenswartz CA, Craske MG: Prevention of panic disorder. Behav Ther 2001;32:725–737.

35 Balle M, Tortella-Feliu M: Efficacy of a brief school-based program for selective prevention of childhood anxiety. Anxiety Stress Coping 2010;23:71–85.

36 Meulenbeek P, Willemse G, Smit F, van Balkom A, Spinhoven Ph, Cuijpers P: Early intervention in panic: pragmatic randomised controlled trial. Br J Psychiatry 2010;196:326–331.

37 Carrera-Arce M, Hoyuela F, Rodriguez-Cabo B: Tratamiento psicológico en las fases tempranas del trastorno de Angustia; in Vázquez-Barquero JL, Herran Gomez A (eds): Las Fases Iniciales de las Enfermedades Mentales: Trastornos de Ansiedad. Barcelona, Elsevier-Masson, 2007, chapter 15, pp 125–131.

38 Bandelow B, Seidler-Brandler U, Becker A, Wedekind D, Rüther E: Meta-analysis of randomized and controlled comparisons of psychopharmacological and psychological treatments of anxiety disorders. World J Biol Psychiatry 2007;8:175–187.

39 McGorry PD: Evidence based reform of mental health care. BMJ 2005;331:586–587.

40 McGorry PD, Hickie IB, Yung AR, Pantelis C, Jackson HJ: Clinical staging of psychiatric disorders: a heuristic framework for choosing earlier, safer and more effective interventions. Aust N Z J Psychiatry 2006;40:616–622.

Dr. Javier Vázquez-Bourgon
Department of Psychiatry, Psychiatric Research Unit of Cantabria
University Hospital Marqués de Valdecilla
Av. Valdecilla s/n, ES– 39008 Santander (Spain)
E-Mail javazquez@humv.es

Baldwin DS, Leonard BE (eds): Anxiety Disorders.
Mod Trends Pharmacopsychiatry. Basel, Karger, 2013, vol 29, pp 111–118 (DOI: 10.1159/000351950)

Duration of Untreated Illness and Duration of Illness in Anxiety Disorders: Assessment and Influence on Outcome

A. Carlo Altamura · Giulia Camuri · Bernardo Dell'Osso

Department of Psychiatry, University of Milan, Fondazione IRCCS Ca' Granda, Ospedale Maggiore Policlinico, Milan, Italy

Abstract

Anxiety disorders are disabling and generally chronic conditions, with a lifetime prevalence of 15–20% in the general population. These disorders are usually associated with early onset and often remain untreated for several years with important consequences on patients' functioning and quality of life. From this perspective, recent literature has considered duration of illness (DI) and duration of untreated illness (DUI), two important variables influencing outcome in many psychiatric conditions including anxiety disorders. The DUI has been defined as the interval between the onset of a specific psychiatric disorder and the subsequent administration of the first adequate pharmacological treatment given at standard dosages and for an adequate period of time in compliant subjects. The DI can be defined as the time elapsing between the onset of a psychiatric disorder and the recovery from the illness. The two variables are likely interrelated, with a longer DUI being a major contributor to a longer DI. A significant body of evidence has shown that prolonged DI and DUI are associated with structural and functional brain abnormalities as well as with poor treatment response, particularly in schizophrenia. More recently, an increasing number of studies have been pointing toward a similar conclusion in affective disorders. As a consequence, the assessment of the latency to treatment (DUI) may represent one of the first steps in order to plan early interventions and reduce the overall DI. The present chapter highlights the role of the DI and latency to treatment in anxiety disorders, focusing on epidemiologic, neuropathological, clinical and prognostic issues.

Anxiety Disorders, Duration of Untreated Illness and Duration of Illness

Anxiety disorders are the most common mental disorders in the general population and are characterized by the presence of impairing anxiety symptoms that vary widely in terms of nature, severity, frequency, persistence and consequences. Anxiety disorders have a similar degree of disability compared to depressive disorders [1] and, therefore, they represent an important public health problem. However, many patients with anxiety disorders do not present to health care systems and/or are not recognized, and the standard of care they receive is often inadequate. As a consequence, they often wait for many years before receiving a proper diagnosis and an adequate pharmacological treatment. From this perspective, it is noteworthy to stress that many patients affected by anxiety disorders often receive benzodiazepines as first pharmacological treatment. However, these should not be considered as adequate treatment when estimating the duration of untreated illness (DUI), being not recommended as monotherapy, particularly in the long-term, in any major treatment guidelines. Recognizing the first adequate treatment for a given anxiety disorder, therefore, represents the first step for correctly computing the real DUI. In fact, according to recent international guidelines [2], selective serotonin reuptake inhibitors (SSRIs) and serotonin-norepinephrine reuptake inhibitors (SNRIs) represent the first-line medication for panic disorder (PD), while tricyclic antidepressants (TCAs) should be considered in cases of non-response. Adequate treatments for generalized anxiety disorder (GAD) comprise SSRIs, SNRIs, TCAs (as second-line treatments), as well as the calcium channel modulator pregabalin, low dosages of atypical antipsychotics (quetiapine) and antihistaminic molecules (hydroxyzine). Obsessive-compulsive disorder (OCD) treatment requires serotonin reuptake inhibitors (SRIs) given at high dosages for a consistent period of time and some patients may also benefit from a low dose of antipsychotic augmentation. SSRIs and venlafaxine are considered as first-line drugs in social phobia (SP). Finally, with respect to posttraumatic stress disorders, SSRIs represent the first-line therapy, and other treatment options include TCAs and the monoamine oxidase inhibitor phenelzine.

From a biological point of view, alterations of different neurotransmitter systems, in particular the noradrenergic, serotoninergic and GABAergic systems, have been involved in the pathogenesis of anxiety disorders. Neuroimaging studies have better clarified the role of different brain areas in the pathogenesis of anxiety showing that the amygdala, the hippocampus and the prefrontal cortex are the most involved areas.

Even though the literature about the role of the DUI in mood and anxiety disorders is less robust when compared to schizophrenia and other psychotic disorders, clinical studies have reported a negative influence over outcome for longer DUI in these conditions as well. It can be hypothesized that chronic untreated anxiety might be responsible for negative sociodemographic consequences, such as greater medical burden, being without a partner, or employment, as well as other socioeconomic disadvantages with negative influence on the long-term course of the illness [3].

Different reasons encourage the study of the latency to treatments in anxiety disorders. These conditions are common, disabling and frequently have an early onset and chronic course, with a negative influence on patients' social and professional functioning. Moreover, these disorders may frequently remain undiagnosed/underdiagnosed and untreated/undertreated with dramatic consequences for this unserved/underserved population. Therefore, assessing the phenomenon of the latency to treat-

Altamura · Camuri · Dell'Osso

ment provides extremely interesting epidemiologic information about major contributors to delayed diagnosis and treatment, the nature of first contact, etc. Finally, the study of the latency to treatment may contribute to better elucidate the pathophysiology and the neurobiological modifications occurring with the progression of illness [4]. Hence, in recent years, the relationship between a prolonged DUI and outcome has also been investigated in the field of affective disorders: in relation to anxiety disorders, specific studies have been conducted in patients affected by SP, PD, GAD and OCD (see chapter on The Early Phases of Anxiety Disorders, pp. 98–110).

Duration of Untreated Illness

The DUI has been defined as the interval between the onset of a specific psychiatric disorder and the subsequent administration of the first pharmacological treatment given at standard dosages and for an adequate period of time in compliant subjects [5]. Practically, the DUI is computed by subtracting the age at onset of a given disorder from the age at first treatment.

Over the last two decades, the DUI has been increasingly investigated as a potential predictor of clinical outcome and course across different psychiatric disorders, particularly in the field of schizophrenia and first-episode psychosis [4]. Converging evidence suggests that a longer DUI is associated with a worse outcome [5]. Most published studies on this topic have focused on the role of the DUI in schizophrenia and other psychotic disorders (duration of untreated psychosis or DUP), documenting a relationship between a long DUP and more severe positive, negative and cognitive symptoms, as well as a greater number of suicide attempts and a higher number of recurrences [6].

Some factors, however, complicate the study of the DUI/DUP. There is no uniform consensus on how to define these variables when looking for associations in relation to outcome and they may be considered either as categorical/dichotomous (i.e. ≤ or >1 year) or continuous variables. In both perspectives, there is a need to define proper threshold values and to define long versus short DUP/DUI [7]. In the case of schizophrenia and psychotic disorders, in general, the term DUI is frequently replaced with DUP, which refers to the time elapsing between the onset of psychotic symptoms and the administration of the first antipsychotic treatment. However, the concept of DUI seems to be more reliable and comprehensive given that psychotic symptoms might not be the first manifestation of a psychotic syndrome (e.g. the first appearance of negative symptoms). Therefore, an investigation that goes beyond psychotic symptoms and incorporates prodromal manifestations that are influenced by the interplay of many individual, familiar and psychosocial factors (such as secretiveness of the illness, parental attitudes, social stigma, treatment related side effects, compliance, etc…), mental health care systems (such as presence and quality of psychiatric services, time to access to first psychiatric visits, secondary care clinicians' versus primary care physicians' ability to make the correct diagnosis and administer an approved treatment) as well as intrinsic features of the disorder (such as an insidious onset, or waning and waxing course) seems to be more accurate and reliable [8]. Certainly, if a biological process – such as progressive neurodegeneration – is traditionally represented as the rationale for the investigation of the DUI/DUP in psychotic disorders in relation to outcome, some differences may also exist in the field of anxiety disorders in relation to latency to treatments. For example, the persistence of untreated anxiety may exert different actions at different time on biological systems. On the other hand, an epidemiologic approach to the field of untreated illness exploring differences in the average time for help seeking, treatment and diagnosis delay contributors may be of even more interest across different anxiety disorders.

Duration of Illness

The duration of illness (DI) can be defined as the time elapsing between the onset of a psychiatric disorder, according to the diagnostic criteria, and the recovery from the illness. Several studies have reported a negative effect of early onset and long DI in terms of outcome across psychiatric disorders [9]. In light of the usual early onset of most psychiatric conditions and their recurring/chronic nature, the concept of DI as a measurable variable affecting outcome is of great clinical interest. For instance, brain imaging studies have shown that prolonged DI in schizophrenia is associated with neurobiological modifications, such as decreased prefrontal grey matter, bilateral insular cortex and temporal lobe [10].

A similar relationship between DI and outcome has been put forward in affective disorders as well, but the association between neurodegenerative changes and DI in patients with mood or anxiety disorders is still debated. In this perspective, a loss of left putaminal gray matter volume has been observed in patients with PD and long DI [11]. Furthermore, DI in patients with OCD has been negatively correlated with hippocampus and amygdala volumes [12], but not with caudate nucleus volume [13].

With respect to outcome, different studies conducted on PD have shown a close relationship between DI and long-term course. In particular, a prolonged DI before the first psychiatric consultation seemed to be a predictor of poor social outcome [14, 15].

Preliminary data indicate a close association between DI and treatment response in anxiety disorders: the longer the DI, the lower level of response to pharmacological treatment is expected. From this perspective, a relationship between early onset, long DI and poor outcome has been found in OCD patients [16]. The majority of patients affected by this condition have an early onset of symptoms and a continuous and chronic course, which are generally related to partial/poor response to standard pharmacological treatments; as many as half of these patients do not fully respond to first-line medications [17]. All these variables – early onset, poor pharmacological response, continuous/chronic course of illness – appear to be related to the DI and seem to be in a relationship of continuous reciprocity and implication rather than in a hierarchical disposition.

The main findings linking a longer DI with a worse outcome in the different anxiety disorders can be summarized as follows. An interesting relationship between PD and OCD has recently been found [18]. In view of a reported association between late-onset OCD and a higher presence of associated panic attacks after the onset of OCD, it could be argued that the presence of panic attacks or PD would delay the onset of OCD and decrease the latency for seeking help and the administration of an effective treatment, resulting in a reduction of the overall DI.

In a naturalistic trial conducted on patients affected by PD, those with a long DI achieved treatment response with higher doses of imipramine in comparison with patients with a short DI [19]. Data from three placebo-controlled multicenter trials showed that DI was a predictor of treatment response also in patients affected by SP [20]. On the other hand, a more recent study did not find a correlation between DI and treatment response in social phobia [21]. Two multicenter double-blind studies conducted on OCD patients have found that response to clomipramine was associated with a short DI [22]; moreover, a short DI seemed to predict early response to antidepressants in OCD patients [23]. GAD is generally considered to follow a chronic course, with fluctuating severity and deteriorations during periods of stress. A preliminary report found that response to venlafaxine was associated with a shorter DI in a sample of 32 GAD patients [24].

Duration of Untreated Illness, Epidemiology and Clinical Outcome in Anxiety Disorders

A naturalistic study was conducted in order to explore the relationship between DUI and outcome in a sample of 96 outpatients with PD who, after receiving an 8-week antidepressant treatment, were divided into 2 subgroups on the basis of a DUI ≤1 or >1 year. Patients with a longer DUI had a higher frequency of comorbid depression with later onset, suggesting that longer DUI may be a predictor of the subsequent development of comorbid depression in PD [25].

With respect to GAD, a study was conducted to assess the influence of the DUI on treatment response and clinical course. The sample included 100 patients treated with SSRIs/venlafaxine for 8 weeks and then subdivided into 2 groups according to DUI (≤ or >1 year): patients with a longer DUI presented an earlier age at onset, a longer DI and a higher rate of comorbidity with onset later than GAD [26].

More recently, a naturalistic study evaluated the influence of the latency to treatment on response and remission rates in a sample of 66 outpatients with OCD who received an open pharmacological treatment for 12 weeks. The sample was divided into 2 groups according to a cutoff for the DUI of 2 years. Results showed that a DUI

<2 years was predictive of a higher rate of treatment response [27]. It is worthwhile to mention that in the majority of the reported studies, a longer DUI was associated with a longer DI suggesting that, understandably, the two variables are strictly interrelated.

Moving from the clinical to an epidemiological viewpoint, a recent study investigated and compared demographic and clinical features in patients with different affective disorders, focusing on age at onset, age at first adequate pharmacological treatment and, ultimately, DUI. The study sample included 729 outpatients affected by major depressive disorder (n = 181), bipolar disorder types I (n = 115) and II (n = 186), GAD (n = 100), PD (n = 96), and OCD (n = 51). With respect to anxiety disorders, patients with PD presented the shortest DUI (44.35 months), whereas patients with OCD showed the longest one (90.57 months). These findings suggest that differences in terms of latency to treatment among diagnostic groups potentially reflect different reasons influencing treatment delay which may be, in general, quantified in years of untreated illness [3]. Another recent article conducted with the same approach in patients with PD, GAD or OCD substantially confirmed the aforementioned values for the DUI in each condition [28].

With respect to SP, there is only one study that examined the cause of delays in reaching primary care and specialist services amongst patients with anxiety disorders (GAD, PD, SP); finding that SP patients had the longest delay (>9 years) when compared with the others [29].

Different hypotheses have been put forward in order to explain the relatively minor DUI in PD, such as the presence of acute and disabling physical symptoms characteristic of panic attacks and the more frequent access to the emergency rooms. By contrast, the longer DUI observed in patients affected by OCD may be explained on the basis of its insidious onset, secretiveness and embarrassment as well as the specific subtypes of the illness. Moreover, some forms of OCD are associated with poor insight, which contributes to delayed diagnosis and treatment.

With respect to GAD, both cited studies have shown the presence of a long DUI (approximately 7 years), though slightly shorter than that observed in OCD. This result may be partially explained by the insidious onset and the gradual impairment of patients' functioning associated with this condition which typically only receives attention after many years.

Conclusion

Anxiety disorders represent an important public health problem. Despite the size, burden and costs of these conditions, many patients remain undiagnosed or undertreated, the standard of care they receive is usually suboptimal and the effectiveness of psychological and pharmacological treatment interventions in clinical practice may be disappointing. Converging evidence suggests that anxiety disorders frequently have an early onset, long DI and long latency to pharmacological treatment. Even though reported studies do not permit definitive conclusions about the relationship between DUI, DI and outcome in anxiety disorders, it can be hypothesized that chronic untreated anxiety reduces quality of life and negatively influences the long-term course of the illness. The majority of patients with anxiety disorders first present to their general practitioner and frequently remain undertreated.

From this perspective it is important to sensitize medical awareness of adequate pharmacological treatment for these conditions. In light of these preliminary data, further investigation in the field is needed in order to better elucidate the nature of this relationship and to better address prevention or early intervention programs [30]. Given that DUI is a potentially modifiable prognostic factor, likely influencing the overall DI, the assessment of the latency to treatment is one of the first steps to introduce early interventions and ameliorate outcome in many aspects [30]. From this perspective, early-onset treatments are aimed at delaying or preventing the onset of the disorder in people with prodromal symptoms and providing effective treatment in the early stages of the disorder. To date, only few studies have evaluated the effect of early interventions in anxiety and mood disorders, mostly in the field of cognitive behavioral therapy, and similar investigations are needed in relation to other treatment approaches.

References

1 Wittchen HU, Jacobi F: Size and burden of mental disorders in Europe – a critical review and appraisal of 27 studies. Eur Neuropsychopharmacol 2005;15: 357–376.

2 Bandelow B, Zohar J, Hollander E, Kasper S, Möller HJ; WFSBP Task Force on Treatment Guidelines for Anxiety, Obsessive-Compulsive and Post-Traumatic Stress Disorders, Zohar J, Hollander E, Kasper S, Möller HJ, Bandelow B, Allgulander C, Ayuso-Gutierrez J, Baldwin DS, Buenvicius R, Cassano G, Fineberg N, Gabriels L, Hindmarch I, Kaiya H, Klein DF, Lader M, Lecrubier Y, Lépine JP, Liebowitz MR, Lopez-Ibor JJ, Marazziti D, Miguel EC, Oh KS, Preter M, Rupprecht R, Sato M, Starcevic V, Stein DJ, van Ameringen M, Vega J: World Federation of Societies of Biological Psychiatry (WFSBP) guidelines for the pharmacological treatment of anxiety, obsessive-compulsive and post-traumatic stress disorders – first revision. World J Biol Psychiatry 2008;9:248–312.

3 Altamura AC, Buoli M, Albano A, Dell'osso B: Age at onset and latency to treatment (duration of untreated illness) in patients with mood and anxiety disorders: a naturalistic study. Int Clin Psychopharmacol 2010;25:172–179.

4 Altamura AC, Bassetti R, Sassella F, Salvatori D, Mundo D: Duration of untreated psychosis as a predictor of outcome in first-episode schizophrenia: a retrospective study. Schizophr Res 2001;52:29–36.

5 Dell'osso B, Altamura AC: Duration of untreated psychosis and duration of untreated illness: new vistas. CNS Spectr 2010;15:238–246.

6 Barnes TR, Leeson VC, Mutsatsa SH, Watt HC, Hutton SB, Joyce EM: Duration of untreated psychosis and social function: 1-year follow-up study of first-episode schizophrenia. Br J Psychiatry 2008;193: 203–209.

7 Barnes TR, Hutton SB, Chapman MJ, Mutsatsa S, Puri BK, Joyce EM: West London first-episode study in schizophrenia. Clinical correlates of duration of untreated psychosis. Br J Psychiatry 2000;177:207–211.

8 Singh SP: Outcome measures in early psychosis; relevance of duration of untreated psychosis. Br J Psychiatry 2007;50:58–63.

9 Altamura AC, Buoli M, Serati M: Duration of illness and duration of untreated illness in relation to drug response in psychiatric disorders. Neuropsychiatry 2011;1:81–90.

10 Velakoulis D, Wood SJ, Smith DJ, Soulsby B, Brewer W, Leeton L, Desmond P, Suckling J, Bullmore ET, McGuire PK, Pantelis C: Increased duration of illness is associated with reduced volume in right medial temporal/anterior cingulate grey matter in patients with chronic schizophrenia. Schizophr Res 2002;57:43–49.

11 Yoo HK, Kim MJ, Kim SJ, Sung YH, Sim ME, Lee YS, Song SY, Kee BS, Lyoo IK: Putaminal gray matter volume decrease in panic disorder: an optimized voxel-based morphometry study. Eur J Neurosci 2005;22:2089–2094.

12 Atmaca M, Yildirim H, Ozdemir H, Ozler S, Kara B, Ozler Z, Kanmaz E, Mermi O, Tezcan E: Hippocampus and amygdalar volumes in patients with refractory obsessive-compulsive disorder. Prog Neuropsychopharmacol Biol Psychiatry 2008;32:1283–1286.

13 Robinson D, Wu H, Munne RA, Ashtari M, Alvir JM, Lerner G, Koreen A, Cole K, Bogerts B: Reduced caudate nucleus volume in obsessive-compulsive disorder. Arch Gen Psychiatry 1995;52:393–398.

14 Shinoda N, Kodama K, Sakamoto T, Yamanouchi N, Takahashi T, Okada S, Noda S, Komatsu N, Sato T: Predictors of 1-year outcome for patients with panic disorder. Compr Psychiatry 1999;40:39–43.

15 Noyes R Jr, Clancy J, Hoenk PR, Slymen DJ: The prognosis of anxiety neurosis. Arch Gen Psychiatry 1980;37:173–178.

16 Stewart SE, Geller DA, Jenike M, Paulus D, Shaw D, Mullin B, Faraone SV: Long-term outcome of pediatric obsessive-compulsive disorder: a meta-analysis and qualitative review of the literature. Acta Psychiatr Scand 2004;110:4–13.

17 Baldwin DS, Allgulander C, Altamura AC, Angst J, Bandelow B, den Boer J, Boyer P, Davies S, Dell'osso B, Eriksson E, Fineberg N, Fredrikson M, Herran A, Maron E, Metspalu A, Nutt D, van der Wee N, Vázquez-Barquero JL, Zohar J: Manifesto for a European anxiety disorders research network. Eur Neuropsychopharmacol 2010;20:426–432.

18 Lensi P, Cassano GB, Correddu G, Ravagli S, Kunovac JL, Akiskal HS: Obsessive-compulsive disorder. Familial-developmental history, symptomatology, comorbidity and course with special reference to gender-related differences. Br J Psychiatry 1996;169:101–107.

19 Marchesi C, Ampollini P, Signifredi R, Maggini C: The treatment of panic disorder in a clinical setting: a 12-month naturalistic study. Neuropsychobiology 1997;36:25–31.

20 Stein DJ, Stein MB, Pitts CD, Kumar R, Hunter B: Predictors of response to pharmacotherapy in social anxiety disorder: an analysis of 3 placebo-controlled paroxetine trials. J Clin Psychiatry 2002;63:152–155.

21 Van Ameringen M, Oakman J, Mancini C, Pipe B, Chung H: Predictors of response in generalized social phobia: effect of age of onset. J Clin Psychopharmacol 2004;24:42–48.

22 DeVeaugh-Geiss J, Katz R, Landau P, Goodman W, Rasmussen S: Clinical predictors of treatment response in obsessive compulsive disorder: exploratory analyses from multicenter trials of clomipramine. Psychopharmacol Bull 1990;26:54–59.

23 Ravizza L, Barzega G, Bellino S, Bogetto F, Maina G: Predictors of drug treatment response in obsessive-compulsive disorder. J Clin Psychiatry 1995;56:368–373.

24 Perugi G, Frare F, Toni C, Ruffolo G, Torti C: Open-label evaluation of venlafaxine sustained release in outpatients with generalized anxiety disorder with comorbid major depression or dysthymia: effectiveness, tolerability and predictors of response. Neuropsychobiology 2002;46:145–149.

25 Altamura AC, Santini A, Salvadori D, Mundo E: Duration of untreated illness in panic disorder: a poor outcome risk factor? Neuropsychiatr Dis Treat 2005;1:345–347.

26 Altamura AC, Dell'Osso B, D'Urso N, Russo M, Fumagalli S, Mundo E: Duration of untreated illness as a predictor of treatment response and clinical course in generalized anxiety disorder. CNS Spectr 2008;13:415–422.

27 Dell'Osso B, Buoli M, Hollander E, Altamura AC: Duration of untreated illness as a predictor of treatment response and remission in obsessive-compulsive disorder. World J Biol Psychiatry 2010;11:59–65.

28 Camuri G, Dell'Osso B, Buoli M, Lietti L, Oldani L, Benatti B, Catenacci E, Bressi C, Altamura AC: Differenze nella durata di malattia non trattata in pazienti con disturbo di panico, disturbo d'ansia generalizzato e disturbo ossessivo compulsivo (poster); in XVII Congresso Nazionale della Società Italiana di Neuropsicofarmacologia, Cagliari, September 2010.

29 Wagner R, Silove D, Marnane C, Rouen D: Delays in referral of patients with social phobia, panic disorder and generalized anxiety disorder attending a specialist anxiety clinic. J Anxiety Disord 2006;20:363–371.

30 Christensen H, Pallister E, Smale S, Hickie IB, Calear AL: Community-based prevention programs for anxiety and depression in youth: a systematic review. J Prim Prev 2010;31:139–170.

Prof. A. Carlo Altamura
Department of Psychiatry, University of Milan
Fondazione IRCCS Ca' Granda, Ospedale Maggiore Policlinico
Via Francesco Sforza 35, IT–20122 Milan (Italy)
E-Mail carlo.altamura@unimi.it

Baldwin DS, Leonard BE (eds): Anxiety Disorders.
Mod Trends Pharmacopsychiatry. Basel, Karger, 2013, vol 29, pp 119–127 (DOI: 10.1159/000351955)

Pharmacotherapy of Generalized Anxiety Disorder

Christer Allgulander[a] · David S. Baldwin[b, c]

[a] Section of Psychiatry, Department of Clinical Neuroscience, Karolinska Institutet, Stockholm, Sweden;
[b] University Department of Psychiatry, University of Southampton, Southampton, UK; [c] Department of
Psychiatry and Mental Health, University of Cape Town, Cape Town, South Africa

Abstract

Generalized anxiety disorder (GAD) is chiefly characterized by a cognitive focus on threats and risks towards the individual and/or the immediate family. It is accompanied by a sense of tension, worry, muscle pain, disturbed sleep and irritability. The condition impairs work capacity, relations, and leisure activities, and aggravates concurrent somatic diseases. Due to its chronic course, GAD increases costs for the individual, the family, and health care services, and reduces work and educational performance. In cardiovascular or cerebrovascular disease, pulmonary disease, diabetes and neurological diseases, GAD is a risk factor for somatic complications and for lowered adherence to somatic treatments. There is evidence that GAD can be treated with cognitive behavioural therapy (CBT), and/or with medications. First-line pharmacotherapies are selective serotonin reuptake inhibitors (SSRIs), serotonin-norepinephrine reuptake inhibitors (SNRIs) and pregabalin. If such therapies fail, one may reconsider the diagnosis, question adherence with the prescribed schedule, and determine the adverse influence of comorbidity (such as depression, substance use, and physical ill-health) as well as the influence of social stressors. Second-line pharmacotherapies are largely not supported by controlled trials, and so leave much to clinical judgment and careful monitoring. One may attempt treatments with benzodiazepine anxiolytics, with quetiapine, or with pregabalin as an adjunct therapy in patients with partial response to SSRI or SNRI treatment. CBT is a valid alternative to pharmacotherapy, depending on patient preference. Copyright © 2013 S. Karger AG, Basel

Clinical Characteristics

Cognition in generalized anxiety is adversely biased towards presumed prospective and potential threats to the individual or the family. Trivially this is called 'worrying', such as in the Penn State Worry Questionnaire, or intolerance of uncertainty, the preferred term in cognition research, or apprehensive expectation as in DSM-IV. Primarily, persons with generalized anxiety disorder (GAD) seek treatment by practitioners *not* for worrying, but instead for symptoms such as poor sleep, muscle tension, dyspepsia, restlessness, fatigue, and irritability. The basic cognitive dysfunction, when paired with secondary somatic anxiety symptoms, impairs the capacity for work, upsets relations, and reduces leisure activities. GAD increases the risk for subsequent depressive episodes, for self-medicating with alcohol, and for complications in concurrent somatic diseases.

GAD patients tend to get caught in distorted risk assessment concerning health, security, and welfare of the individual and next of kin. This bias towards anticipated untoward future events is different from the cognitive dysfunction seen in depression, which mainly focuses on past failures and mistakes, causing ruminations, a sense of guilt and feelings of worthlessness. The cognitive bias seen in GAD also differs from that in obsessive-compulsive disorder that is chiefly concerned with symmetry, contamination, and ambivalence in moral issues.

GAD patients worry prospectively about hazards: *what if* our business goes bankrupt, *what if* our daughter is run over on her way from day care, *what if* we get robbed on our summer trip or we have an accident far away from home. Workmates and family members testify that a person with GAD exaggerates concerns over potential events in ordinary life, that the person is a 'born worrier'.

Imaging of the amygdala and associated neuronal circuits shows an enhanced base activity, as well as an increased reactivity to stimuli, interpreted as deficits in emotional processing of which the individual is unaware [1–3]. In a pilot study, medication reduced this excessive state of alertness parallel to a reduction in reported anxiety symptoms [1]. The reduction in sympathetic activity that occurs normally during night-time remained high in a laboratory study of GAD patients [4]. Inhaling air enriched with carbon dioxide resulted in anxiety symptoms and activation in GAD patients [5, 6].

Among psychological theories regarding the cause and maintenance of worry, Borkovec and Roemer [7] hypothesize that the function of worry is to avoid, thereby causing ineffective problem solving. Accordingly, worry about imagined events suppresses negative thoughts and images and strengthens avoidance behaviour. Another theory stresses the concept of intolerance of uncertainty, with worry being caused by not trusting information [8]. Thirdly, there is meta-cognition, by which worrying prevents catastrophes [9]. There is extensive research into how GAD patients manage information by cognitive schemata and selective bias towards threats [10]. A prospective study of Dutch teenagers provided support for the notion that worry is a trait rather than a state condition [11].

Prevalence of Generalized Anxiety Disorder in Population Samples and in Primary Care

European and US prevalence studies show similar rates of GAD in the adult population. A representative sample of Swedes aged 55–74 years was interviewed about GAD symptomatology [12]. The lifetime risk of GAD was estimated to be 3.95% in women, and 1.74% in men. The genetic contribution was 27%, and individual environmental factors 72%: only 1% was accounted for by shared environment, such as parenting. A British population study found that 3% of those interviewed had GAD by ICD-10 criteria, though only 8% of those diagnosed were undergoing treatment with medications or psychotherapy [13].

Turning to GAD in health care settings, Ansseau et al. [14] found that 8.3% of a sample of patients in primary care in Belgium in 2001 had a diagnosis of GAD according to DSM-IV criteria. Additional patients had comorbid major depression, and only a minority received proper pharmacotherapy. The chances of identifying the disorder are influenced by comorbidity. Secondary depression is common in GAD, as shown in prospective and longitudinal studies [15]. This is usually the time when a GAD patient first seeks help, after several years of trying to cope with worrying and mounting adverse social consequences. General practitioners more easily recognize GAD patients who appear with secondary depression, and are more likely to institute treatment in that group [16, 17]. On a typical working day in 2001, 648 general practitioners in Sweden and their patients participated in a comprehensive survey to identify cases of GAD in primary care [18]. The age-standardized rate of GAD was 4.1–6.0% among men, and 3.7–7.1% among women.

Cultural aspects influence the symptomatology of anxiety disorders, with a shift towards somatizing in Asians, sometimes called 'distress syndromes' [19, 20]. Illness attribution and illness presentations need to be considered when treating patients in their own ethnic environment or in those who migrate to western society. The pharmacodynamics and pharmacokinetics of medications for GAD, usually assessed in western populations, may also be influenced by pharmacogenetic factors [21, 22].

Somatic Comorbidity

The course of neurological, cardiovascular, pulmonary, dermatological, and endocrine diseases can be adversely modified by anxiety [23]. Anxiety can arise when patients are given a diagnosis of a serious somatic disease such as diabetes or AIDS. It may be a consequence of stroke or traumatic brain injury, and is an independent risk factor for cardiac events. Parkinson's disease and epilepsy are both accompanied by anxiety [24, 25]. It may also be a primary concurrent anxiety disorder. A well-designed Norwegian study showed that the risk of contracting type 2 diabetes was increased by baseline anxiety or depression, even when adjusting for other well-known diabetic risk factors [26].

Anxiety is an independent risk factor for cardiac events: for example, significantly more cardiac events occurred within an 8-year period in patients with coronary heart disease in those who were anxious at baseline when compared to those were not [27]. A study of 913,570 of anxiety disorder cases in Taiwan treated with psychotropic medications during a 4-year period evaluated the rate of ischemic heart disease and hypertension [28], and found the relative risk of having treatment for ischemic heart disease to be increased 10-fold in treated anxiety subjects below age 20 years, and increased 5-fold among those treated for hypertension. These risks decreased substantially with age in the study, as cardiovascular disease became more common in the matched population. A similar study of 9,641 probands with panic disorder in Taiwan concluded that they were more likely at baseline to have hypertension, hyperlipidemia and coronary heart disease and less likely to have diabetes and renal disease; a subsequent first myocardial infarction occurred in 5% of the probands and 3% of the controls, yielding a hazard ratio of 1.8 [29].

Pain and anxiety are closely related entities [30]. Chronic neuropathic pain, affecting a large portion of elderly people, is strongly associated with depression and anxiety. Pain often precedes and accompanies a diagnosis of GAD [31, 32]. Interestingly, pregabalin is approved by the European regulatory authority for both neuropathic pain and GAD, while in the US it is approved for fibromyalgia – another pain disorder that is associated with GAD [33]. In addition, duloxetine, approved for GAD in Europe and in the US, is also approved for fibromyalgia in the US.

How does a practitioner best determine whether a patient suffers from GAD? Screening instruments may be helpful – such as the GAD-7, recommended by the DSM 5 committee for GAD www.dsm5.org [34]. A diagnosis can then be confirmed with the aid of the MINI Neuropsychiatric Interview (www.medical-outcomes.com). A medical examination and history should include tests for substance use, particularly alcohol and caffeine, as well as screen for thyroid disease. Prominent gastrointestinal symptoms may be due to irritable bowel syndrome, which is common among patients with GAD, as well as signs of an incipient neurological disease. Beta-stimulant medications, corticosteroids, and several other medications may cause anxiety symptoms. Pain can be assessed using a visual analogue scale, the scores of which can be monitored during treatment intervention.

Insomnia in Generalized Anxiety Disorder

At least every other GAD patient reports reduced sleep quality, reduced total sleep time, and less time in deep sleep [35]. A Swedish study of GAD patients in specialized outpatient care found that a high proportion received hypnotics, in addition to maintenance treatment with serotonergic drugs, particularly in the elderly [36]. The prognosis in anxiety disorders, particularly PTSD, is influenced by addressing sleep problems [37]. One study noted that the treatment response in GAD patients was greater if poor sleep was ameliorated by hypnotic usage in addition to anxiolytic therapy [38].

Table 1. Medications approved by regulatory authorities for treating patients with GAD

Generic name	Trade names	GAD dosing, mg
Venlafaxine	Effexor XR, Faxine, Efexor	75–375
Paroxetine	Seroxat, Eutimil, Paxil, Deroxat	20–50
Duloxetine	Cymbalta, Xeristar	(30–) 60–120
Pregabalin	Lyrica	150–600
Escitalopram	Cipralex, Sipralex, Lexapro, Entact	10–20

Cost of Illness Studies

Since GAD is a chronic disorder and the most frequent anxiety disorder in health care, it is important to realize its costs for society and for the individual – even more so in view of the demographic shift towards the elderly in many societies. According to a European study of disorders of the brain, GAD incurred substantial direct health care costs, as well as indirect costs for work absenteeism and burden to others [39]. A recent review on the burden of GAD in society confirms these data [40].

Evidence-Based Generalized Anxiety Disorder Treatments

The medications approved by European regulatory authorities for GAD, based on extensive phase III studies, are escitalopram, venlafaxine, duloxetine, paroxetine, and pregabalin (table 1).

The most recent international and independent guideline for pharmacotherapy of GAD was published in October 2008 [41]. First-line treatment choices for GAD included a serotonin-norepinephrine reuptake inhibitor (SNRI), a selective serotonin reuptake inhibitor (SSRI) medication, or pregabalin. Consideration was not given to cost of treatment as this varies between countries. The updated consensus guideline for pharmacotherapy of anxiety disorders by the British Association for Psychopharmacology is to become available early in 2014 (www.bap.org.uk).

In 2010, the Swedish national board of health and welfare issued similar guidelines, adding benzodiazepines as a potential third-line treatment option. Cognitive behavioural therapy (CBT) was also a recommended treatment for GAD, although the board accepted that the studies were generally small and of varying quality [42–44]. Fifty per cent of those who completed CBT and 40% of those who started CBT in controlled studies accomplished an improved functioning. The CBT approach involves psychoeducation, acceptance, time to control and to master worry, and advice on how to avoid relapse. Studies of Internet-mediated CBT are ongoing.

With regard to combining CBT with pharmacotherapy, a pragmatic study found that few patients accepted the offer of add-on CBT, and that no measurable added benefit could be demonstrated [45]. A recent Dutch study compared the effectiveness of meta-cognitive therapy and intolerance-of-uncertainty therapy with a delayed-treatment condition (waiting list) in a total of 126 consecutive cases, and found substantial improvements in GAD symptomatology in both active groups [46].

With the waxing and waning course of GAD, expert opinion recommends that if a patient responds to pharmacotherapy, it should be continued for at least 1 year in order to optimize the chance for remission and restoration of function [47, 48]. Naturally, adverse drug effects may call for a change of dosing or medication. In spite of pharmacogenetic population differences, as well as differences in illness attribution, duloxetine proved efficacious in a study of patients in Chinese patients with GAD [49]. Generally, the risks of not treating anxiety, particularly the risk of cardiovascular consequences, type 2 diabetes, secondary depressive episodes, and self-medication with alcohol, outweigh the risks of drug adverse effects. This general policy may include pregnancy, as there are consequences of untreated anxiety not only for the mother but for the developing foetus [50, 51]; fluoxetine and sertraline are preferred drugs in pregnancy as these medications have been used extensively.

GAD patients who do not respond to first-line treatment can be offered benzodiazepines or an antipsychotic drug; quetiapine has shown efficacy in several short-term studies [52], and pregabalin has been found efficacious as an adjunct therapy in patients with partial response to SSRI or SNRI treatment [53]. The clinician must rely on clinical experience as second- and third-line treatments, including adjunct combinations, have not been sufficiently evaluated in controlled trials [54]. European psychiatrists, according to a recent survey, found that most of their referred GAD patients had already been prescribed benzodiazepines by other physicians: the psychiatrists' first-line treatments were an SSRI, an SNRI, or pregabalin [55]. One may consider reasons for failing to respond, such as substance use, personality disorder, and not adhering to dosing regimens.

Taken together, GAD is a common and costly anxiety disorder tending to persist over many years; it increases the risk of somatic and psychiatric comorbidity, and requires maintenance treatment in many patients. The demographic changes in many societies will increase the number of elderly patients in need of treatment [56]. Since elderly patients are excluded from most phase 3 trials, we currently have little knowledge on how to manage them, especially considering the effects of somatic comorbidity and potential for interaction with other medications.

Disclosure Statement

Christer Allgulander is an advisor for Pfizer Sweden and a speaker for Pfizer, H. Lundbeck, and Servier. David Baldwin has acted as a consultant to and holds or has held research grants (on behalf of his employer) from a number of companies with an interest in anxiety and depressive disorders (Asahi, AstraZeneca, Cephalon, Eli Lilly, Grunenthal, GSK, Lundbeck, Organon, Pharmacia, Pierre Fabre, Pfizer, Roche, Servier, Sumitomo, and Wyeth).

References

1 Nitschke JB, Sarinopoulos I, Oathes DJ, Johnstone T, Whalen PJ, Davidson RJ, Kalin NH: Anticipatory activation in the amygdala and anterior cingulate in generalized anxiety disorder and prediction of treatment response. Am J Psychiatry 2009;166:302–310.

2 Etkin A, Prater KE, Hoeft F, Menon V, Schatzberg AF: Failure of anterior cingulate activation and connectivity with the amygdala during implicit regulation of emotional processing in generalized anxiety disorder. Am J Psychiatry 2010;167:545–554.

3 Brambilla P, Como G, Isola M, Taboga F, Zuliani R, Goljevscek S, Ragogna M, et al: White-matter abnormalities in the right posterior hemisphere in generalized anxiety disorder: a diffusion imaging study. Psychol Med 2011, DOI:10.1017/S0033291711001255.

4 Roth WT, Doberenz S, Dietel A, Conrad A, Mueller A, Wollburg E, Meuret AE, Taylor CB, Kim S: Sympathetic activation in broadly defined generalized anxiety disorder. J Psychiatry Res 2008;42:205–212.

5 Seddon K, Morris K, Bailey J, Potokar J, Rich A, Wilson S, Bettica P, Nutt DJ: Effects of 7.5% CO_2 challenge in generalized anxiety disorder. J Psychopharmacol 2011;25:43–51.

6 Bailey JE, Dawson GR, Dourish CT, Nutt DJ: Validating the inhalation of 7.5% CO_2 in healthy volunteers as a human experimental medicine: a model of generalized anxiety disorder (GAD). J Psychopharmacol 2011;25:1192–1198.

7 Borkovec TD, Roemer L: Perceived functions of worry among generalized anxiety disorder subjects: distraction from more emotionally distressing topics? J Behav Ther Exp Psychiatry 1995;26:25–30.

8 Ladouceur R, Gosselin P, Dugas MJ: Experimental manipulation of intolerance of uncertainty: a study of a theoretical model of worry. Behav Res Ther 2000;38:933–941.

9 MacLeod C, Rutherford E: Information-processing approaches. Assessing the selective, functioning of attention, interpretation, and retrieval; in Heimberg RG, Turk CL, Mennin DS (eds): Generalized Anxiety Disorder. Advances in Research and Practice. New York, Guilford Press, 2004, pp 109–142.

10 Heimberg RG, Turk CL, Mennin DS (eds): Generalized Anxiety Disorder. Advances in Research and Practice. New York, Guilford Press, 2004.

11 Hale WW, Klimstra TA, Meeus WHJ: Is the generalized anxiety disorder symptom of worry just another form of neuroticism? A 5-year longitudinal study of adolescents from the general population. J Clin Psychiatry 2010;71:942–948.

12 Mackintosh MA, Gatz M, Wetherell JL, Pedersen NL: A twin study of lifetime generalized anxiety disorder (GAD) in older adults: genetic and environmental influences shared by neuroticism and GAD. Twin Res Hum Genet 2006;9:30–37.

13 Bebbington PE, Brugha TS, Meltzer H, Jenkins R, Ceresa C, Farrell M, Lewis G: Neurotic disorders and the receipt of psychiatric treatment. Psychol Med 2000;30:1369–1376.

14 Ansseau M, Fischler B, Dierick M, Mignon A, Leyman S: Prevalence and impact of generalized anxiety disorder and major depression in primary care in Belgium and Luxemburg: the GADIS study. Eur Psychiatry 2005;20:229–235.

15 Moffitt TE, Harrington H, Caspi A, Kim-Cohen J, Goldberg D, Gregory AM, Poulton R: Depression and generalized anxiety disorder: cumulative and sequential comorbidity in a birth cohort followed prospectively to age 32 years. Arch Gen Psychiatry 2007; 64:651–660.

16 Weiller E, Bisserbe JC, Maier W, Lecrubier Y: Prevalence and recognition of anxiety syndromes in five European primary care settings. A report from the WHO study on Psychological Problems in General Health Care. Br J Psychiatry Suppl 1998;34:18–23.

17 Fernández A, Rubio-Valera M, Bellón JA, et al: Recognition of anxiety disorders by the general practitioner: results from the DASMAP Study. Gen Hosp Psychiatry 2012;34:227–233.

18 Munk-Jörgensen P, Allgulander C, Dahl AA, Foldager L, Holm M, Rasmussen I, Virta A, Huuhtanen M-J, Wittchen H-U: Prevalence of generalized anxiety disorder in general practice in Denmark, Finland, Norway, and Sweden. Psychiatr Serv 2006;57:1738–1744.

19 Hinton DE, Park L, Hsia C, Hofmann S, Pollack MH: Anxiety disorder presentations in Asian populations: a review. CNS Neurosci Ther 2009;15:295–303.

20 Marques L, Robinaugh DJ, LeBlanc NJ, Hinton D: Cross-cultural variations in the prevalence and presentation of anxiety disorders. Expert Rev Neurother 2011;11:313–322.

21 Chen P-Y, Wang S-C, Poland RE, Lin K-M: Biological variations in depression and anxiety between East and West. CNS Neurosci Therap 2009;15:283–294.

22 Perlis RH, Fijal B, Dharia S, Houston JP: Pharmacogenetic investigation of response to duloxetine treatment in generalized anxiety disorder. Pharmacogenomics J 2013;13:280–285.

23 Allgulander C: Morbid anxiety as a risk factor in patients with somatic diseases: a review of recent findings. J Psychiatry 2010;1:11–19.

24 Shiba M, Bower JH, Maraganore DM, McDonnell SK, Peterson BJ, Ahlskog JE, Schaid DJ, Rocca WA: Anxiety disorders and depressive disorders preceding Parkinson's disease: a case-control study. Mov Disord 2000;15:669–677.

25 Johnson EK, Jones JE, Sidenberg M, Hermann BP: The relative impact of anxiety, depression, and clinical seizure features on health-related quality of life, in epilepsy. Epilepsia 2004;45:544–550.

26 Engum A: The role of depression and anxiety in onset of diabetes in a large population-based study. J Psychosom Res 2007;62:31–38.

27 Martens EJ, de Jonge P, Na B, Cohen BE, Lett H, Whooley MA: Scared to death? Generalized anxiety disorder and cardiovascular events in patients with stable coronary heart disease. Arch Gen Psychiatry 2010;67:750–758.

28 Huang KL, Su TP, Chen TJ, Chou YH, Bai YM: Comorbidity of cardiovascular diseases with mood and anxiety disorder: a population based 4-year study. Psychiatry Clin Neurosci 2009;63:401–409.

29 Chen Y-H, Tsai S-Y, Lee H-C, Lin H-C: Increased risk of acute myocardial infarction for patients with panic disorder: a nationwide population study. Psychosom Med 2009;71:798–804.

30 Elman I, Zubieta J-K, Borsook D: The missing P in psychiatric training. Arch Gen Psychiatry 2011;68:12–20.

31 Beesdo K, Hoyer J, Jacobi F, Low NC, Höfler M, Wittche HU: Association between generalized anxiety levels and pain in a community sample: evidence for diagnostic specificity. J Anxiety Disord 2009;23:684–693.

32 Romera I, Férnandez-Pérez S, Montego ÁL, Caballero F, Caballero L, Arbesú JÁ, Delgado-Cohen H, et al: Generalized anxiety disorder, with or without comorbid major depressive disorder, in primary care: prevalence of painful somatic symptoms, functioning and health status. J Affect Disord 2010;127:160–168.

33 Raphale KG, Janal MN, Nayak S, Schwartz JE, Gallagher M: Psychiatric comorbidities in a community sample of women with fibromyalgia. Pain 2006;124:117–125.

34 Benjamin S, Herr NR, McDuffie J, Nagi A, Williams JW: Performance characteristics of self-report instruments for diagnosing generalized anxiety and panic disorders in primary care: a systematic review. VA Evidence-Based Synthesis Program Reports. Washington, Department of Veterans Affairs, August 2011.

35 Monti JM, Monti D: Sleep disturbance in generalized anxiety disorder and its treatment. Sleep Med Rev 2000;4:263–276.

36 Sandelin R, Kowalski J, Ahnemark E, Allgulander C: Generalized anxiety disorder treatments in a cohort of all 3,701 cases in psychiatric care in 2006, Sweden. Eur Psychiatry 2012;28:125–133.

37 Marcks BA, Weisberg RB, Edelen MO, Keller MB: The relationship between sleep disturbance and the course of anxiety disorders in primary care patients. Psychiatry Res 2010;178:487–492.

38 Pollack M, Kinrys G, Krystal A, McCall WV, Roth T, Schaefer K, Rubens R, et al: Eszopiclone coadministered with escitalopram in patients with insomnia and comorbid generalized anxiety disorder. Arch Gen Psychiatry 2008;65:551–562.

39 Andlin-Sobocki P, Wittchen HU: Cost of anxiety disorders in Europe. Eur J Neurol 2005;12:39–44.

40 Revicki DA, Travers K, Wyrwich KW, Svedsäter H, Locklear J, Mattera MS, Sheehan DV, Montgomery S: Humanistic and economic burden of generalized anxiety disorder in North America and Europe. J Affect Disord 2012;140:103–112.

41 Bandelow B, Zohar J, Hollander E, Kasper S, Möller HJ, WFSBP Task Force on Treatment Guidelines for Anxiety Obsessive-Compulsive Post-Traumatic Stress Disorders: World Federation of Societies of Biological Psychiatry (WFSBP) guidelines for the pharmacological treatment of anxiety, obsessive-compulsive and post-traumatic stress disorders – 1st revision. World J Biol Psychiatry 2008;9:248–312.

42 Hoyer J, Gloster AT: Psychotherapy for generalized anxiety disorder: don't worry, it works! Psychiatr Clin North Am 2009;32:629–640.

43 Leichsenring F, Salzer S, Jaeger U, Kachele H, Kreische R, Leweke F, Rüger U, Winkelbach C, Leibing E: Short-term psychodynamic psychotherapy and cognitive-behavioral therapy in generalized anxiety disorder: a randomized, controlled trial. Am J Psychiatry 2009;166:875–881.

44 Robinson E, Titov N, Andrews G, McIntyre K, Schwencke G, Solley K: Internet treatment for generalized anxiety disorder: a randomized controlled trial comparing clinician vs. technician assistance. PLoS One 2010;5:e10942.

45 Crits-Christoph P, Newman MG, Rickels K, Gallop R, Connolly Gibbons MB, Hamilton JL, Ring-Kurtz S, Pastva AM: Combined medication and cognitive therapy for generalized anxiety disorder. J Anxiety Disord 2011;25:1087–1094.

46 van der Heiden C, Muris P, van der Molen HT: Randomized controlled trial on the effectiveness of metacognitive therapy and intolerance-of-uncertainty therapy for generalized anxiety disorder. Behav Res Ther 2012;50:100–109.

47 Rickels K, Etemad B, Khalid-Khan S, Lohoff FW, Rynn MA, Gallop RJ: Time to relapse after 6 and 12 months' treatment of generalized anxiety disorder with venlafaxine extended release. Arch Gen Psychiatry 2010;67:1274–1281.

48 Reinhold JA, Mandos LA, Rickels K, Lohoff FW: Pharmacological treatment of generalized anxiety disorder. Expert Opin Pharmacother 2011;12:2457–2467.

49 Wu W, Wang G, Ball SG, Desaiah D, Ang Q: Duloxetine versus placebo in the treatment of patients with generalized anxiety disorder in China. Chin Med J 2011;124:3260–3268.

50 Ross LE, McLean LM: Anxiety disorders during pregnancy and the postpartum period: a systematic review. J Clin Psychiatry 2006;67:1285–1298.

51 Stein A, Craske MG, Lehtonen A, Harvey A, et al: Maternal cognitions and mother-infant interaction in postnatal depression and generalized anxiety disorder. J Abnorm Psychol 2012;121:795–809.

52 Stein DJ, Bandelow B, Merideth C, Olausson B, Szamosi J, Eriksson H: Efficacy and tolerability of extended release quetiapine fumarate (quetiapine XR) monotherapy in patients with generalised anxiety disorder: an analysis of pooled data from three 8-week placebo-controlled studies. Hum Psychopharmacol 2011;26:616–628.

53 Rickels K, Shiovitz TM, Ramey TS, Weaver JJ, Knapp LE, Miceli JJ: Adjunctive therapy with pregabalin in generalized anxiety disorder patients with partial response to SSRI or SNRI treatment. Int Clin Psychopharmacol 2012;27:142–150.

54 Pollack MH: Refractory generalized anxiety disorder. J Clin Psychiatry 2009;70(suppl 2):32–38.

55 Baldwin DS, Allgulander C, Bandelow B, Ferre F, Pallanti S: An international survey of reported prescribing practice in the treatment of patients with generalised anxiety disorder. World J Biol Psychiatry November 2012;13:510–516.

56 Porensky EK, Dew MA, Karp JF, Skidmore E, Rollman BL, Shear MK, Lenze EJ: The burden of late-life generalized anxiety disorder: effects on disability, health-related quality of life, and healthcare utilization. Am J Geriatr Psychiatry 2009;17:473–482.

57 Smoller JW, Block SR, Young MM: Genetics of anxiety disorders: the complex road from DSM to DNA. Depress Anxiety 2009;26:965–975.

Christer Allgulander, MD
Karolinska Institutet, Department of Clinical Neuroscience
Section of Psychiatry, Karolinska University Hospital Huddinge
SE–141 86 Huddinge (Sweden)
E-Mail Christer.Allgulander@ki.se

Baldwin DS, Leonard BE (eds): Anxiety Disorders.
Mod Trends Pharmacopsychiatry. Basel, Karger, 2013, vol 29, pp 128–143 (DOI: 10.1159/000351953)

Pharmacological Treatment of Panic Disorder

Borwin Bandelow[a] · David S. Baldwin[c, d] · Peter Zwanzger[b]

[a]Department of Psychiatry and Psychotherapy, University of Göttingen, Göttingen, and
[b]Department of Psychiatry and Psychotherapy, University of Münster, Münster, Germany;
[c]Clinical and Experimental Sciences, Faculty of Medicine, University of Southampton, Southampton, UK;
[d]Department of Psychiatry and Mental Health, University of Cape Town, Cape Town, South Africa

Abstract

A comprehensive database has developed and precise recommendations can be provided for treating patients with panic disorder. Selective serotonin reuptake inhibitors and serotonin-norepinephrine reuptake inhibitors are standard treatments for panic disorder. Tricyclic antidepressants are as effective as modern antidepressants, but less well tolerated. For short-term treatment and in nonresponsive cases, benzodiazepines such as alprazolam may be used when the patient does not have a history of dependency and tolerance. Combining drug treatment with cognitive behaviour therapy is the most successful treatment strategy for panic disorder. This chapter also includes treatment recommendations for pregnant or lactating women, children, adolescents, elderly patients, and patients who are non-responsive to standard treatments.   Copyright © 2013 S. Karger AG, Basel

Pharmacological treatment of panic disorder emerged in 1959, when Donald F. Klein established the beneficial effects of the tricyclic antidepressant (TCA) imipramine [1]. The first benzodiazepine chlordiazepoxide was introduced in 1960. The selective serotonin reuptake inhibitors (SSRIs) have been used in the treatment of patients with panic disorder since the 1980s [2, 3], followed by the dual reuptake inhibitor venlafaxine in the subsequent decade. The effectiveness of pharmacotherapy for panic disorder has been established through a series of randomized placebo-controlled studies. A comprehensive database has developed, and precise recommendations can be provided for treating patients with panic disorder (table 1). According to the principles of evidence-based medicine, this chapter focuses on the results from randomized double-blind placebo- and comparator-controlled trials [4, 5]. There is only limited evi-

Table 1. Recommendations for drug treatment of panic disorder

Treatment	Examples	Recommended daily dose for adults, mg
Treatment of acute panic attacks		
Benzodiazepines, e.g.	Alprazolam	0.5–2
	Lorazepam melting tablets	1–2.5
Standard treatment		
SSRIs, e.g.	Citalopram	20–40
	Escitalopram	10–20
	Fluoxetine	20–40
	Fluvoxamine	100–300
	Paroxetine	20–60
	Sertraline	50–200
SNRI	Venlafaxine	75–225
TCA, e.g.	Clomipramine	75–250
	Imipramine	75–250
When other treatment strategies are not effective or not tolerated:		
Benzodiazepines, e.g.	Alprazolam	1.5–8
	Clonazepam	1–4
MAOI	Phenelzine	45–90
NASSA	Mirtazapine	45
RIMA	Moclobemide	300–600

These recommendations are based on randomized, double-blind clinical studies published in peer-reviewed journals. Not all of the recommended drugs are licensed for these indications in every country. MAOI = Monoamine oxidase inhibitor; NASSA = noradrenergic and specific serotonergic antidepressant.

dence for the superiority of certain medications in terms of efficacy, but the available drugs differ in their side effect profile, making some medications more or less suitable for particular patient groups.

Selective Serotonin Reuptake Inhibitors

The efficacy of SSRIs in the acute treatment in panic disorder has been established through many controlled studies, and most authorities consider them to be the first-line drugs for this disorder. Efficacy has been shown for citalopram in a placebo- and comparator-controlled trial [6] and through comparison with fluoxetine [7]; and in a relapse prevention study, citalopram was as effective as clomipramine and superior to placebo [8]. Escitalopram has been found superior to placebo and citalopram [9, 10]; as escitalopram is an enantiomer of the racemic mixture citalopram, studies with citalopram are also relevant for escitalopram. Although findings are mixed, fluvoxamine has been found efficacious in a number of double-blind, placebo-controlled studies [11–

16]. In one, fluvoxamine and the comparator drug imipramine were both superior to placebo, and similarly effective [17]. A small study did not find fluvoxamine to be superior to placebo on the main efficacy measure, but on some other instruments [18], whereas another found no evidence of efficacy for fluvoxamine, but a strong effect for imipramine when compared to placebo [19]. Fluoxetine has been found effective in placebo- [20, 21] and comparator-controlled trials [7, 22, 23]; in a 26-week study, it was similarly effective as imipramine [23], and in a 52-week study it was similarly effective as the reversible inhibitor of monoamine oxidase-A (RIMA) moclobemide [24]. Paroxetine has shown efficacy in placebo-controlled trials [25–28] and in comparator-controlled studies [25, 29–33]. In a relapse prevention study, paroxetine was similarly effective as the TCA clomipramine [34]. Sertraline has been found efficacious in placebo-controlled studies [35–37] and in one comparator-controlled trial [31], although another study found no evidence of superiority to placebo [38]. As regards long-term treatment, in a 26-week relapse prevention study, followed by open treatment over one year, sertraline was found superior to placebo [39]; but in a second relapse prevention study, sertraline was not superior to placebo on the primary efficacy measure [40]; and in a long-term study in patients with panic disorder and co-morbid major depression, sertraline was superior to placebo and similarly effective as imipramine [41].

Anxiolytic effects typically start after 2–4 weeks, but in some patients beneficial effects may emerge after 6 or 8 weeks. Doses are typically given in the morning or mid-day, except in patients reporting daytime sedation. Treatment with SSRIs is reasonably well tolerated, but restlessness, jitteriness, and increase in anxiety symptoms and insomnia in the first days or weeks of treatment may cause some patients to stop treatment. Lowering the starting dose of SSRIs may reduce this overstimulation. Side effects which are more troublesome over the long-term include fatigue, dizziness, nausea, and reduced appetite or weight gain. Sexual dysfunction (reduced libido, erectile or ejaculatory disturbances, anorgasmia) may be troublesome [42], and discontinuation syndromes have been reported [43, 44].

Serotonin-Noradrenaline Reuptake Inhibitors

The efficacy of venlafaxine was established in randomized placebo-controlled studies [45, 46]. In one [47], venlafaxine was not superior to placebo in the proportion of patients becoming free from full-symptom panic attacks, but was superior in reducing panic attack frequency in the proportion becoming free from limited-symptom panic attacks, in response and remission rates, and in reductions in the severity of anticipatory anxiety, fear and avoidance. In addition, venlafaxine was found superior to placebo and similarly effective as paroxetine [32, 47]; and in a relapse prevention study, it was superior to placebo [48]. The side effect profile of venlafaxine is broadly similar to that of the SSRIs, though excessive perspiration may be more frequent. When using higher doses (that is a dosage of 300 mg/day or more), blood pressure should be monitored regularly.

Tricyclic Antidepressants

Imipramine has been found efficacious in placebo-controlled [49–51] and comparator-controlled studies [19, 52–54]. In relapse prevention studies, it was superior to placebo and similarly effective as alprazolam [55]; although similarly effective as alprazolam in an 8-week acute treatment study, it was found less effective than alprazolam in a 26-week extension [56]; and in a another long-term study, it was similarly effective as fluoxetine [23].

The tricyclic clomipramine has also been found efficacious in placebo- [57, 58] and comparator-controlled studies [6, 30, 59–61], and in a relapse prevention trial was similarly effective as paroxetine [34]. In one study, desipramine was found superior to placebo [62], and lofepramine was also found efficacious in a placebo- and comparator controlled study with clomipramine as an active comparator [61].

Treatment adherence with tricyclic drugs may be affected by adverse effects such as an initial increase in 'nervousness', dry mouth, postural hypotension, tachycardia, sedation, and sexual dysfunction. Psychomotor function can be impaired affecting car driving safety, and weight gain may be troublesome over long-term treatment. The frequency of adverse events is generally considered to be higher for tricyclics than with newer antidepressants such as SSRIs [6, 17, 22, 23, 29, 34]; for example, in an SSRI-TCA comparison, adverse events occurred in 73.2% of paroxetine-treated but 89.2% of clomipramine-treated patients [34]. As such, most authorities recommend that better tolerated drugs should be tried before TCAs are used. In addition, the dosage should be titrated steadily until dosage is as high as in the treatment of depression. Patients should be made aware that the onset of the anxiolytic effect of the drug generally takes between 2 to 4 weeks (but in some patients up to 6 or 8 weeks may pass before beneficial effects are seen).

Benzodiazepines

A number of benzodiazepines have been found efficacious in the treatment of panic disorder. Alprazolam has been found superior to placebo and as effective as comparator drugs in a number of acute treatment studies [52, 54, 63–66]. In relapse prevention studies, it was found superior to placebo and similarly effective as imipramine [55]; and although similarly effective as imipramine in an acute treatment study, alprazolam was more effective than imipramine in a long-term extension [56]. Clonazepam has been found efficacious in placebo-controlled studies [67–70] and in one placebo- and comparator-controlled study [71]. Diazepam was found superior to placebo and similarly effective as alprazolam in 2 studies [65, 72]. Lorazepam was found to be similarly effective as alprazolam in 2 studies, and both drugs were found superior to placebo [73, 74].

Anxiolytic effects of benzodiazepines often start soon after oral or parenteral administration. Unlike antidepressants, benzodiazepines are not associated with an initial increase in 'nervousness', and in general have a reasonable record of safety. However due to central depressant effects benzodiazepines may be associated with sedation, dizziness, an increase in reaction times, and driving skills may be affected. Long-term treatment with benzodiazepines (e.g. over 4–8 months), may be complicated by the development of dependence in some patients [75–81], especially in those who are predisposed [82], though tolerance seems to be uncommon [83]. Benzodiazepine treatment hence requires a careful weighing of potential risks and benefits. In patients in whom other treatments have not proved effective or were poorly tolerated due to side effects, year-long treatment with benzodiazepines may be justified: but patients with a history of benzodiazepine abuse should not be exposed again. Cognitive-behavioural interventions may help patients withdraw from benzodiazepine treatment [84, 85]. Unlike antidepressants, benzodiazepines do not treat conditions that are comorbid with panic disorder, such as major depression or obsessive-compulsive disorder.

In clinical practice, benzodiazepines are often combined with antidepressants. A study of combined treatment with paroxetine and clonazepam found the combination resulted in more rapid response than was seen with paroxetine alone, but there was no evidence of added benefit after the first few weeks of treatment [86]. Similar placebo-controlled studies have examined the combination of imipramine with alprazolam [87], and sertraline with clonazepam [88], both showing a faster response with the combination than with imipramine or sertraline plus placebo, respectively.

Monoamine Oxidase Inhibitors

Although the monoamine oxidase inhibitor phenelzine is often used in the treatment of patients with panic disorder, the evidence for efficacy derives from a single study [89], in which it was found superior to placebo and similarly effective (or superior) to imipramine on some measures. Because of its often poor tolerability and the risk of interactions with other drugs or food components, phenelzine is not considered a first-line drug, and should be reserved for use by experienced psychiatrists, when other treatment modalities have proved unhelpful. Phenelzine is rather alerting; so, to avoid overstimulation and insomnia, doses should be given in the morning and certainly by midday.

Other Medications

Some other drugs have shown preliminary evidence of efficacy, or mixed results. These drugs may be considered for 'off-label' use in patients who have not responded to standard treatments. For the RIMA moclobemide, results have been inconsistent: it was similarly effective as fluoxetine [24] or clomipramine [90], but it was not found superior to placebo in a double-blind study [91]; and in another study, it was superior to placebo in only the more severely ill patients [92]. Side effects include restlessness, insomnia, dry mouth, and headache; and as with phenelzine, doses should be given in the morning and midday to avoid insomnia. The noradrenaline reuptake inhibitor reboxetine was found efficacious in a placebo-controlled study [93], and in a single-blind study reboxetine was similarly effective as fluvoxamine [94], but less effective than paroxetine [95]. In a small double-blind comparison involving the $\alpha_2/5$-$HT_2/5$-HT_3 blocker mirtazapine and fluvoxamine, no differences were found in effectiveness, though the sample size of the study was probably too small for a non-inferiority comparison [96]; in an open evaluation, mirtazapine [97] appeared beneficial. Although efficacious in generalized anxiety disorder, the $5HT_{1A}$ agonist buspirone was not found superior to placebo [53, 98], and was less effective than imipramine [53], clorazepate [99] and alprazolam [98] in patients with panic disorder.

Medications which may have a role in some patients include the norepinephrine/dopamine reuptake inhibitor bupropion, which was not found effective in a small controlled study [100], but showed some effect in a small open-label evaluation [101]. Beta-blockers can reduce the intensity of autonomic anxiety symptoms – such as palpitations and tremor – and so have been used in the treatment of panic disorder; however, propranolol was not found superior to placebo [102] and was less effective than comparator drugs [102, 103]. In another placebo-controlled study, propranolol was not substantially different to alprazolam, although the benzodiazepine had a more rapid onset of effect [104]. The anticonvulsant valproate (valproic acid) was found efficacious in a small crossover study [105], and beneficial in open evaluations [106–108]. The γ-aminobutyric acid reuptake inhibitor tiagabine showed beneficial effects in a case series [109]; the irreversible inhibitor of GABA transaminase vigabatrin was used in a small case series [110]; and in a placebo-controlled study, gabapentin was only found to be superior to placebo in the more severely ill patients [111]. The intracellular second-messenger precursor inositol was found superior to placebo in a small study [112], and similarly effective as fluvoxamine [113]. The 5-HT_3 antagonist ondansetron was also found beneficial in an open evaluation [114].

Long-Term Treatment

Panic disorder tends to run a waxing and waning course, and as such treatment should continue for many months after symptomatic remission in order to reduce the risk of relapse. The benefit of long-term treatment has been assessed through a series of continuation studies which compare a drug and placebo over a long period (between 26–60 weeks), and through relapse prevention studies in which patients receive initial treatment with the study drug for a shorter period, after which responders are randomized to receive either continued drug treatment or placebo for 6 months or longer. Some SSRIs, venlafaxine, some TCAs and moclobemide have all shown long-term efficacy in these studies. Expert consensus conferences have generally recommended a duration of continuation treatment of at least 12–24 months [115], though other guidelines have suggested a treatment for at least 6 months after symptom remission has occurred. The same doses of SSRIs are usually prescribed in the maintenance phase and the acute treatment phase, but to our knowledge, there are no studies examining reduction in dosage in maintenance treatment. In an open study with imipramine, patients who had stabilized received further treatment with half their previous dosage, and did not show evidence of relapse or sustained worsening [116].

Comparisons between Drugs in the Treatment of Panic Disorder

No differences were found in terms of efficacy between SSRIs and TCA type drugs in a series of evaluations [6, 17, 22, 23, 29, 34, 117], with the exception of maprotiline, which had no beneficial effect, in contrast to the SSRI fluvoxamine [3]. However, in most comparisons, SSRIs were better tolerated than TCAs. An investigation in patients with comorbid panic disorder and major depressive disorder, found that both sertraline and imipramine were effective, though sertraline had significantly greater tolerability and improved compliance in comparison with imipramine [41]. Comparisons between SSRIs do not reveal differences with regard to efficacy [31, 118], but in a post hoc analysis escitalopram was found superior to citalopram on some outcome measures [10]. There are no direct comparisons between SSRIs and benzodiazepines, but a meta-analysis found that the effect sizes for the SSRIs were higher than the effect size for the benzodiazepine alprazolam [119]. In a number of studies, alprazolam has been compared to imipramine [52, 54, 66, 120–123], but no differences could be found in terms of global improvement. The relative advantages and drawbacks of differing medications are summarized in table 2.

Practical Guidelines for Treatment

Recommended dosages are shown in table 1. SSRIs have a generally flat response curve, but for paroxetine, a dosage of 40 mg/day was more effective than 20 mg/day. Patients with panic disorder are sensitive to the adverse effects of antidepressants and may easily discontinue treatment because of initial jitteriness and nervousness, so in some patients, treatment may be started at half the recommended dose in the first days or weeks. For TCAs, the drug should be started at a low dose, then increased every 3–5 days. The antidepressant dose should be increased to the highest recommended and tolerated level when initial treatment with a low or medium dosage fails. In order to enhance treatment adherence, it is often helpful to give all the antidepressant medication in a single dose, depending on overall tolerability. Benzodiazepine dosage should be kept as low as possible but as high as needed to achieve an optimal treatment effect.

Table 2. Advantages and disadvantages of antianxiety drugs

Medication class	Advantages	Disadvantages
SSRIs	No dependency Sufficient evidence from clinical studies Favourable side effect profile Relatively safe in overdose	Latency of effect 2–6 weeks Initial jitteriness, nausea, restlessness, sexual dysfunctions and other side effects
SNRIs	No dependency Sufficient evidence from clinical studies Favourable side effect profile Relatively safe in overdose	Latency of effect 2–6 weeks Initial jitteriness, nausea, restlessness, sexual dysfunctions, increase of blood pressure in high doses and other side effects
TCAs	No dependency Sufficient evidence from clinical studies	Latency of effect 2–6 weeks Anticholinergic effects, cardiovascular side effects, weight gain and other side effects, sexual dysfunctions May be lethal in overdose
Benzodiazepines	Rapid onset of action Sufficient evidence from clinical studies Generally favourable side effect profile (with the exception of addiction potential) Relatively safe in overdose	Dependency possible; sedation, slow reaction time and other side effects

Particular Patient Populations

In pregnant women, the risks of drug treatment have to be weighed against the risk of untreated panic disorder. The use of SSRIs or TCAs probably carries no increased risk for fetal malformations [124–136], but some reports have raised concerns about fetal cardiac effects, newborn persistent pulmonary hypertension, and other effects [137]. Preschool age children who had been exposed to fluoxetine in utero show no significant neurobehavioural abnormalities [138], and the findings of a prospective controlled study suggest that long-term prenatal exposure to TCAs or fluoxetine did not adversely affect cognition, language development or temperament [139]. Although there is no consistent proof that benzodiazepines may be hazardous, an association between the use of benzodiazepines and congenital malformations has been reported [140]. It has been suggested that it may be prudent to avoid treatment with alprazolam during pregnancy [141].

In lactating women, SSRIs and TCAs are excreted into breast milk, and low levels have been found in infant serum [133, 142, 143]. In mothers taking TCAs (with the exception of doxepin, which is very sedative), it seems unwarranted to recommend that breastfeeding should be discontinued. Fluoxetine should probably be avoided during lactation [143], but treatment with other SSRIs seems to be broadly compatible with breastfeeding, although this view should be regarded as preliminary due to a lack of substantial data [143, 144]. During maternal treatment with all psychotropic drugs, infants should be observed for signs of sedation, lethargy, poor suckling, and weight loss, and if high doses have to be used and long-term treatment is needed, breastfeeding should probably be discontinued [141, 143].

In children and adolescents, panic disorder is uncommon, the average age at onset of panic disorder being between 23 and 28 years [145]. There are no double-blind treatment studies in younger age groups, and experience with the pharmacological treatment of anxiety disorders in children and adolescents is derived mainly from studies in patients with obsessive-compulsive disorder, data suggesting that SSRIs can be a first-line treatment [135]. However, treatment with SSRIs and serotonin-norepinephrine reuptake inhibitors (SNRIs) has been associated with suicidal ideation and suicide attempts, so the risks and benefits of drug treatment should be weighed carefully in this age group. It may be best to reserve pharmacological treatment for patients who have not responded to psychological approaches.

Panic disorder is relatively rare in elderly patients as symptoms of panic disorder tend to decrease after the age of 45–50 years; however, panic attacks are not uncommon in elderly depressed patients. Few studies have examined the effect of treatment of anxiety disorders in elderly patients, though escitalopram and citalopram appeared effective in reducing panic attack frequency in a small sample of elderly patients with recurrent panic attacks associated with a range of anxiety disorders [146]. Elderly patients have an increased sensitivity for anticholinergic properties of drugs, an increased sensitivity for extrapyramidal symptoms, an increased risk for orthostatic hypotension and ECG changes, and possibly greater risk of paradoxical reactions to benzodiazepines. As such, treatment with TCAs or benzodiazepines is probably less favourable, whilst SSRIs and SNRIs appear relatively safe.

Management of Treatment-Resistant Panic Disorder

Many patients continue to experience recurrent panic attacks, agoraphobic avoidance, or continuing distress and impairment despite undergoing evidence-based pharmacological treatment. Around 20–40% of the patients treated with standard approaches remain symptomatic [14, 31]. In non-responding patients, the first steps are to ascertain that the diagnosis is correct, the patient is adherent to treatment, the dosage prescribed is therapeutic, and the treatment period has been sufficiently long. Some concomitantly prescribed drugs may interfere with efficacy through metabolic effects. Some patients metabolize drugs very fast, and although the determination of plasma levels is not used routinely due to a low correlation between oral dose and plasma level or between plasma level and clinical effect, this may be helpful in identifying patients who are non-compliant or who are fast metabolizers. Unresolved psychosocial difficulties also reduce the likelihood of a treatment response, as does the presence of comorbidity for other axis I and axis II disorders.

Data from controlled clinical studies do not easily transfer to the management of treatment-resistant patients. Pindolol can augment the effect of fluoxetine [147], but this strategy is rarely used in practice. A small single-blind crossover study in non-responders showed that switching to citalopram or reboxetine may be worthwhile [94]. A small open study involving the addition of fluoxetine to patients taking a TCA, or vice versa, found some evidence of benefit [148]. Sodium valproate and clonazepam have been combined in the treatment of patients who proved resistant to several previous anti-panic drug treatments [149]. In a single case report, the addition of lithium to clomipramine was found successful [150], as has the addition of 5–12.5 mg olanzapine to various drug combinations [151, 152]. Finally, some drugs may be tried which have been investigated in other anxiety disorders, such as buspirone, the SNRI duloxetine, the calcium channel modulator pregabalin [153, 154], and the antipsychotic quetiapine [155]. Psychological treatments such as cognitive behaviour therapy (CBT) have to be considered in all patients, and the addition of group CBT may be beneficial in non-responders to pharmacological approaches [156–158].

References

1 Klein DF, Fink M: Psychiatric reaction patterns to imipramine. Am J Psychiatry 1962;119:432–438.
2 Evans L, Kenardy J, Schneider P, Hoey H: Effect of a selective serotonin uptake inhibitor in agoraphobia with panic attacks. A double-blind comparison of zimeldine, imipramine and placebo. Acta Psychiatr Scand 1986;73:49–53.
3 den Boer JA, Westenberg HG: Effect of a serotonin and noradrenaline uptake inhibitor in panic disorder; a double-blind comparative study with fluvoxamine and maprotiline. Int Clin Psychopharmacol 1988;3:59–74.
4 Baldwin DS, Anderson IM, Nutt DJ, Bandelow B, Bond A, Davidson JR, den Boer JA, Fineberg NA, Knapp M, Scott J, Wittchen HU: Evidence-based guidelines for the pharmacological treatment of anxiety disorders: recommendations from the British Association for Psychopharmacology. J Psychopharmacol 2005;19:567–596.
5 Bandelow B, Zohar J, Hollander E, et al: World Federation of Societies of Biological Psychiatry (WFSBP) guidelines for the pharmacological treatment of anxiety, obsessive-compulsive and post-traumatic stress disorders – first revision. World J Biol Psychiatry 2008;9:248–312.
6 Wade AG, Lepola U, Koponen HJ, Pedersen V, Pedersen T: The effect of citalopram in panic disorder. Br J Psychiatry 1997;170:549–553.
7 Amore M, Magnani K, Cerisoli M, Ferrari G: Short-term and long-term evaluation of selective serotonin reuptake inhibitors in the treatment of panic disorder: fluoxetine vs citalopram. Hum Psychopharmacol 1999;14:435–440.
8 Lepola UM, Wade AG, Leinonen EV, Koponen HJ, Frazer J, Sjodin I, Penttinen JT, Pedersen T, Lehto HJ: A controlled, prospective, 1-year trial of citalopram in the treatment of panic disorder. J Clin Psychiatry 1998;59:528–534.
9 Stahl SM, Gergel I, Li D: Escitalopram in the treatment of panic disorder: a randomized, double-blind, placebo-controlled trial. J Clin Psychiatry 2003;64: 1322–1327.
10 Bandelow B, Stein DJ, Dolberg OT, Andersen HF, Baldwin DS: Improvement of quality of life in panic disorder with escitalopram, citalopram, or placebo. Pharmacopsychiatry 2007;40:152–156.
11 Asnis GM, Hameedi FA, Goddard AW, Potkin SG, Black D, Jameel M, Desagani K, Woods SW: Fluvoxamine in the treatment of panic disorder: a multicenter, double-blind, placebo-controlled study in outpatients. Psychiatry Res 2001;103:1–14.
12 den Boer JA, Westenberg HG: Serotonin function in panic disorder: a double blind placebo controlled study with fluvoxamine and ritanserin. Psychopharmacology (Berl) 1990;102:85–94.

13 Hoehn-Saric R, McLeod DR, Hipsley PA: Effect of fluvoxamine on panic disorder. J Clin Psychopharmacol 1993;13:321–326.

14 Black DW, Wesner R, Bowers W, Gabel J: A comparison of fluvoxamine, cognitive therapy, and placebo in the treatment of panic disorder. Arch Gen Psychiatry 1993;50:44–50.

15 Pols H, Zandergen J, de Loof C, Fernandez I, Griez E: Clinical effects of fluvoxamine on panic symptomatology. Acta Psychiatr Belg 1993;93:169–177.

16 de Beurs E, van Balkom AJ, Lange A, Koele P, van Dyck R: Treatment of panic disorder with agoraphobia: comparison of fluvoxamine, placebo, and psychological panic management combined with exposure and of exposure in vivo alone. Am J Psychiatry 1995;152:683–691.

17 Bakish D, Hooper CL, Filteau MJ, Charbonneau Y, Fraser G, West DL, Thibaudeau C, Raine D: A double-blind placebo-controlled trial comparing fluvoxamine and imipramine in the treatment of panic disorder with or without agoraphobia. Psychopharmacol Bull 1996;32:135–141.

18 Sandmann J, Lorch B, Bandelow B, Hartter S, Winter P, Hiemke C, Benkert O: Fluvoxamine or placebo in the treatment of panic disorder and relationship to blood concentrations of fluvoxamine. Pharmacopsychiatry 1998;31:117–121.

19 Nair NP, Bakish D, Saxena B, Amin M, Schwartz G, West TE: Comparison of fluvoxamine, imipramine, and placebo in the treatment of outpatients with panic disorder. Anxiety 1996;2:192–198.

20 Michelson D, Allgulander C, Dantendorfer K, Knezevic A, Maierhofer D, Micev V, Paunovic VR, Timotijevic I, Sarkar N, Skoglund L, Pemberton SC: Efficacy of usual antidepressant dosing regimens of fluoxetine in panic disorder: randomised, placebo-controlled trial. Br J Psychiatry 2001;179:514–518.

21 Michelson D, Lydiard RB, Pollack MH, Tamura RN, Hoog SL, Tepner R, Demitrack MA, Tollefson GD: Outcome assessment and clinical improvement in panic disorder: Evidence from a randomized controlled trial of fluoxetine and placebo. The fluoxetine panic disorder study group. Am J Psychiatry 1998; 155:1570–1577.

22 Bystritsky A, Rosen RM, Murphy KJ, Bohn P, Keys SA, Vapnik T: Double-blind pilot trial of desipramine versus fluoxetine in panic patients. Anxiety 1994;1:287–290.

23 Amore M, Magnani K, Cerisoli M, Casagrande C, Ferrari G: Panic disorder. A long-term treatment study: fluoxetine vs imipramine. Hum Psychopharmacol 1999;14:429–434.

24 Tiller JW, Bouwer C, Behnke K: Moclobemide and fluoxetine for panic disorder. International panic disorder study group. Eur Arch Psychiatry Clin Neurosci 1999;249(suppl 1):S7–S10.

25 Oehrberg S, Christiansen PE, Behnke K, Borup AL, Severin B, Soegaard J, Calberg H, Judge R, Ohrstrom JK, Manniche PM: Paroxetine in the treatment of panic disorder. A randomised, double-blind, placebo-controlled study. Br J Psychiatry 1995;167:374–379.

26 Ballenger JC, Wheadon DE, Steiner M, Bushnell W, Gergel IP: Double-blind, fixed-dose, placebo-controlled study of paroxetine in the treatment of panic disorder. Am J Psychiatry 1998;155:36–42.

27 Pollack MH, Doyle AC: Treatment of panic disorder: focus on paroxetine. Psychopharmacol Bull 2003; 37(suppl 1):53–63.

28 Sheehan DV, Burnham DB, Iyengar MK, Perera P: Efficacy and tolerability of controlled-release paroxetine in the treatment of panic disorder. J Clin Psychiatry 2005;66:34–40.

29 Bakker A, van Dyck R, Spinhoven P, van Balkom A: Paroxetine, clomipramine, and cognitive therapy in the treatment of panic disorder. J Clin Psychiatry 1999;60:831–838.

30 Lecrubier Y, Bakker A, Dunbar G, Judge R: A comparison of paroxetine, clomipramine and placebo in the treatment of panic disorder. Collaborative paroxetine panic study investigators. Acta Psychiatr Scand 1997;95:145–152.

31 Bandelow B, Behnke K, Lenoir S, Hendriks GJ, Alkin T, Goebel C, Clary CM: Sertraline versus paroxetine in the treatment of panic disorder: an acute, double-blind noninferiority comparison. J Clin Psychiatry 2004;65:405–413.

32 Pollack MH, Lepola U, Koponen H, Simon NM, Worthington JJ, Emilien G, Tzanis E, Salinas E, Whitaker T, Gao B: A double-blind study of the efficacy of venlafaxine extended-release, paroxetine, and placebo in the treatment of panic disorder. Depress Anxiety 2007;24:1–14.

33 Wedekind D, Broocks A, Weiss N, Engel K, Neubert K, Bandelow B: A randomized, controlled trial of aerobic exercise in combination with paroxetine in the treatment of panic disorder. World J Biol Psychiatry 2010;11:904–913.

34 Lecrubier Y, Judge R: Long-term evaluation of paroxetine, clomipramine and placebo in panic disorder. Collaborative paroxetine panic study investigators. Acta Psychiatr Scand 1997;95:153–160.

35 Londborg PD, Wolkow R, Smith WT, DuBoff E, England D, Ferguson J, Rosenthal M, Weise C: Sertraline in the treatment of panic disorder. A multisite, double-blind, placebo-controlled, fixed-dose investigation. Br J Psychiatry 1998;173:54–60.

36 Pollack MH, Otto MW, Worthington JJ, Manfro GG, Wolkow R: Sertraline in the treatment of panic disorder: a flexible-dose multicenter trial. Arch Gen Psychiatry 1998;55:1010–1016.

37 Pohl RB, Wolkow RM, Clary CM: Sertraline in the treatment of panic disorder: a double-blind multicenter trial. Am J Psychiatry 1998;155:1189–1195.

38 Koszycki D, Taljaard M, Segal Z, Bradwejn J: A randomized trial of sertraline, self-administered cognitive behavior therapy, and their combination for panic disorder. Psychol Med 2011;41:373–383.

39 Rapaport MH, Wolkow R, Rubin A, Hackett E, Pollack M, Ota KY: Sertraline treatment of panic disorder: results of a long-term study. Acta Psychiatr Scand 2001;104:289–298.

40 Kamijima K, Kuboki T, Kumano H, Burt T, Cohen G, Arano I, Hamasaki T: A placebo-controlled, randomized withdrawal study of sertraline for panic disorder in Japan. Int Clin Psychopharmacol 2005;20: 265–273.

41 Lepola U, Arato M, Zhu Y, Austin C: Sertraline versus imipramine treatment of comorbid panic disorder and major depressive disorder. J Clin Psychiatry 2003;64:654–662.

42 Baldwin DS: Sexual dysfunction associated with antidepressant drugs. Expert Opin Drug Saf 2004;3: 457–470.

43 Price JS, Waller PC, Wood SM, MacKay AV: A comparison of the post-marketing safety of four selective serotonin re-uptake inhibitors including the investigation of symptoms occurring on withdrawal. Br J Clin Pharmacol 1996;42:757–763.

44 Stahl MMS, Lindquist M, Pettersson M, Edwards IR, Sanderson JH, Taylor NFA, Fletcher AP, Schou JS: Withdrawal reactions with selective serotonin re-uptake inhibitors as reported to the who system. Eur J Clin Pharmacol 1997;53:163–169.

45 Pollack MH, Worthington JJ 3rd, Otto MW, Maki KM, Smoller JW, Manfro GG, Rudolph R, Rosenbaum JF: Venlafaxine for panic disorder: results from a double-blind, placebo-controlled study. Psychopharmacol Bull 1996;32:667–670.

46 Bradwejn J, Ahokas A, Stein DJ, Salinas E, Emilien G, Whitaker T: Venlafaxine extended-release capsules in panic disorder: flexible-dose, double-blind, placebo-controlled study. Br J Psychiatry 2005;187:352–359.

47 Pollack M, Mangano R, Entsuah R, Tzanis E, Simon NM, Zhang Y: A randomized controlled trial of venlafaxine ER and paroxetine in the treatment of outpatients with panic disorder. Psychopharmacology 2007;194:233–242.

48 Ferguson JM, Khan A, Mangano R, Entsuah R, Tzanis E: Relapse prevention of panic disorder in adult outpatient responders to treatment with venlafaxine extended release. J Clin Psychiatry 2007;68:58–68.

49 Klein DF: Delineation of two drug-responsive anxiety syndromes. Psychopharmacologia 1964;5:397–408.

50 Zitrin CM, Klein DF, Woerner MG: Treatment of agoraphobia with group exposure in vivo and imipramine. Arch Gen Psychiatry 1980;37:63–72.

51 Zitrin CM, Klein DF, Woerner MG, Ross DC: Treatment of phobias. I. Comparison of imipramine hydrochloride and placebo. Arch Gen Psychiatry 1983; 40:125–138.

52 Uhlenhuth EH, Matuzas W, Glass RM, Easton C: Response of panic disorder to fixed doses of alprazolam or imipramine. J Affect Disord 1989;17:261–270.

53 Sheehan DV, Raj AB, Sheehan KH, Soto S: Is buspirone effective for panic disorder? J Clin Psychopharmacol 1990;10:3–11.

54 CNCPS: Cross-national collaborative panic study. Drug treatment of panic disorder. Comparative efficacy of alprazolam, imipramine, and placebo. Br J Psychiatry 1992;160:191–202.

55 Curtis GC, Massana J, Udina C, Ayuso JL, Cassano GB, Perugi G: Maintenance drug therapy of panic disorder. J Psychiatr Res 1993;27(suppl 1):127–142.

56 Rickels K, Schweizer E: Panic disorder: Long-term pharmacotherapy and discontinuation. J Clin Psychopharmacol 1998;18:12S–18S.

57 Johnston DG, Troyer IE, Whitsett SF: Clomipramine treatment of agoraphobic women. An eight-week controlled trial. Arch Gen Psychiatry 1988;45:453–459.

58 Bandelow B, Broocks A, Pekrun G, George A, Meyer T, Pralle L, Bartmann U, Hillmer-Vogel U, Ruther E: The use of the panic and agoraphobia scale (P & A) in a controlled clinical trial. Pharmacopsychiatry 2000;33:174–181.

59 Cassano GB, Petracca A, Perugi G, Nisita C, Musetti L, Mengali F, McNair DM: Clomipramine for panic disorder. I. The first 10 weeks of a long-term comparison with imipramine. J Affect Disord 1988;14: 123–127.

60 Modigh K, Westberg P, Eriksson E: Superiority of clomipramine over imipramine in the treatment of panic disorder: a placebo-controlled trial. J Clin Psychopharmacol 1992;12:251–261.

61 Fahy TJ, O'Rourke D, Brophy J, Schazmann W, Sciascia S: The Galway study of panic disorder. I. Clomipramine and lofepramine in DSM III-R panic disorder: a placebo controlled trial. J Affect Disord 1992;25:63–75.

62 Lydiard RB, Morton WA, Emmanuel NP, Zealberg JJ, Laraia MT, Stuart GW, O'Neil PM, Ballenger JC: Preliminary report: placebo-controlled, double-blind study of the clinical and metabolic effects of desipramine in panic disorder. Psychopharmacol Bull 1993;29:183–188.

63 Ballenger JC, Burrows GD, DuPont RL Jr, Lesser IM, Noyes R Jr, Pecknold JC, Rifkin A, Swinson RP: Alprazolam in panic disorder and agoraphobia: results from a multicenter trial. I. Efficacy in short-term treatment. Arch Gen Psychiatry 1988;45:413–422.

64 Lydiard RB, Lesser IM, Ballenger JC, Rubin RT, Laraia M, DuPont R: A fixed-dose study of alprazolam 2 mg, alprazolam 6 mg, and placebo in panic disorder. J Clin Psychopharmacol 1992;12:96–103.

65 Noyes R Jr, Burrows GD, Reich JH, Judd FK, Garvey MJ, Norman TR, Cook BL, Marriott P: Diazepam versus alprazolam for the treatment of panic disorder. J Clin Psychiatry 1996;57:349–355.

66 Andersch S, Rosenberg NK, Kullingsjo H, Ottosson JO, Bech P, Bruun-Hansen J, Hanson L, Lorentzen K, Mellergard M, Rasmussen S, et al: Efficacy and safety of alprazolam, imipramine and placebo in treating panic disorder. A Scandinavian multicenter study. Acta Psychiatr Scand Suppl 1991;365:18–27.

67 Dyukova GM, Shepeleva IP, Vorob'eva OV: Treatment of negative crises (panic attacks). Neurosci Behav Physiol 1992;22:343–345.

68 Beauclair L, Fontaine R, Annable L, Holobow N, Chouinard G: Clonazepam in the treatment of panic disorder – a double-blind, placebo-controlled trial investigating the correlation between clonazepam concentrations in plasma and clinical-response. J Clin Psychopharmacol 1994;14:111–118.

69 Moroz G, Rosenbaum JF: Efficacy, safety, and gradual discontinuation of clonazepam in panic disorder: a placebo-controlled, multicenter study using optimized dosages. J Clin Psychiatry 1999;60:604–612.

70 Rosenbaum JF, Moroz G, Bowden CL: Clonazepam in the treatment of panic disorder with or without agoraphobia: a dose-response study of efficacy, safety, and discontinuance. Clonazepam panic disorder dose-response study group. J Clin Psychopharmacol 1997;17:390–400.

71 Tesar GE, Rosenbaum JF, Pollack MH, Otto MW, Sachs GS, Herman JB, Cohen LS, Spier SA: Double-blind, placebo-controlled comparison of clonazepam and alprazolam for panic disorder. J Clin Psychiatry 1991;52:69–76.

72 Dunner DL, Ishiki D, Avery DH, Wilson LG, Hyde TS: Effect of alprazolam and diazepam on anxiety and panic attacks in panic disorder: a controlled study. J Clin Psychiatry 1986;47:458–460.

73 Charney DS, Woods SW: Benzodiazepine treatment of panic disorder: a comparison of alprazolam and lorazepam. J Clin Psychiatry 1989;50:418–423.

74 Schweizer E, Pohl R, Balon R, Fox I, Rickels K, Yeragani VK: Lorazepam vs alprazolam in the treatment of panic disorder. Pharmacopsychiatry 1990;23:90–93.

75 Schweizer E, Rickels K, Case WG, Greenblatt DJ: Long-term therapeutic use of benzodiazepines. II. Effects of gradual taper. Arch Gen Psychiatry 1990; 47:908–915.

76 Rickels K, Schweizer E, Case WG, Greenblatt DJ: Long-term therapeutic use of benzodiazepines. I. Effects of abrupt discontinuation. Arch Gen Psychiatry 1990;47:899–907, erratum Arch Gen Psychiatry 1991;48:51.

77 Smith DE, Landry MJ: Benzodiazepine dependency discontinuation: focus on the chemical dependency detoxification setting and benzodiazepine-polydrug abuse. J Psychiatr Res 1990;24(suppl 2):145–156.

78 Bradwejn J: Benzodiazepines for the treatment of panic disorder and generalized anxiety disorder: clinical issues and future directions. Can J Psychiatry 1993;38(suppl 4):S109–S113.

79 Shader RI, Greenblatt DJ: Use of benzodiazepines in anxiety disorders. N Engl J Med 1993;13:1398–1405.

80 Livingston MG: Benzodiazepine dependence. Br J Hosp Med 1994;51:281–286.

81 Nelson J, Chouinard G: Guidelines for the clinical use of benzodiazepines: pharmacokinetics, dependency, rebound and withdrawal. Canadian Society for Clinical Pharmacology. Can J Clin Pharmacol 1999;6:69–83.

82 Schweizer E, Rickels K, De Martinis N, Case G, Garcia-Espana F: The effect of personality on withdrawal severity and taper outcome in benzodiazepine dependent patients. Psychol Med 1998;28:713–720.

83 Rickels K: Benzodiazepines in the treatment of anxiety. Am J Psychother 1982;36:358–370.

84 Otto MW, Pollack MH, Sachs GS, Reiter SR, Meltzer-Brody S, Rosenbaum JF: Discontinuation of benzodiazepine treatment: efficacy of cognitive-behavioral therapy for patients with panic disorder. Am J Psychiatry 1993;150:1485–1490.

85 Spiegel DA: Psychological strategies for discontinuing benzodiazepine treatment. J Clin Psychopharmacol 1999;19:17S–22S.

86 Pollack MH, Simon NM, Worthington JJ, Doyle AL, Peters P, Toshkov F, Otto MW: Combined paroxetine and clonazepam treatment strategies compared to paroxetine monotherapy for panic disorder. J Psychopharmacol (Oxford) 2003;17:276–282.

87 Woods SW, Nagy LM, Koleszar AS, Krystal JH, Heninger GR, Charney DS: Controlled trial of alprazolam supplementation during imipramine treatment of panic disorder. J Clin Psychopharmacol 1992;12: 32–38.

88 Goddard AW, Brouette T, Almai A, Jetty P, Woods SW, Charney D: Early coadministration of clonazepam with sertraline for panic disorder. Arch Gen Psychiatry 2001;58:681–686.

89 Sheehan DV, Ballenger J, Jacobsen G: Treatment of endogenous anxiety with phobic, hysterical, and hypochondriacal symptoms. Arch Gen Psychiatry 1980;37:51–59.

90 Kruger MB, Dahl AA: The efficacy and safety of moclobemide compared to clomipramine in the treatment of panic disorder. Eur Arch Psychiatry Clin Neurosci 1999;249(suppl 1):S19–S24.

91 Loerch B, Graf-Morgenstern M, Hautzinger M, Schlegel S, Hain C, Sandmann J, Benkert O: Randomised placebo-controlled trial of moclobemide, cognitive-behavioural therapy and their combination in panic disorder with agoraphobia. Br J Psychiatry 1999;174:205–212.

92 Uhlenhuth EH, Warner TD, Matuzas W: Interactive model of therapeutic response in panic disorder: moclobemide, a case in point. J Clin Psychopharmacol 2002;22:275–284.

93 Versiani M, Cassano G, Perugi G, Benedetti A, Mastalli L, Nardi A, Savino M: Reboxetine, a selective norepinephrine reuptake inhibitor, is an effective and well-tolerated treatment for panic disorder. J Clin Psychiatry 2002;63:31–37.

94 Seedat S, van Rheede van Oudtshoorn E, Muller JE, Mohr N, Stein DJ: Reboxetine and citalopram in panic disorder: a single-blind, cross-over, flexible-dose pilot study. Int Clin Psychopharmacol 2003; 18:279–284.

95 Bertani A, Perna G, Migliarese G, Di Pasquale D, Cucchi M, Caldirola D, Bellodi L: Comparison of the treatment with paroxetine and reboxetine in panic disorder: a randomized, single-blind study. Pharmacopsychiatry 2004;37:206–210.

96 Ribeiro L, Busnello JV, Kauer-Sant'Anna M, Madruga M, Quevedo J, Busnello EA, Kapczinski F: Mirtazapine versus fluoxetine in the treatment of panic disorder. Braz J Med Biol Res 2001;34:1303–1307.

97 Carpenter LL, Leon Z, Yasmin S, Price LH: Clinical experience with mirtazapine in the treatment of panic disorder. Ann Clin Psychiatry 1999;11:81–86.

98 Sheehan DV, Raj AB, Harnett-Sheehan K, Soto S, Knapp E: The relative efficacy of high-dose buspirone and alprazolam in the treatment of panic disorder: a double-blind placebo-controlled study. Acta Psychiatr Scand 1993;88:1–11.

99 Schweizer E, Rickels K: Buspirone in the treatment of panic disorder: a controlled pilot comparison with clorazepate (letter). J Clin Psychopharmacol 1988;8:303.

100 Sheehan DV, Davidson J, Manschreck T, Van Wyck Fleet J: Lack of efficacy of a new antidepressant (bupropion) in the treatment of panic disorder with phobias. J Clin Psychopharmacol 1983;3:28–31.

101 Simon NM, Emmanuel N, Ballenger J, Worthington JJ, Kinrys G, Korbly NB, Farach FJ, Pollack MH: Bupropion sustained release for panic disorder. Psychopharmacol Bull 2003;37:66–72.

102 Munjack DJ, Crocker B, Cabe D, Brown R, Usigli R, Zulueta A, McManus M, McDowell D, Palmer R, Leonard M: Alprazolam, propranolol, and placebo in the treatment of panic disorder and agoraphobia with panic attacks. J Clin Psychopharmacology 1989;9:22–27.

103 Noyes R Jr, Anderson DJ, Clancy J, Crowe RR, Slymen DJ, Ghoneim MM, Hinrichs JV: Diazepam and propranolol in panic disorder and agoraphobia. Arch Gen Psychiatry 1984;41:287–292.

104 Ravaris CL, Friedman MJ, Hauri PJ, McHugo GJ: A controlled study of alprazolam and propranolol in panic-disordered and agoraphobic outpatients. J Clin Psychopharmacol 1991;11:344–350.

105 Lum M, Fontaine R, Elie R, Ontiveros A: Divalproex sodium's antipanic effect in panic disorder: a placebo-controlled study. Biol Psychiatry 1990;27:164A–165A.

106 Primeau F, Fontaine R, Beauclair L: Valproic acid and panic disorder. Can J Psychiatry 1990;35:248–250.

107 Keck PE Jr, Taylor VE, Tugrul KC, McElroy SL, Bennett JA: Valproate treatment of panic disorder and lactate-induced panic attacks. Biol Psychiatry 1993;33:542–546.

108 Woodman CL, Noyes R Jr: Panic disorder: treatment with valproate. J Clin Psychiatry 1994;55:134–136.

109 Zwanzger P, Baghai TC, Schule C, Minov C, Padberg F, Moller HJ, Rupprecht R: Tiagabine improves panic and agoraphobia in panic disorder patients. J Clin Psychiatry 2001;62:656–657.

110 Zwanzger P, Baghai T, Boerner RJ, Moller HJ, Rupprecht R: Anxiolytic effects of vigabatrin in panic disorder. J Clin Psychopharmacol 2001;21:539–540.

111 Pande AC, Pollack MH, Crockatt J, Greiner M, Chouinard G, Lydiard RB, Taylor CB, Dager SR, Shiovitz T: Placebo-controlled study of gabapentin treatment of panic disorder. J Clin Psychopharmacol 2000;20:467–471.

112 Benjamin J, Levine J, Fux M, Aviv A, Levy D, Belmaker RH: Double-blind, placebo-controlled, crossover trial of inositol treatment for panic disorder. Am J Psychiatry 1995;152:1084–1086.

113 Palatnik A, Frolov K, Fux M, Benjamin J: Double-blind, controlled, crossover trial of inositol versus fluvoxamine for the treatment of panic disorder. J Clin Psychopharmacol 2001;21:335–339.

114 Schneier FR, Garfinkel R, Kennedy B, Campeas R, Fallon B, Marshall R, O'Donnell L, Hogan T, Liebowitz MR: Ondansetron in the treatment of panic disorder. Anxiety 1996;2:199–202.

115 American Psychiatric Association: Practice guideline for the treatment of patients with panic disorder. Work group on panic disorder. American Psychiatric Association. Am J Psychiatry 1998;155:1–34.

116 Mavissakalian M, Perel JM: Clinical experiments in maintenance and discontinuation of imipramine therapy in panic disorder with agoraphobia. Arch Gen Psychiatry 1992;49:318–323.

117 Cavaljuga S, Licanin I, Kapic E, Potkonjak D: Clomipramine and fluoxetine effects in the treatment of panic disorder. Bosn J Basic Med Sci 2003;3:27–31.

118 Perna G, Bertani A, Caldirola D, Smeraldi E, Bellodi L: A comparison of citalopram and paroxetine in the treatment of panic disorder: a randomized, single-blind study. Pharmacopsychiatry 2001;34:85–90.

119 Boyer W: Serotonin uptake inhibitors are superior to imipramine and alprazolam in alleviating panic attacks: a meta-analysis. Int Clin Psychopharmacol 1995;10:45–49.

120 Rizley R, Kahn RJ, McNair DM, Frankenthaler LM: A comparison of alprazolam and imipramine in the treatment of agoraphobia and panic disorder. Psychopharmacol Bull 1986;22:167–172.

121 Charney DS, Woods SW, Goodman WK, Rifkin B, Kinch M, Aiken B, Quadrino LM, Heninger GR: Drug treatment of panic disorder: the comparative efficacy of imipramine, alprazolam, and trazodone. J Clin Psychiatry 1986;47:580–586.

122 Lepola U, Heikkinen H, Rimon R, Riekkinen P: Clinical evaluation of alprazolam in patients with panic disorder a double-blind comparison with imipramine. Hum Psychopharmacol 1990;5:159–163.

123 Taylor CB, Hayward C, King R, Ehlers A, Margraf J, Maddock R, Clark D, Roth WT, Agras WS: Cardiovascular and symptomatic reduction effects of alprazolam and imipramine in patients with panic disorder: results of a double-blind, placebo-controlled trial. J Clin Psychopharmacol 1990;10:112–118.

124 Alwan S, Reefhuis J, Rasmussen SA, Olney RS, Friedman JM: Use of selective serotonin-reuptake inhibitors in pregnancy and the risk of birth defects. N Engl J Med 2007;356:2684–2692.

125 Kallen BA, Otterblad Olausson P: Maternal use of selective serotonin re-uptake inhibitors in early pregnancy and infant congenital malformations. Birth Defects Res A Clin Mol Teratol 2007;79:301–308.

126 Malm H, Klaukka T, Neuvonen PJ: Risks associated with selective serotonin reuptake inhibitors in pregnancy. Obstet Gynecol 2005;106:1289–1296.

127 Lattimore KA, Donn SM, Kaciroti N, Kemper AR, Neal CR Jr, Vazquez DM: Selective serotonin reuptake inhibitor (SSRI) use during pregnancy and effects on the fetus and newborn: a meta-analysis. J Perinatol 2005;25:595–604.

128 Nordeng H, Spigset O: Treatment with selective serotonin reuptake inhibitors in the third trimester of pregnancy: effects on the infant. Drug Saf 2005;28:565–581.

129 Koren G, Matsui D, Einarson A, Knoppert D, Steiner M: Is maternal use of selective serotonin reuptake inhibitors in the third trimester of pregnancy harmful to neonates? CMAJ 2005;172:1457–1459.

130 Hogberg U, Wang M: Depression and pregnancy – may selective serotonin reuptake inhibitors be associated to behavioural teratogenicity? Comment on 'The obstetrician and depression during pregnancy' by Campagne DM [Eur J Obstet Gynecol Reprod Biol 2004;116:125–130]. Eur J Obstet Gynecol Reprod Biol 2005;120:123–124.

131 Austin MPV, Mitchell PB: Psychotropic medications in pregnant women: treatment dilemmas. Med J Aust 1998;169:428–431.

132 Ericson A, Kallen B, Wiholm BE: Delivery outcome after the use of antidepressants in early pregnancy. Eur J Clinl Pharmacol 1999;55:503–508.

133 Misri S, Kostaras D, Kostaras X: The use of selective serotonin reuptake inhibitors during pregnancy and lactation: current knowledge. Can J Psychiat 2000;45:285–287.

134 Misri S, Burgmann A, Kostaras D: Are SSRIs safe for pregnant and breastfeeding women? Can Fam Physician 2000;46:626–628, 631–623.

135 Emslie G, Judge R: Tricyclic antidepressants and selective serotonin reuptake inhibitors: use during pregnancy, in children/adolescents and in the elderly. Acta Psychiatr Scand 2000;101:26–34.

136 Altshuler LL, Cohen LS, Moline ML, Kahn DA, Carpenter D, Docherty JP: The Expert Consensus Guideline Series. Treatment of depression in women. Postgrad Med 2001(Spec No):1–107.

137 ACOG Committee on Obstetric Practice: ACOG Committee Opinion No. 354: Treatment with selective serotonin reuptake inhibitors during pregnancy. Obstet Gynecol 2006;108:1601–1603.

138 Goldstein DJ, Sundell K: A review of the safety of selective serotonin reuptake inhibitors during pregnancy. Hum Psychopharmacol 1999;14:319–324.

139 Nulman I, Rovet J, Stewart DE, Wolpin J, Pace-Asciak P, Shuhaiber S, Koren G: Child development following exposure to tricyclic antidepressants or fluoxetine throughout fetal life: a prospective, controlled study. Am J Psychiatry 2002;159:1889–1895.

140 Laegreid L, Olegard R, Conradi N, Hagberg G, Wahlstrom J, Abrahamsson L: Congenital malformations and maternal consumption of benzodiazepines: a case-control study. Dev Med Child Neurol 1990;32:432–441.

141 Iqbal MM, Sobhan T, Ryals T: Effects of commonly used benzodiazepines on the fetus, the neonate, and the nursing infant. Psychiatr Serv 2002;53:39–49.

142 Simpson K, Noble S: Fluoxetine – a review of its use in women's health. CNS Drugs 2000;14:301–328.

143 Spigset O, Hägg S: Excretion of psychotropic drugs into breast milk – pharmacokinetic overview and therapeutic implications. CNS Drugs 1998;9:111–134.

144 Gentile S, Rossi A, Bellantuono C: SSRIs during breastfeeding: spotlight on milk-to-plasma ratio. Arch Womens Ment Health 2007;10:39–51.

145 Bandelow B: Epidemiology of depression and anxiety; in Kasper S, den Boer JA, Sitsen AJM (eds): Handbook on Depression and Anxiety. New York, M Dekker, 2003, pp 49–68.

146 Rampello L, Alvano A, Raffaele R, Malaguarnera M, Vecchio I: New possibilities of treatment for panic attacks in elderly patients: escitalopram versus citalopram. J Clin Psychopharmacol 2006;26: 67–70.

147 Hirschmann S, Dannon PN, Iancu I, Dolberg OT, Zohar J, Grunhaus L: Pindolol augmentation in patients with treatment-resistant panic disorder: a double-blind, placebo-controlled trial. J Clin Psychopharmacol 2000;20:556–559.

148 Tiffon L, Coplan JD, Papp LA, Gorman JM: Augmentation strategies with tricyclic or fluoxetine treatment in seven partially responsive panic disorder patients. J Clin Psychiatry 1994;55:66–69.

149 Ontiveros A, Fontaine R: Sodium valproate and clonazepam for treatment-resistant panic disorder. J Psychiatry Neurosci 1992;17:78–80.

150 Cournoyer J: Rapid response of a disorder to the addition of lithium carbonate: panic resistant to tricyclic antidepressants (in French). Can J Psychiatry 1986;31:335–338.

151 Etxebeste M, Aragüés E, Malo P, Pacheco L: Olanzapine and panic attacks. Am J Psychiatry 2000; 157:659–660.

152 Khaldi S, Kornreich C, Dan B, Pelc I: Usefulness of olanzapine in refractory panic attacks. J Clin Psychopharmacol 2003;23:100–101.

153 Baldwin DS, Ajel K: The role of pregabalin in the treatment of generalized anxiety disorder. Neuropsychiatr Dis Treat 2007;3:185–191.

154 Bandelow B, Wedekind D, Leon T: Pregabalin for the treatment of generalized anxiety disorder: a novel pharmacologic intervention. Expert Rev Neurother 2007;7:769–781.

155 Bandelow B, Chouinard G, Bobes J, Ahokas A, Eggens I, Liu S, Eriksson H: Extended-release quetiapine fumarate (quetiapine XR): a once-daily monotherapy effective in generalized anxiety disorder. Data from a randomized, double-blind, placebo- and active-controlled study. Int J Neuropsychopharmacol 2010;13:305–320.

156 Pollack MH, Otto MW, Kaspi SP, Hammerness PG, Rosenbaum JF: Cognitive behavior therapy for treatment-refractory panic disorder. J Clin Psychiatry 1994;55:200–205.

157 Otto MW, Pollack MH, Penava SJ, Zucker BG: Group cognitive-behavior therapy for patients failing to respond to pharmacotherapy for panic disorder: a clinical case series. Behav Res Ther 1999;37: 763–770.

158 Heldt E, Manfro GG, Kipper L, Blaya C, Maltz S, Isolan L, Hirakata VN, Otto MW: Treating medication-resistant panic disorder: predictors and outcome of cognitive-behavior therapy in a Brazilian public hospital. Psychother Psychosom 2003;72: 43–48.

Prof. Dr. Borwin Bandelow
Department of Psychiatry and Psychotherapy, University of Göttingen
von-Siebold-Strasse 5
DE–37075 Göttingen (Germany)
E-Mail sekretariat.bandelow@med.uni-goettingen.de

Baldwin DS, Leonard BE (eds): Anxiety Disorders.
Mod Trends Pharmacopsychiatry. Basel, Karger, 2013, vol 29, pp 144–153 (DOI: 10.1159/000351960)

Pharmacological Treatment of Social Anxiety Disorder

Vasilios G. Masdrakis[a] · Darko Turic[b] · David S. Baldwin[b, c]

[a]First Department of Psychiatry, Eginition Hospital, Athens University Medical School, Athens, Greece;
[b]Clinical and Experimental Sciences Academic Unit, Faculty of Medicine, University of Southampton,
Southampton, UK; [c]Department of Psychiatry and Mental Health, University of Cape Town, Cape Town,
South Africa

Abstract

Social anxiety disorder (social phobia) is a common and typically long-standing medical condition, characterized by an excessive fear of being observed or evaluated negatively in social or performance situations. Efficacious interventions in acute treatment include cognitive behavioural therapy and a range of medications including many antidepressants, some benzodiazepines and anticonvulsants, and the antipsychotic olanzapine. Most studies report no significant differences in overall efficacy or tolerability between active compounds. Responders to previous acute treatment benefit from continuing active medication for 6 months. Evidence of a dose-response relationship with antidepressant drugs is inconsistent, though only higher doses of pregabalin are efficacious. Switching between treatments with proven efficacy may be helpful. Augmentation of a selective serotonin reuptake inhibitor with buspirone or clonazepam can be beneficial. It is unlikely that combining pharmacotherapy with psychotherapy results in greater overall efficacy compared to either treatment given alone. Proof-of-concept and other preliminary studies suggest the efficacy of psychotherapy can be enhanced through prior administration of D-cycloserine, cannabidiol, or oxytocin.

Clinical Features

Social anxiety disorder (SAD) is characterized by a marked, persistent and unreasonable fear of being observed or evaluated negatively by other people in social or performance situations, which is associated with physical and psychological anxiety symptoms. Feared situations (such as speaking to unfamiliar people or eating in public) are either avoided or are endured with significant personal distress (avoidance must be prominent for ICD-10 diagnosis). Epidemiological studies in the general population indicate that it has a 12-month prevalence of between 1.1 and 4.4% [1]. The disorder tends to run a chronic course in primary [2] and secondary medical care settings [3, 4].

Recognition and Diagnosis

Social phobia is often not recognized in primary medical care [5], but detection can be enhanced through the use of screening questionnaires in psychologically distressed primary care patients [6, 7]. Social phobia is often misconstrued as mere 'shyness' but can be distinguished from shyness by the higher levels of personal distress, more severe symptoms and greater impairment [8, 9]. The generalized subtype is associated with greater disability and higher comorbidity, but patients with the non-generalized subtype can be substantially impaired [10, 11]. Social phobia is hard to distinguish from avoidant personality disorder, which may represent a more severe form of the same condition [12]. Patients with social phobia often present with symptoms arising from comorbid conditions (especially depression), rather than with anxiety symptoms and avoidance of social and performance situations [13]. There are strong, and possibly two-way, associations between social phobia and dependence on alcohol and cannabis [14, 15].

Social Anxiety and Psychosis

SAD is more frequent in patients with schizophrenia than in controls [16, 17], and social anxiety may arise as a consequence of psychosis in some individuals [18]. A meta-analysis of 52 studies in patients (n = 4,032) with schizophrenia or related disorders found it to be the anxiety disorder most often (14.9%) comorbid with psychosis [19]. Reported point prevalence varies between 8.2% in inpatients [20] and 36.3% in outpatients [21]. An investigation in patients with first-episode psychosis found that 25% met the criteria for SAD, with a further 11.6% having problems in social interactions that warrant clinical intervention; social anxiety is not necessarily related to 'positive' psychotic symptoms [22]. Social anxiety symptoms are associated with greater illness severity and adversely affect the course of schizophrenia [23], with positive correlations between the presence of comorbidity and Positive and Negative Syndrome Scale (PANSS) total score, between social anxiety fear symptoms and PANSS positive subscales, and between social anxiety avoidance symptoms and 'negative' symptoms [24]. Individuals with poor interpersonal skills are less likely to be successful in social encounters and are less likely to be motivated to engage in them [25]. Unfortunately, comorbid SAD is often not recognized in patients with schizophrenia, perhaps due to a common misconception that social withdrawal is either due to negative symptoms or to the behavioural consequences of positive symptoms [26, 27]; the use of the Liebowitz Social Anxiety Scale can be helpful in identifying the co-morbid condition [21, 27].

Presumed Neuropsychobiology

As with other anxiety disorders, many influences are likely to be involved in the development and maintenance of social anxiety symptoms in an affected individual, and the aetiology of the condition probably involves an interplay of multiple factors. For example, possession of the short allele of the human serotonin transporter gene promoter polymorphism is associated with greater activity in the right amygdala during a public speech test [28], and with a poorer response to treatment with a selective serotonin reuptake inhibitor (SSRI) [29]. The efficacy of a range of SSRIs in treating SAD [30, 31], and the finding of lower $5\text{-}HT_{1A}$ receptor binding potential [32] together suggest that serotonergic neurotransmission may be attenuated. Parkinson's disease is associated with an increased risk of SAD [33], and patients with social anxiety have shown both significantly lower striatal dopamine D_2 receptor binding [34] and a significantly lower response in the left caudate nucleus during a striatal-dependent learning task [35]. However, not all evidence is suggestive of perturbed dopaminergic neurotransmission, as others have reported similar D_2 receptor binding potential and amphetamine-induced decrease in D_2 receptor binding in patients with SAD and controls [36]. Dysregulation of the HPA axis is probably limited to a subgroup of patients (for example those who endured child abuse during childhood) [37].

Patients with more severe forms of illness show evidence of higher plasma levels of oxytocin (a neuropeptide thought to be involved in social behaviour) [38].

Neuroimaging studies suggest a greater 'threat-signalling' faces-induced activation of the amygdala and other limbic and paralimbic regions, which is attenuated after treatment [39]. This amygdala excitability may partly result from the 'failure' of the prefrontal or anterior cingulate cortex to exert sufficient inhibitory influence through balanced cognitive evaluation of feared social cues; or conversely by excessive activity in frontocortical regions, corresponding to social anxiety-related cognitions [40]. The insula is also thought to play a key role in 'interoceptive awareness', and its hyperactivity may relate to the enhanced self-focus on SAD-specific bodily sensations which is known to characterize the condition [41].

Acute Treatment

The findings of meta-analyses and randomized placebo-controlled treatment studies indicate that a range of approaches are efficacious in acute treatment [31]. Cognitive behavioural therapy is efficacious in adults [42] and children [43]. Cognitive therapy appears superior to exposure therapy [44]. The evidence for the efficacy of social skill training is not strong [45]. Antidepressant drugs with proven efficacy include the SSRIs escitalopram, fluoxetine, fluvoxamine, paroxetine, and sertraline, the serotonin-noradrenaline reuptake inhibitor venlafaxine, the monoamine oxidase inhibitor phenelzine, and the reversible inhibitor of monoamine oxidase type A moclobemide; however, nefazodone is not efficacious, and the evidence for mirtazapine is inconsistent [46]. The potential efficacy of tricyclic antidepressants is unknown. Some benzodiazepines (bromazepam and clonazepam, but not alprazolam) and anticonvulsants (gabapentin and pregabalin, but not levetiracetam), and the antipsychotic olanzapine also appear efficacious [31]. Neither the 5-HT$_{1A}$ partial agonist buspirone nor the beta-blocker atenolol are efficacious in generalized social phobia [31], but the findings of small single-dose placebo-controlled crossover studies together suggest that beta-blockers can reduce anxiety symptoms in individuals with 'performance anxiety' (which overlaps with mild non-generalized social phobia) [31].

There have been few randomized comparator-controlled studies and most find no significant differences in overall efficacy or tolerability between active compounds. In randomized placebo- and comparator-controlled studies, phenelzine was superior to placebo, but atenolol was not [47]; phenelzine was superior to placebo, but alprazolam was not [48], and escitalopram was found superior to paroxetine [49]. Venlafaxine and paroxetine had similar overall efficacy in 2 randomized placebo-controlled studies [50, 51]. The findings of a meta-analytic review demonstrate that pharmacological and psychological treatments, when delivered singly, have broadly similar efficacy in acute treatment [52]. However, acute treatment with cognitive therapy (group or individual) is possibly associated with a reduced risk of symptomatic relapse at follow-up [52]. It is unlikely that the combination of pharmacological and psychological treatments is associated with greater overall efficacy than with either treatment when given alone as only 1 of 4 studies of the relative efficacy of combination treatment found evidence for superior efficacy [53].

Longer-Term Treatment

The proportion of responding patients increases steadily over time in acute treatment studies [31], and double-blind studies indicate that continuing SSRI or SNRI treatment from 12 weeks to 24 weeks is associated with an increase in overall treatment response rates [49, 54, 55]. A post hoc analysis of the clinical trial database with paroxetine indicates that many non-responders to treatment at 8 weeks become responders with a further 4 weeks of double-blind treatment [56]; however, a post hoc analysis of the clinical trial database for escitalopram suggests that a response is unlikely if there is no onset of clinical effect within the first 4 weeks of treatment [57]. The findings of randomized placebo-controlled relapse-prevention studies in patients who have responded to previous acute treatment show there is a significant advantage for staying on active medication (clonazepam, escitalopram, paroxetine, pregabalin, sertraline) for up to 6 months [31].

Further Management after Non-Response to Initial Treatment

The findings of fixed-dose randomized controlled trials do not provide consistent evidence of a dose-response relationship with antidepressant drugs; but a fixed-dose study of pregabalin found that only the higher daily dosage was efficacious [58]. A double-blind randomized controlled dosage escalation trial found no advantage for increasing to a higher daily dosage (120 mg) of duloxetine, when compared to continuing treatment with a lower (60 mg) dosage [59]. Switching between treatments with proven efficacy may be helpful [31]. An uncontrolled study of augmentation of SSRI treatment with buspirone found some evidence of beneficial effects [60]; but a placebo-controlled crossover study of the augmentation of paroxetine with pindolol found no evidence of efficacy [61]. A small placebo-controlled study of the augmentation of paroxetine with clonazepam found the combination was marginally short of superiority, when compared to paroxetine alone [62].

Treatment of Social Anxiety Symptoms in Psychosis

Maladaptive cognitions relating to social interactions are associated with worse social functioning in patients experiencing a first episode of psychotic illness [63], and social anxiety symptoms can worsen after discharge from hospital [64]. Fortunately, social anxiety symptoms in patients with psychotic illness are amenable to psychological interventions. Group-based cognitive behaviour therapy, comprising exposure and cognitive techniques and 'homework' assignments was found beneficial in 20 patients undergoing weekly 2-hour sessions over 8 weeks [65], and in 33 patients after 12 sessions [66]. The effects of pharmacological treatments are less certain; switching to aripiprazole was found beneficial in a small (n = 16) sample of patients, with some evidence of persistent benefit at 1-year follow-up [67]; clozapine treatment may worsen social anxiety symptoms, though these can be reduced through treatment with fluoxetine [68].

Potential Novel Pharmacological Treatments

Potential new pharmacological treatments may derive from the observations of studies examining the effects of D-cycloserine (DCS), oxytocin, and cannabidiol (CBD). For example, the extinction of conditioned fear is mediated by N-methyl-D-aspartate

(NMDA) receptors in the amygdala and medial prefrontal cortex, and accordingly the NMDA partial agonist DCS may hasten the onset of effect of exposure therapy [69]. In SAD, two randomized, double-blind, placebo-controlled trials suggest that DCS (50 mg) administered adjunctively to exposure therapy is associated with beneficial effects in reducing symptom severity, altering dysfunctional cognitions and reducing overall impairment [70, 71]. In individuals with specific phobia, augmentation of exposure therapy with DCS (50 mg) was found to lead to changes in prefrontal (especially ventromedial) cortex response to phobic stimuli [72], but these findings may not necessarily translate to patients with SAD.

Oxytocin nasal administration reduces social threat perception and enhances trust, empathy, attention and the encoding of positive social cues [73]. Two randomized, double-blind, placebo-controlled studies have evaluated the efficacy of intranasal oxytocin (24 IU = 40.32 µg) when administered as an adjunct to exposure therapy in individuals with social anxiety, and found evidence for enhanced positive evaluations of appearance and speech performance, although overall treatment outcome was not significantly affected [74]. Oxytocin administration in patients with generalized SAD was associated with attenuation of the heightened amygdala reactivity to fearful faces, and to normalization of amygdala hyperactivity [75].

CBD, a major constituent of *Cannabis sativa*, is thought to have anxiolytic properties. In a randomized, double-blind, placebo-controlled trial in patients with generalized SAD, pretreatment with CBD (600 mg) significantly reduced symptoms in a public speech simulation test, leading to a pattern of response that was similar to that with healthy controls [76]. In addition, neuroimaging studies suggest that a reduction of SAD-related anxiety in CBD (400 mg)-treated patients is associated with the effects of CBD on limbic and paralimbic areas (including the left parahippocampal gyrus, hippocampus, inferior temporal gyrus and right posterior cingulate gyrus) [77].

Conclusions

A range of pharmacological and psychological interventions are available for the treatment of patients with SAD. It remains uncertain whether combining current evidence-based pharmacological and psychological treatments is superior to giving either intervention alone. As with other anxiety disorders, overall response rates in real-world clinical practice can be disappointing, and it is not possible to reliably predict the likelihood of response in an individual patient. In addition, many patients experience unwanted side effects of treatment, and others experience a relapse of symptoms despite adhering to treatment. Little is known about the further management of patients who have not responded to first-line treatments, and about the management of patients in whom social phobia is a comorbid condition. There is much room for improvement in developing novel treatments with enhanced effectiveness and greater acceptability when compared to existing medications [78].

Acknowledgements

Secretarial and administrative assistance in writing this chapter was provided by Miss Magda Nowak, herself supported through a grant to the Anxiety Disorders Research Network from the European College of Neuropsychopharmacology Network Initiative.

References

1 Wittchen HU, Jacobi F, Rehm J, Gustavsson A, Svensson M, Jonsson B, Olesen J, Allgulander C, Alonso J, Faravelli C, Fratiglioni L, Jennum P, Lieb R, Maercker A, van Os J, Preisig M, Salvador-Carulla L, Simon R, Steinhausen HC: The size and burden of mental disorders and other disorders of the brain in Europe 2010. Eur Neuropsychopharmacol 2011; 21:655–679.

2 Beard C, Moitra E, Weisberg RB, Keller MB: Characteristics and predictors of social phobia course in a longitudinal study of primary-care patients. Depress Anxiety 2010;27:839–845.

3 Bruce SE, Yonkers KA, Otto MW, Eisen JL, Weisberg RB, Pagano M, Shea MT, Keller MB: Influence of psychiatric comorbidity on recovery and recurrence in generalized anxiety disorder, social phobia, and panic disorder: a 12-year prospective study. Am J Psychiatry 2005;162:1179–1187.

4 Ramsawh HJ, Raffa SD, Edelen MO, Rende R, Keller MB: Anxiety in middle adulthood: effects of age and time on the 14-year course of panic disorder, social phobia and generalized anxiety disorder. Psychol Med 2009;39:615–624.

5 Weiller E, Bisserbe C, Boyer P, Lepine JP, Lecrubier Y: Social phobia in general health care – an unrecognised undertreated disabling disorder. Br J Psychiatry 1996;168:169–174.

6 Terluin B, Brouwers EPM, van Marwijk HWJ, Verhaak PFM, van der Horst HE: Detecting depressive and anxiety disorders in distressed patients in primary care; comparative diagnostic accuracy of the Four-Dimensional Symptom Questionnaire (4DSQ) and the Hospital Anxiety and Depression Scale (HADS). BMC Fam Pract 2009;10:58.

7 Donker T, Comijs H, Cuijpers P, Terluin B, Nolen W, Zitman F, Penninx B: The validity of the Dutch K10 and extended K10 screening scales for depressive and anxiety disorders. Psychiatry Res 2010;176: 45–50.

8 Heiser NA, Turner SM, Beidel DC, Roberson-Nay R: Differentiating social phobia from shyness. J Anxiety Disord 2009;23:469–476.

9 Burstein M, Ameli-Grillon L, Merikangas KR: Shyness versus social phobia in US youth. Pediatrics 2011;128:917–925.

10 Wong N, Sarver DE, Beidel DC: Quality of life impairments among adults with social phobia: the impact of subtype. J Anxiety Disord 2012;26:50–57.

11 Aderka IM, Hofmann SG, Nickerson A, Hermesh H, Gilboa-Schechtman E, Marom S: Functional impairment in social anxiety disorder. J Anxiety Disord 2012;26:393–400.

12 Reich J: Avoidant personality disorder and its relationship to social phobia. Curr Psychiatry Rep 2009; 11:89–93.

13 Stein MB, McQuaid JR, Laffaye C, McCahill ME: Social phobia in the primary care medical setting. J Fam Pract 1999;48:514–519.

14 Buckner JD, Schmidt NB, Lang AR, Small JW, Schlauch RC, Lewinsohn PM: Specificity of social anxiety disorder as a risk factor for alcohol and cannabis dependence. J Psychiatry Res 2008;42:230–239.

15 Robinson J, Sareen J, Cox BJ, Bolton JM, Longitudinal I: Role of self-medication in the development of comorbid anxiety and substance use disorders a longitudinal investigation. Arch Gen Psychiatry 2011; 68:800–807.

16 Pilkonis PA, Feldman H, Himmelhoch J, Cornes C: Social anxiety and psychiatric diagnosis. J Nerv Ment Dis 1980;168:13–18.

17 Braga RJ, Petrides G, Figueira I: Anxiety disorders in schizophrenia. Compr Psychiatry 2004;45:460–468.

18 Birchwood M, Trower P: The future of cognitive-behavioural therapy for psychosis: not a quasi-neuroleptic. Br J Psychiatry 2006;188:107–108.

19 Achim A, Maziade M, Raymond E, Olivier D, Mérette C, Roy M: How prevalent are anxiety disorders in schizophrenia? A meta-analysis and critical review on a significant association. Schizophr Bull 2011;37:811–821.

20 Goodwin G: Evidence-based guidelines for treating bipolar disorder: recommendations from the British association for psychopharmacology. J Psychopharmacol 2003;17:149–173.

21 Pallanti S, Quercioli L, Hollander E: Social anxiety in outpatients with schizophrenia: a relevant cause of disability. Am J Psychiatry 2004;161:53–58.

22 Michail M, Birchwood M: Social anxiety disorder in first-episode psychosis: incidence, phenomenology and relationship with paranoia. Br J Psychiatry 2009; 195:234–241.

23 Ciapparelli A, Paggini R, Marazziti D, Carmassi C, Bianchi M, Taponecco C, Consoli G, Lombardi V, Massimetti G, Dell'Osso L: Comorbidity with axis I anxiety disorders in remitted psychotic patients 1 year after hospitalization. CNS Spectr 2007;12:913–919.

24 Mazeh D, Bodner E, Weizman R, Delayahu Y, Cholostoy A, Martin T, Barak Y: Co-morbid social phobia in schizophrenia. Int J Soc Psychiatry 2009;55: 198–202.

25 Barrowclough C, Tarrier N, Humphreys L, Ward J, Gregg L, Andrews B: Self-esteem in schizophrenia: relationships between self-evaluation, family attitudes, and symptomatology. J Abnorm Psychol 2003; 112:92–99.

26 Cosoff SJ, Hafner RJ: The prevalence of comorbid anxiety in schizophrenia, schizoaffective disorder and bipolar disorder. Aust N Z J Psychiatry 1998;32: 67–72.

27 Romm KL, Rossberg JI, Berg AO, Hansen CF, Andreassen OA, Melle I: Assessment of social anxiety in first episode psychosis using the Liebowitz Social Anxiety Scale as a self-report measure. Eur Psychiatry 2011;26:115–121.

28 Furmark T, Tillfors M, Garpenstrand H, Marteinsdottir I, Langstrom B, Oreland L, Fredrikson M: Serotonin transporter polymorphism related to amygdala excitability and symptom severity in patients with social phobia. Neurosci Lett 2004;362:189–192.

29 Stein MB, Seedat S, Gelernter J: Serotonin transporter gene promoter polymorphism predicts SSRI response in generalized social anxiety disorder. Psychopharmacology 2006;187:68–72.

30 Ipser JC, Kariuki CM, Stein DJ: Pharmacotherapy for social anxiety disorder: a systematic review. Expert Rev Neurother 2008;8:235–257.

31 Blanco C, Bragdon LB, Schneier FR, Liebowitz MR: The evidence-based pharmacotherapy of social anxiety disorder. Int J Neuropsychopharmacol 2013;16: 235–249.

32 Lanzenberger RR, Mitterhauser M, Spindelegger C, Wadsak W, Klein N, Mien L-K, Holik A, Attarbaschi T, Mossaheb N, Sacher J, Geiss-Granadia T, Kletter K, Kasper S, Tauscher J: Reduced serotonin-1a receptor binding in social anxiety disorder. Biol Psychiatry 2007;61:1081–1089.

33 Richard IH, Schiffer RB, Kurlan R: Anxiety and Parkinson's disease. J Neuropsychiatry Clin Neurosci 1996;8:383–392.

34 Schneier FR, Liebowitz MR, Abi-Dargham A, Zea-Ponce Y, Lin SH, Laruelle M: Low dopamine D-2 receptor binding potential in social phobia. Am J Psychiatry 2000;157:457–459.

35 Sareen J, Campbell DW, Leslie WD, Malisza KL, Stein MB, Paulus MP, Kravetsky LB, Kjernisted KD, Walker JR, Reiss JP: Striatal function in generalized social phobia: a functional magnetic resonance imaging study. Biol Psychiatry 2007;61:396–404.

36 Schneier FR, Abi-Dargham A, Martinez D, Slifstein M, Hwang D-R, Liebowitz MR, Laruelle M: Dopamine transporters, D2 receptors, and dopamine release in generalized social anxiety disorder. Depress Anxiety 2009;26:411–418.

37 Phan K, Klumpp H: Neuroendocrinology and neuroimaging studies of social anxiety disorder; in Hofmann S, DiBartolo P (eds): Social Anxiety: Clinical, Developmental, and Social Perspectives. London, Elsevier, 2010, pp 273–312.

38 Hoge EA, Pollack MH, Kaufman RE, Zak PJ, Simon NM: Oxytocin levels in social anxiety disorder. CNS Neurosci Ther 2008;14:165–170.

39 Freitas-Ferrari MC, Hallak JEC, Trzesniak C, Santos Filho A, Machado-de-Sousa JP, Chagas MHN, Nardi AE, Crippa JAS: Neuroimaging in social anxiety disorder: a systematic review of the literature. Prog Neuropsychopharmacol Biol Psychiatry 2010;34: 565–580.

40 Furmark T: Neurobiological aspects of social anxiety disorder. Isr J Psychiatry Relat Sci 2009;46:5–12.

41 Etkin A, Wager TD: Functional neuroimaging of anxiety: a meta-analysis of emotional processing in PTSD, social anxiety disorder, and specific phobia. Am J Psychiatry 2007;164:1476–1488.

42 Hofmann SG, Smits JAJ: Cognitive-behavioral therapy for adult anxiety disorders: a meta-analysis of randomized placebo-controlled trials. J Clin Psychiatry 2008;69:621–632.

43 James A, Soler A, Weatherall R: Cognitive behavioural therapy for anxiety disorders in children and adolescents. Cochrane Database Syst Rev 2005; CD004690.

44 Ougrin D: Efficacy of exposure versus cognitive therapy in anxiety disorders: systematic review and meta-analysis. BMC Psychiatry 2011;11:200.

45 Ponniah K, Hollon SD: Empirically supported psychological interventions for social phobia in adults: a qualitative review of randomized controlled trials. Psychol Med 2008;38:3–14.

46 de Menezes GB, Freire Coutinho ES, Fontenelle LF, Vigne P, Figueira I, Versiani M: Second-generation antidepressants in social anxiety disorder: meta-analysis of controlled clinical trials. Psychopharmacology (Berl) 2011;215:1–11.

47 Liebowitz MR, Schneier F, Campeas R, Hollander E, Hatterer J, Fyer A, Gorman J, Papp L, Davies S, Gully R, Klein DF: Phenelzine vs atenolol in social phobia – a placebo-controlled comparison. Arch Gen Psychiatry 1992;49:290–300.

48 Gelernter CS, Uhde TW, Cimbolic P, Arnkoff DB, Vittone BJ, Tancer ME, Bartko JJ: Cognitive-behavioural and pharmacological treatment of social phobia – a controlled study. Arch Gen Psychiatry 1991; 48:938–945.

49 Lader M, Stender K, Burger V, Nil R: Efficacy and tolerability of escitalopram in 12-and 24-week treatment of social anxiety disorder: randomised, double-blind, placebo-controlled, fixed-dose study. Depress Anxiety 2004;19:241–248.

50 Allgulander C, Mangano R, Zhang J, Dahl AA, Lepola U, Sjodin I, Emilien G, Grp SADS: Efficacy of Venlafaxine ER in patients with social anxiety disorder: a double-blind, placebo-controlled, parallel-group comparison with paroxetine. Hum Psychopharmacol 2004;19:387–396.

51 Liebowitz MR, Gelenberg AJ, Munjack D: Venlafaxine extended release vs placebo, and paroxetine in social anxiety disorder. Arch Gen Psychiatry 2005;62:190–198.

52 Canton J, Scott KM, Glue P: Optimal treatment of social phobia: systematic review and meta-analysis. Neuropsychiatr Dis Treat 2012;8:203–215.

53 Blanco C, Heimberg RG, Schneier FR, Fresco DM, Chen HN, Turk CL, Vermes D, Erwin BA, Schmidt AB, Juster HR, Campeas R, Liebowitz MR: A placebo-controlled trial of phenelzine, cognitive behavioral group therapy, and their combination for social anxiety disorder. Arch Gen Psychiatry 2010;67:286–295.

54 Stein DJ, Westenberg HGM, Yang HC, Li D, Barbato LM: Fluvoxamine CR in the long-term treatment of social anxiety disorder: the 12- to 24-week extension phase of a multicentre, randomized, placebo-controlled trial. Int J Neuropsychopharmacol 2003;6:317–323.

55 Stein DJ, Andersen EW, Lader M: Escitalopram versus paroxetine for social anxiety disorder: an analysis of efficacy for different symptom dimensions. Eur Neuropsychopharmacol 2006;16:33–38.

56 Stein DJ, Versiani M, Hair T, Kumar R: Efficacy of paroxetine for relapse prevention in social anxiety disorder – a 24-week study. Arch Gen Psychiatry 2002;59:1111–1118.

57 Baldwin DS, Stein DJ, Dolberg OT, Bandelow B: How long should a trial of escitalopram treatment be in patients with major depressive disorder, generalised anxiety disorder or social anxiety disorder? An exploration of the randomised controlled trial database. Hum Psychopharmacol 2009;24:269–275.

58 Pande AC, Feltner DE, Jefferson JW, Davidson JRT, Pollack M, Stein MB, Lydiard RB, Futterer R, Robinson P, Slomkowski M, DuBoff E, Phelps M, Janney CA, Werth JL: Efficacy of the novel anxiolytic pregabalin in social anxiety disorder – a placebo-controlled, multicenter study. J Clin Psychopharmacol 2004;24:141–149.

59 Simon NM, Worthington JJ, Moshier SJ, Marks EH, Hoge EA, Brandes M, Delong H, Pollack MH: Duloxetine for the treatment of generalized social anxiety disorder: a preliminary randomized trial of increased dose to optimize response. CNS Spectr 2010;15:367–373.

60 Van Ameringen M, Mancini C, Wilson C: Buspirone augmentation of selective serotonin reuptake inhibitors (SSRIs) in social phobia. J Affect Disord 1996;39:115–121.

61 Stein MB, Sareen J, Hami S, Chao J: Pindolol potentiation of paroxetine for generalized social phobia: a double-blind, placebo-controlled, crossover study. Am J Psychiatry 2001;158:1725–1727.

62 Seedat S, Stein MB: Double-blind, placebo-controlled assessment of combined clonazepam with paroxetine compared with paroxetine monotherapy for generalized social anxiety disorder. J Clin Psychiatry 2004;65:244–248.

63 Voges M, Addington J: The association between social anxiety and social functioning in first episode psychosis. Schizophr Res 2005;76:287–292.

64 Kumazaki H, Kobayashi H, Niimura H, Kobayashi Y, Ito S, Nemoto T, Sakuma K, Kashima H, Mizuno M: Lower subjective quality of life and the development of social anxiety symptoms after the discharge of elderly patients with remitted schizophrenia: A 5-year longitudinal study. Compr Psychiatry 2012;53:946–951.

65 Halperin S, Nathan P, Drummond P, Castle D: A cognitive-behavioural, group-based intervention for social anxiety in schizophrenia. Aust N Z J Psychiatry 2000;34:809–813.

66 Kingsep P, Nathan P, Castle D: Cognitive behavioural group treatment for social anxiety in schizophrenia. Schizophr Res 2003;63:121–129.

67 Stern RG, Petti TA, Bopp K, Tobia A: Aripiprazole for the treatment of schizophrenia with co-occurring social anxiety an open-label cross-taper study. J Clin Psychopharmacol 2009;29:206–209.

68 Pallanti S, Quercioli L, Rossi A, Pazzagli A: The emergence of social phobia during clozapine treatment and its response to fluoxetine augmentation. J Clin Psychiatry 1999;60:819–823.

69 Davis M: NMDA receptors and fear extinction: implications for cognitive behavioral therapy. Dialogues Clin Neurosci 2011;13:463–474.

70 Hofmann SG, Meuret AE, Smits JAJ, Simon NM, Pollack MH, Eisenmenger K, Shiekh M, Otto MW: Augmentation of exposure therapy with D-cycloserine for social anxiety disorder. Arch Gen Psychiatry 2006;63:298–304.

71 Guastella AJ, Richardson R, Lovibond PF, Rapee RM, Gaston JE, Mitchell P, Dadds MR: A randomized controlled trial of D-cycloserine enhancement of exposure therapy for social anxiety disorder. Biol Psychiatry 2008;63:544–549.

72 Nave AM, Tolin DF, Stevens MC: Exposure therapy, D-cycloserine, and functional magnetic resonance imaging in patients with snake phobia: a randomized pilot study. J Clin Psychiatry 2012;73:1179–1186.

73 Guastella AJ, MacLeod C: A critical review of the influence of oxytocin nasal spray on social cognition in humans: evidence and future directions. Horm Behav 2012;61:410–418.

74 Guastella AJ, Howard AL, Dadds MR, Mitchell P, Carson DS: A randomized controlled trial of intranasal oxytocin as an adjunct to exposure therapy for social anxiety disorder. Psychoneuroendocrinology 2009;34:917–923.

75 Labuschagne I, Phan KL, Wood A, Angstadt M, Chua P, Heinrichs M, Stout JC, Nathan PJ: Oxytocin attenuates amygdala reactivity to fear in generalized social anxiety disorder. Neuropsychopharmacology 2010;35:2403–2413.

76 Bergamaschi MM, Costa Queiroz RH, Nisihara Chagas MH, Gomes de Oliveira DC, De Martinis BS, Kapczinski F, Quevedo J, Roesler R, Schroeder N, Nardi AE, Martin-Santos R, Cecilio Hallak JE, Zuardi AW, Crippa JAS: Cannabidiol reduces the anxiety induced by simulated public speaking in treatment-naive social phobia patients. Neuropsychopharmacology 2011;36:1219–1226.

77 Crippa JAS, Derenusson GN, Ferrari TB, Wichert-Ana L, Duran FLS, Martin-Santos R, Simoes MV, Bhattacharyya S, Fusar-Poli P, Atakan Z, Filho AS, Freitas-Ferrari MC, McGuire PK, Zuardi AW, Busatto GF, Cecilio Hallak JE: Neural basis of anxiolytic effects of cannabidiol (CBD) in generalized social anxiety disorder: a preliminary report. J Psychopharmacol 2011;25:121–130.

78 Baldwin DS: Room for improvement in the pharmacological treatment of anxiety disorders. Curr Pharm Des 2008;14:3482–3491.

Vasilios G. Masdrakis
First Department of Psychiatry, Eginition Hospital, Athens University Medical School
Eginition Hospital, 74 Vas. Sofias Avenue
GR–11528 Athens (Greece)
E-Mail vmasdrakis@med.uoa.gr

Baldwin DS, Leonard BE (eds): Anxiety Disorders.
Mod Trends Pharmacopsychiatry. Basel, Karger, 2013, vol 29, pp 154–163 (DOI: 10.1159/000353540)

Pharmacotherapy of Posttraumatic Stress Disorder

Anthony Koller · Dan J. Stein

Department of Psychiatry, University of Cape Town, Cape Town, South Africa

Abstract

Advances in the basic neuroscience of fear conditioning and extinction, as well as in the clinical neuroscience of posttraumatic stress disorder (PTSD), have laid the foundations for research on the pharmacotherapy of PTSD. Clinical trials have ranged from early work on tricyclic antidepressants and benzodiazepines through to more recently introduced antidepressants, and on to a range of other psychotropic agents. Despite the growing database of trials, the area remains a controversial one insofar as key systematic reviews in the field have emphasized the methodological limitations of existing work. Here, we briefly review the existing literature on the pharmacotherapy of PTSD, attempting to highlight key clinical lessons, and important areas for future research.

Copyright © 2013 S. Karger AG, Basel

Posttraumatic stress disorder (PTSD) is a common and disabling condition that by definition occurs after exposure to a traumatic event. Kessler et al. [1, 2], in the United States, estimated the 12-month prevalence of PTSD to be 3.5%, and the lifetime prevalence to be approximately 6.8%. Similar prevalence estimates have been obtained in other contexts [3]. Early views were that PTSD was a 'normal' reaction to abnormal stressors. However, subsequent work emphasized that given that the vast majority of people are exposed to traumatic events during their lifetime, and that only 5–9% develop the symptoms of PTSD, this condition is best understood as an 'abnormal' response to common events [1, 4].

Indeed, there has been a good deal of interest in both the basic and clinical neuroscience of PTSD. The symptom clusters of PTSD include reexperiencing/ intrusion, avoidance, negative alterations in cognition and mood, and hyperarousal symptoms. In DSM-5 [5], once these symptoms persist for longer than 1 month after the traumatic experience, a diagnosis of PTSD can be made. Animal studies have focused on the neurobiology of specific processes thought relevant to these clusters, e.g. fear conditioning, while clinical studies have focused on particular neurocircuitry and neurotransmitters that may be relevant.

Pharmacotherapy should also address the many associated features of PTSD. These include both the morbidity that emerges from PTSD (e.g. social and occupational dysfunctioning, reduced resilience) as well as the comorbidity that is associated with this condition (e.g. depressive symptoms, panic or anxiety, obsessional thoughts and substance abuse or dependency, aggression). There is increasing interest in whether dissociative PTSD involves a different psychobiology and deserves different treatment [6].

Clinical trials have ranged from early tricyclic agents and benzodiazepines, through to more recently introduced antidepressants, and on to a range of other psychotropic agents. Here, we briefly review the existing literature on the pharmacotherapy of PTSD, attempting to highlight key clinical lessons, and important areas for future research. We begin by briefly covering some basic and clinical neuroscience that may help inform pharmacotherapy.

Psychobiology of Posttraumatic Stress Disorder

Psychobiological disruptions have been shown to occur in PTSD, and these may provide both an understanding of why certain medications work, as well as therapeutic targets for future interventions [7, 8]. Particular psychobiological abnormalities can be linked theoretically to one or more clinical manifestations of PTSD or its associated symptoms [9, 10]. Dysregulation of the hypothalamic-pituitary-adrenocortical axis, for example, with possibly increased negative feedback, could be linked to decreased stress tolerance. Conversely, an increase in corticotropin-releasing factor could be linked to hyperarousal, reexperiencing and comorbid anxiety or panic [6, 10]. Opioid dysregulation could lead to numbing [6]. Disruption of the serotonergic system could result in a broad range of symptoms including reexperiencing, avoidance, hyperarousal, decreased stress tolerance and other associated symptoms [4–6]. A disruption of noradrenergic functioning could lead to re-experiencing, hyperarousal, dissociation, rage, disruption in information and memory function, and anxiety [5, 6]. Disruption of glutamatergic processing could contribute to dissociation, impaired information and memory processing and resistance to extinction of conditioned fear, while GABAergic underactivity could lead to hyperarousal and stress intolerance [6].

Overview of the Pharmacotherapy of Posttraumatic Stress Disorder

Rationale for Pharmacotherapy

Besides the theorized psychobiological basis of PTSD, there are other factors providing a rationale for pharmacotherapy. The common comorbidities of PTSD, including major depressive disorder, anxiety disorders like panic disorder, and substance abuse may respond to pharmacotherapy. Besides full comorbid disorders, associated features such as impulsivity, mood lability, irritability, aggression or suicidality can co-occur in PTSD. These, too, can be targeted by pharmacotherapy.

When discussing pharmacotherapy with a patient, it may be particularly important to ascertain their explanatory model of symptoms, and to negotiate a shared understanding of pharmacotherapy as contributing to symptom reduction and building resilience. Thus, the goals of pharmacotherapy are to reduce the core symptoms of PTSD, to treat comorbid conditions when present, to treat associated symptoms, and to increase resilience. Nevertheless, pharmacotherapy takes place within a broader clinician-patient relationship, which is paramount.

Evidence Base for Pharmacotherapy of Posttraumatic Stress Disorder

Clinical trials in PTSD have ranged from the early tricyclic agents, monoamine oxidase inhibitors (MAOIs), and benzodiazepines, through to more recently introduced antidepressants, and on to a range of other psychotropic agents. Given the growing database of trials, and the importance of evidence-based pharmacotherapy, several treatment guidelines have reviewed the existing literature; these include those of the National Institute for Clinical Excellence [11], the Institute of Medicine [12], the American Psychiatric Association [13], the US Department of Veterans Health Administration/Department of Defense [14], the International Psychopharmacology Algorithm Project [15], the British Association for Psychopharmacology [16], the Canadian Psychiatric Association [17] and the World Federation of Societies of Biological Psychiatry [18].

The general consensus of these guidelines is that there is a large enough evidence base of randomized controlled trials (RCTs) to conclude that pharmacotherapy in general and selective serotonin reuptake inhibitors (SSRIs) in particular can be considered first-line agents in the treatment of PTSD. It is notable, however, that some exceptions exist. The NICE guidelines [11] recommended that mirtazapine should be the first-line agent as SSRIs did not meet the predetermined threshold for significance of an effect size greater than 0.5. Similarly, the Institute of Medicine [12] concluded that the evidence base for pharmacotherapy was too inadequate to make a recommendation on the efficacy of psychotropic medications in PTSD; indeed, although there has been progress in this area, much further work is needed.

Determinants of Study Outcomes in Posttraumatic Stress Disorder

A particular area of controversy has been the question of whether some subtypes of PTSD, or some groups of PTSD patients are particularly nonresponsive to medication. Negative trials of SSRIs in combat veterans [19] have suggested the possibility that combat veterans do not respond well to pharmacotherapy. Nevertheless, given that some groups of combat veterans (e.g. World War II veterans) do appear to respond to medication, it has been suggested that Vietnam veterans in particular are less responsive to pharmacotherapy.

Another area of controversy is that surrounding complex PTSD or PTSD associated with early sexual trauma. There is an argument that patients with dissociative symptoms are less likely to respond to pharmacotherapy, and that patients with early trauma require more psychotherapeutic interventions. On the other hand, there are data suggesting that pharmacotherapy is equally effective in PTSD patients with and without early trauma [20]. Once again, further research is needed to fully delineate subtypes of PTSD and predictors of response.

Brief Review of the Evidence of Pharmacotherapy in Posttraumatic Stress Disorder

Early Trials

Tricyclic Antidepressants
An early RCT of desipramine in 18 combat veterans with PTSD failed to show superiority over placebo [21]. Nevertheless, subsequent trials have indicated that the tricyclic antidepressants (TCAs) are efficacious in PTSD. Davidson et al. [22] conducted an RCT on 46 subjects over 8 weeks in which amitriptyline was found superior to placebo. In an RCT using imipramine, phenelzine and placebo in 60 veterans, imipramine was shown to be superior to placebo [23].

Monoamine Oxidase Inhibitors
Data with classical MAOIs are also somewhat inconsistent, again perhaps reflecting methodological weaknesses in early studies (e.g. short duration, lack of standardized symptom severity scales). A 5-week crossover RCT found no differences between phenelzine and placebo [24]. The study had a high dropout rate with over 50% (7/13) of participants receiving phenelzine withdrawing. However, Kosten et al. [23], in an RCT of phenelzine in 60 combat veterans found a significant decrease in symptoms after phenelzine compared to placebo, and phenelzine had a higher response rate than imipramine (44 vs. 25%).

Brofaromine is a reversible inhibitor of monoamine oxidase A, and also has weak serotonin reuptake properties. Katz et al. [25] conducted a 14-week RCT of brofaromine and found no significant decrease on the Clinician-Administered PTSD Scale

(CAPS). Similarly, Baker et al. [26] conducted an RCT of brofaromine using 118 participants and did not detect a difference on the CAPS after 12 weeks.

Benzodiazepines
Evidence does not support the use of benzodiazepines in PTSD. An RCT of alprazolam showed no reduction in core symptoms of PTSD [27]. Cates et al. [28] used clonazepam in a single-blind crossover study specifically for sleep disturbances in PTSD and showed negative findings on all measures.

Selective Serotonin Reuptake Inhibitors

Paroxetine
Paroxetine is licensed by the Food and Drug Administration (FDA) for the short-term treatment of PTSD. There have been 3 published RCTs of paroxetine in PTSD all with positive results. Marshall et al. [29] conducted an RCT using fixed doses of paroxetine (20 vs. 40 mg/day), which showed a significant difference in the CAPS by 4 weeks and efficacy in all three symptom clusters. In their RCT, Tucker et al. [30] also demonstrated a significant decrease in CAPS by 12 weeks. Marshall et al. [31] conducted an RCT in which a significant difference was detected on the CGI-I by 10 weeks and one third of patients responded to treatment.

Sertraline
Sertraline is licensed by the FDA both for the short-term and the long-term treatment of PTSD. There have been 7 published RCTs of sertraline so far. Two had positive results and 5 were unable to find a significant difference in response. Londborg et al. [32] studied 128 patients who had completed a 12-week RCT of sertraline in a 24-week open-label continuation phase study. They obtained good results with 92% of responders in the acute phase maintaining their response and 54% of acute phase nonresponders converting to response during the continuation phase. Davidson et al. [33] conducted a 28-week relapse prevention study in patients who had completed 12-week acute treatment RCT and a subsequent 24-week open-label extension phase study. Patients were then randomized to placebo or sertraline for a further 28 weeks. The study had positive results, showing a significant difference in relapse rates between sertraline and placebo (5 vs. 26%).

Fluoxetine
Although fluoxetine is not licensed for PTSD, it was one of the first SSRIs to be brought onto the market and was used in the first published RCT of an SSRI for PTSD. It has been extensively investigated in 6 randomized controlled acute-phase studies that have been published to date and one randomized controlled relapse prevention study. Results have been mixed with the acute-phase RCTs. Three found fluoxetine superior

to placebo and the other 3 failed to detect a significant difference. Martenyi et al. [34] conducted a 28-week relapse prevention study using responders from a 12-week acute-phase RCT of fluoxetine, with favorable results. There was a significant difference in time to relapse between the fluoxetine and placebo groups.

Newer Agents

Venlafaxine Extended Release
In two large RCTs, the SNRI venlafaxine has been shown to be superior to placebo, and also appears comparable to sertraline [35, 36]. This provides good evidence to recommend venlafaxine as a first-line agent along with the SSRIs.

Mirtazapine
In a small 8-week RCT, mirtazapine was found to be superior to placebo in PTSD response rate [37].

Nefazodone
Nefazodone, a serotonin antagonist reuptake inhibitor, was found superior to placebo in an RCT conducted by Davis et al. [38]. However, nefazodone has been withdrawn from the market due to its risk of hepatotoxicity.

Prazosin
Prazosin is an α_1-adrenergic antagonist. Taylor et al. [39] conducted an RCT with 13 subjects on sleep disturbances in PTSD, and found that this agent significantly reduced trauma-related nightmares. Similarly, Raskind et al. [40] in a 20-week crossover placebo-controlled trial in 10 veterans with sleep disturbances in PTSD found that prazosin reduced occurrences of nightmares, and Raskind et al. [41] in an RCT in 40 veterans with sleep disturbances and PTSD also found a significant reduction in trauma-related nightmares.

Anticonvulsants
There is relatively little support for using anticonvulsants in PTSD. An RCT using lamotrigine showed superiority over placebo for reexperiencing and avoidance/numbing symptoms [42]. However, tiagabine, a GABA reuptake inhibitor, failed to separate from placebo in a large RCT [43]. Further, in an RCT of topiramate, lack of efficacy over placebo was seen on most measures [44]. Finally, an RCT of divalproex found no superiority over placebo on all outcome measures [45].

Antipsychotics
Trials have been conducted of antipsychotic agents in PTSD as both monotherapy and as augmentation therapy. Reich et al. [46] found risperidone superior to placebo in an

RCT of risperidone augmentation. Similarly, Bartzokis et al. [47] showed positive results for the use of adjunctive risperidone in a double-blind placebo-controlled study with 73 participants. Finally, Padala et al. [48] found risperidone monotherapy superior to placebo in reducing core PTSD symptoms. Although olanzapine monotherapy was unsuccessful in a small trial [49], it was found efficacious in a larger trial [50].

Other Agents

Two RCTs have been conducted on guanfacine, both with negative results. Neylan et al. [51] completed an RCT in veterans and obtained negative results. Similarly, Davis et al. [52] also completed an RCT in veterans, and showed no significant differences in CAPS or other measures.

An RCT of inositol by Kaplan et al. [53] did not show efficacy. Similarly, an RCT of cyproheptadine for sleep disturbances in PTSD did not show efficacy [54].

Conclusion

Advances in the basic and clinical neuroscience of PTSD, have emphasized the role of particular neurocircuitry in fear conditioning (e.g. amygdala, hippocampus) and fear extinction (e.g. prefrontal cortex), as well as component neurotransmitters (e.g. serotonin, glutamate). A range of clinical trials have studied psychotropic medications that act on these neurocircuits and neurotransmitters.

Early trials with the TCAs and MAOIs were not entirely consistent, but provided some evidence that these agents are effective for PTSD. Subsequent trials with SSRIs were useful in driving the field forward, with a good deal of evidence indicating that these agents are both effective and well tolerated. Agents within this class remain the only ones that have been approved by both the FDA and European Medicines Agency (EMA) for the treatment of PTSD.

Nevertheless, significant concerns have been raised. The database remains relatively small, methodological problems are particularly apparent in early trials of TCAs and MAOIs, and effect sizes remain relatively small in the later trials of SSRIs. Clearly much additional research is required to further strengthen the existing database and to find novel agents for the treatment of PTSD.

Basic and clinical research provides several targets for such future work. Studies demonstrating the role of cycloserine in augmenting cognitive behavioral therapy, for example, deserve to be further expanded in PTSD. Work on the molecular science of neuroplasticity may be particularly relevant to intervention in PTSD. Given the growing understanding of biological alterations in the immediate aftermath of trauma exposure, there is also growing attention to the possibility of clinical PTSD prophylaxis.

References

1 Kessler R, Berglund P, Demler O, Jin R, Merikangas K, Walters E: Lifetime prevalence and age-of-onset distributions of DSM-IV disorders in the National Comorbidity Survey Replication. Arch Gen Psychiatry 2005;62:593–602.

2 Kessler RC, Chiu WT, Demler O, Walters EE: Prevalence, severity, and comorbidity of 12-month DSM-IV disorders in the National Comorbidity Survey Replication. Arch Gen Psychiatry 2005;62: 617–627.

3 Frans O, Rimmo PA, Aberg L, Fredrikson M: Trauma exposure and post-traumatic stress disorder in the general population. Acta Psychiatry Scand 2005; 111:291–299.

4 Yehuda R, Kahana B, Binderbrynes K, Southwick SM, Mason JW, Giller EL: Low urinary cortisol excretion in Holocaust survivors with posttraumatic stress disorder. Am J Psychiatry 1995;152: 982–986.

5 American Psychiatric Association: Diagnostic and Statistical Manual of Mental Disorders, ed 4, DSM-IV-TR. Washington, American Psychiatric Association, 2000.

6 Lanius R: Complex adaptations to traumatic stress: from neurobiological to social and cultural aspects. Am J Psychiatry 2007;164:1628–1630.

7 Charney DS: Psychobiological and vulnerability: implications for successful adaptation to extreme stress. Am J Psychiatry 2004;161:195–216.

8 Southwick SM, Davis LD, Aikins DE, Rasmusson A, Barron J, Morgan CA: Neurobiological alterations associated with PTSD; in Friedman MJ, Keane TM, Resick PA (eds): Handbook of PTSD: Science and Practice. New York, The Guilford Press, 2007.

9 Stein D, Cloitre M, Nemeroff C, Nutt D, Seedat S, Shalev A, Wittchen H, Zohar J: Cape Town consensus on posttraumatic stress disorder. CNS Spectr 2009;14:52–58.

10 Nemeroff CB, Bremner JD, Foa EB, Mayberg HS, North CS, Stein MB: Posttraumatic stress disorder: a state-of-the-science review. J Psychiatry Res 2006;40: 1–21.

11 National Institute for Clinical Excellence (NICE): Post-Traumatic Stress Disorder (PTSD): The Management of PTSD in Adults and Children in Primary and Secondary Care. NICE Guideline 26. London, National Institute for Clinical Excellence, 2005.

12 Institute of Medicine: Treatment of Posttraumatic Stress Disorder: An Assessment of the Evidence. Washington, National Academies Press, 2007.

13 Ursano RJ, Bell C, Eth S, Friedman M, Norwood A, Pfefferbaum B, Pynoos JDRS, Zatzick DF, Benedek DM, McIntyre JS, Charles SC, Altshuler K, Cook I, Cross CD, Mellman L, Moench LA, Norquist G, Twemlow SW, Woods S, Yager J, Work Group on ASD, PTSD, Steering Committee on Practice G: Practice guideline for the treatment of patients with acute stress disorder and posttraumatic stress disorder. Am J Psychiatry 2004;161:3–31.

14 Susskind O, Ruzek JI, Friedman MJ: The VA/DOD Clinical Practice Guideline for Management of Post-Traumatic Stress (update 2010): development and methodology. J Rehabil Res Dev 2012;49:xvii–xxviii.

15 The International Psychopharmacology Algorithm Project (IPAP): International Psychopharmacology Algorithm Project: Post-Traumatic Stress Disorder (PTSD) Algorithm IPAP. 2005. http://www.ipap.org/ptsd/ (accessed June 6, 2013).

16 Baldwin D, Anderson I, Nutt D, Bandelow B, Bond A, Davidson J, et al: Evidence-based guidelines for the pharmacological treatment of anxiety disorders: recommendations from the British Association for Psychopharmacology. J Psychopharmacol 2005;19: 567–596.

17 Canadian Psychiatric Association: Clinical practice guidelines. Management of anxiety disorders. Can J Psychiatry 2006;51:9S–91S.

18 Bandelow B, Zohar J, Hollander E, et al: World Federation of Societies of Biological Psychiatry (WFSBP) guidelines for the pharmacological treatment of anxiety, obsessive-compulsive and post-traumatic stress disorders-first revision. World J Biol Psychiatry 2008;9:248–312.

19 Friedman MJ, Marmar CR, Baker DG, Sikes CR, Farfel GM: Randomized, double-blind comparison of sertraline and placebo for posttraumatic stress disorder in a Department of Veterans Affairs setting. J Clin Psychiatry 2007;68:711–720.

20 Ipser JC, Stein DJ: Evidence-based pharmacotherapy of post-traumatic stress disorder (PTSD). Int J Neuropsychopharmacol 2012;15:825–840.

21 Reist C, Kauffmann CD, Haier RJ, Sangdahl C, Demet EM, Chiczdemet A, Nelson JN: A controlled trial of desipramine in 18 men with posttraumatic stress disorder. Am J Psychiatry 1989;146:513–516.

22 Davidson J, Kudler H, Smith R, Mahorney SL, Lipper S, Hammett E, Saunders WB, Cavenar JO: Treatment of posttraumatic stress disorder with amitriptyline and placebo. Arch Gen Psychiatry 1990;47: 259–266.

23 Kosten TR, Frank JB, Dan E, McDougle CJ, Giller EL: Pharmacotherapy for posttraumatic stress disorder using phenelzine or imipramine. J Nerv Ment Dis 1991;179:366–370.

24 Shestatzky M, Greenberg D, Lerer B: A controlled trial of phenelzine in posttraumatic stress disorder. Psychiatry Res 1988;24:149–155.

25 Katz R, Lott MH, Arbus P, Crocq L, Herlobsen P, Lingjaerde O, Lopez G, Loughrey GC, Macfarlane DJ, McIvor R, Mehlum L, Nugent D, Turner SW, Weisaeth L, Yule W: Pharmacotherapy of post-traumatic stress disorder with a novel psychotropic. Anxiety 1994;1:169–174.

26 Baker DG, Diamond BI, Gillette G, Hamner M, Katzelnick D, Keller T, Mellman TA, Pontius E, Rosenthal M, Tucker P, vanderKolk BA, Katz R: A double-blind, randomized, placebo-controlled, multi-center study of brofaromine in the treatment of post-traumatic stress disorder. Psychopharmacology 1995;122:386–389.

27 Braun P, Greenberg D, Dasberg H, Lerer B: Core symptoms of posttraumatic stress disorder unimproved by alprazolam treatment. J Clin Psychiatry 1990;51:236–238.

28 Cates ME, Bishop MH, Davis LL, Lowe JS, Woolley TW: Clonazepam for treatment of sleep disturbances associated with combat-related posttraumatic stress disorder. Ann Pharmacother 2004;38:1395–1399.

29 Marshall RD, Beebe KL, Oldham M, Zaninelli R: Efficacy and safety of paroxetine treatment for chronic PTSD: a fixed-dose, placebo-controlled study. Am J Psychiatry 2001;158:1982–1988.

30 Tucker P, Zaninelli R, Yehuda R, Ruggiero L, Dillingham K, Pitts CD: Paroxetine in the treatment of chronic posttraumatic stress disorder: results of a placebo-controlled, flexible-dosage trial. J Clin Psychiatry 2001;62:860–868.

31 Marshall RD, Lewis-Fernandez R, Blanco C, Simpson HB, Lin S-H, Vermes D, Garcia W, Schneier F, Neria Y, Sanchez-Lacay A, Liebowitz MR: A controlled trial of paroxetine for chronic PTSD, dissociation, and interpersonal problems in mostly minority adults. Depress Anxiety 2007;24:77–84.

32 Londborg PD, Hegel MT, Goldstein S, Goldstein D, Himmelhoch JM, Maddock R, Patterson WM, Rausch J, Farfel GM: Sertraline treatment of posttraumatic stress disorder: results of 24 weeks of open-label continuation treatment. J Clin Psychiatry 2001;62:325–331.

33 Davidson J, Pearlstein T, Londborg P, Brady KT, Rothbaum B, Bell J, Maddock R, Hegel MT, Farfel G: Efficacy of sertraline in preventing relapse of posttraumatic stress disorder: results of a 28-week double-blind, placebo-controlled study. Am J Psychiatry 2001;158:1974–1981.

34 Martenyi F, Brown EB, Zhang H, Koke SC, Prakash A: Fluoxetine v. placebo in prevention of relapse in post-traumatic stress disorder. Br J Psychiatry 2002;181:315–320.

35 Davidson J, Baldwin D, Stein DJ, Kuper E, Benattia I, Ahmed S, Pedersen R, Musgnung J: Treatment of posttraumatic stress disorder with venlafaxine extended release – a 6-month randomized controlled trial. Arch Gen Psychiatry 2006;63:1158–1165.

36 Davidson J, Rothbaum BO, Tucker P, Asnis G, Benattia I, Musgnung JJ: Venlafaxine extended release in posttraumatic stress disorder – a sertraline- and placebo-controlled study. J Clin Psychopharmacol 2006;26:259–267.

37 Davidson JRT, Weisler RH, Butterfield MI, Casat CD, Connor KM, Barnett S, van Meter S: Mirtazapine vs. placebo in posttraumatic stress disorder: a pilot trial. Biol Psychiatry 2003;53:188–191.

38 Davis LL, Jewell ME, Ambrose S, Farley J, English B, Bartolucci A, Petty F: A placebo-controlled study of nefazodone for the treatment of chronic posttraumatic stress disorder – a preliminary study. J Clin Psychopharmacol 2004;24:291–297.

39 Taylor FB, Martin P, Thompson C, Williams J, Mellman TA, Gross C, Peskind ER, Raskind MA: Prazosin effects on objective sleep measures and clinical symptoms in civilian trauma posttraumatic stress disorder: a placebo-controlled study. Biol Psychiatry 2008;63:629–632.

40 Raskind MA, Peskind ER, Kanter ED, Petrie EC, Radant A, Thompson CE, Dobie DJ, Hoff D, Rein RJ, Straits-Troster K, Thomas RG, McFall MM: Reduction of nightmares and other PTSD symptoms in combat veterans by prazosin: a placebo-controlled study. Am J Psychiatry 2003;160:371–373.

41 Raskind MA, Peskind ER, Hoff DJ, Hart KL, Holmes HA, Warren D, Shofer J, O'Connell J, Taylor F, Gross C, Rohde K, McFall ME: A parallel group placebo controlled study of prazosin for trauma nightmares and sleep disturbance in combat veterans with post-traumatic stress disorder. Biol Psychiatry 2007;61:928–934.

42 Hertzberg MA, Butterfield MI, Feldman ME, Beckham JC, Sutherland SM, Connor KM, Davidson JRT: A preliminary study of lamotrigine for the treatment of posttraumatic stress disorder. Biol Psychiatry 1999;45:1226–1229.

43 Davidson JRT, Brady K, Mellman TA, Stein MB, Pollack MH: The efficacy and tolerability of tiagabine in adult patients with post-traumatic stress disorder. J Clin Psychopharmacol 2007;27:85–88.

44 Tucker P, Trautman RP, Wyatt DB, Thompson J, Wu S-C, Capece JA, Rosenthal NR: Efficacy and safety of topiramate monotherapy in civilian posttraumatic stress disorder: a randomized, double-blind, placebo-controlled study. J Clin Psychiatry 2007;68:201–206.

45 Davis LL, Davidson JRT, Ward LC, Bartolucci A, Bowden CL, Petty F: Divalproex in the treatment of posttraumatic stress disorder – a randomized, double-blind, placebo-controlled trial in a veteran population. J Clin Psychopharmacol 2008;28:84–88.

46 Reich DB, Winternitz S, Hennen J, Watts T, Stan-
culescu C: A preliminary study of risperidone in the
treatment of posttraumatic stress disorder related to
childhood abuse in women. J Clin Psychiatry 2004;
65:1601–1606.

47 Bartzokis G, Lu PH, Turner J, Mintz J, Saunders CS:
Adjunctive risperidone in the treatment of chronic
combat-related posttraumatic stress disorder. Biol
Psychiatry 2005;57:474–479.

48 Padala PR, Madison J, Monnahan M, Marcil W, Price
P, Ramaswamy S, Din AU, Wilson DR, Petty F: Risperidone monotherapy for post-traumatic stress disorder related to sexual assault and domestic abuse in
women. Int Clin Psychopharmacol 2006;21:275–280.

49 Butterfield MI, Becker ME, Connor KM, Sutherland
S, Churchill LE, Davidson JRT: Olanzapine in the
treatment of post-traumatic stress disorder: a pilot
study. Int Clin Psychopharmacol 2001;16:197–203.

50 Carey P, Suliman S, Ganesan K, Seedat S, Stein DJ:
Olanzapine monotherapy in postraumatic stress disorder: efficacy in a randomized, double-blind, placebo-controlled study. Hum Psychopharm Clin 2012;
27:386–391.

51 Neylan TC, Lenoci M, Samuelson KW, Metzler TJ,
Henn-Haase C, Hierholzer RW, Lindley SE, Otte C,
Schoenfeld FB, Yesavage JA, Marmar CR: No improvement of posttraumatic stress disorder symptoms with guanfacine treatment. Am J Psychiatry
2006;163:2186–2188.

52 Davis L, Ward LC, Rasmusson A, Newell JM, Frazier
E, Southwick SM: A placebo-controlled trial of guanfacine for the treatment of posttraumatic stress disorder in veterans. Psychopharmacol Bull 2008;41:
8–18.

53 Kaplan Z, Amir M, Swartz M, Levine J: Inositol treatment of post-traumatic stress disorder. Anxiety
1996;2:51–52.

54 Jacobs-Rebhun S, Schnurr PP, Friedman MJ, Peck R,
Brophy M, Fuller D: Posttraumatic stress disorder
and sleep difficulty. Am J Psychiatry 2000;157:1525–
1526.

Anthony Koller
UCT Dept. of Psychiatry, Groote Schuur Hospital J2
Anzio Rd., Observatory 7925
Cape Town (South Africa)
E-Mail KLLANT005@myuct.ac.za

Baldwin DS, Leonard BE (eds): Anxiety Disorders.
Mod Trends Pharmacopsychiatry. Basel, Karger, 2013, vol 29, pp 164–177 (DOI: 10.1159/000353618)

Evidence-Based Treatment Pathways for Translational Studies in Obsessive-Compulsive Disorders

N.A. Fineberg[a–c] · S. Pallanti[d, e] · S. Reghunandanan[a]

[a]National Obsessive Compulsive Disorders Specialist Service, Hertfordshire Partnership University NHS Foundation Trust, Queen Elizabeth II Hospital, Welwyn Garden City, [b]Postgraduate Medical School, University of Hertfordshire, College Lane, Hatfield, and [c]University of Cambridge School of Clinical Medicine, Addenbrooke's Hospital, Cambridge, UK; [d]University of Florence, Florence, Italy; [e]Mount Sinai Hospital Medical School, New York, N.Y., USA

Abstract

Obsessive-compulsive disorder (OCD) and related disorders are costly and burdensome long-term illnesses. Whilst evidence-based pharmacological and psychological treatments are available for OCD, a significant proportion of OCD patients fail to respond and for many of the OCD-related disorders no validated treatments are as yet recognised. In addition, predictors of treatment response/non-response to guide clinicians in the management of individual patients are lacking. The introduction of personalised medicine to psychiatry is expected to offer the novel prospect of identifying the most effective treatment for a patient in a timely and cost-effective way. Translational research that investigates endophenotype predictors of treatment response in OCD and related disorders may pave the way toward personalised medicine. Such research is likely to require multidisciplinary collaboration between neuroscientists and clinicians, so that the right clinical questions are addressed, and large datasets, entailing multinational, multicentre sampling. In order to facilitate the translational investigation of the key aspects of the treatment response, these studies would require access to standardised treatment paradigms that are internationally recognised. In this chapter, we introduce some of the most important outstanding questions for personalised medicine that translational research could be expected to address within the next 10 years. We review the available tools and techniques for standardised clinical assessment and the criteria that are used to define the degree of therapeutic response (response, remission, relapse, resistance) that would naturally dictate the direction of treatment. We also present a series of consecutive stepped treatment algorithms based on evidence-based practice and modelled on naturalistic care that we believe could be adapted to multicentre settings as a template for the translational researcher to aid in the design of pragmatic treatment trials that are capable of identifying biomarkers of treatment response or non-response at each key stage of the evidence-based canon.

Copyright © 2013 S. Karger AG, Basel

Obsessive-compulsive disorder (OCD) is a disabling neuropsychiatric disorder. Whilst pharmacological treatment with selective serotonin reuptake inhibitors (SSRIs) and clomipramine and cognitive behaviour therapy (CBT) with exposure and response prevention (ERP) are known to be effective in roughly 60% cases entering treatment trials, a large proportion of individuals either do not respond to treatment at all or continue to present with persistent fluctuating symptoms severe enough to lead to chronic functional disability [1, 2]. In SSRI non-responders, approximately one third of patients experience clinical improvement with further treatment with adjunctive dopamine antagonists [1]. For the more highly treatment-refractory patient, a range of potentially effective experimental treatments are available, including the use of novel pharmacological agents, intensive inpatient CBT [3] and somatic treatments such as ablative neurosurgery and deep brain stimulation [4].

OCD is associated with a considerable cost and burden, arising at least in part from the direct medical costs associated with the use of unsuccessful treatment [5] as well as the indirect costs on the individual and society associated with living and caring for someone with chronic mental illness. There is increasing interest in advancing the role of personalised medicine for psychiatric disorders, so that the individual patient can be offered the treatment that is most likely to be effective for him or her in a timely and cost-effective way [6]. In the case of OCD and the related disorders, there are no existing accurate or reliable objective predictors of treatment response (or non-response) to guide the clinician and patient through the various stages of treatment. However, it is recognised that an extended duration of OCD is associated with a poor response to established treatments including CBT and an overall poor prognosis [7], emphasising the importance of intervening early in the course of the illness using a treatment with a high chance of success. Translational research that aims to identify clinical and neurobiological markers (biomarkers) that might predict a priori which patients are most likely to respond to specific drug or CBT treatments, would therefore represent a welcome advance in the field [8]. Such research is likely to require multidisciplinary collaboration between neuroscientists and clinicians, so that the right clinical questions are addressed, and large datasets, sometimes entailing multinational, multicentre sampling. In order to facilitate the translational investigation of the key aspects of the treatment response, these studies would require access to standardised treatment paradigms that are internationally recognised.

In this chapter, we summarise the internationally recognised evidence-based treatment recommendations for OCD to determine a rational stepped care treatment pathway from treatment-naïve through to treatment-resistant cases. We introduce some of the most important outstanding questions for personalised medicine that translational research could be expected to address within the next 10 years. We review the available tools and techniques for standardised clinical assessment and the criteria that are used to define the degree of therapeutic response (response, remission, relapse, resistance) that would naturally dictate the direction of treatment. We also present a series of consecutive stepped treatment algorithms based on evidence-based practice and modelled on naturalistic care that we believe could be adapted to multicentre settings as a template for the translational researcher to aid in the design of pragmatic treatment trials that are capable of identifying biomarkers of treatment response or non-response at each key stage of the evidence-based canon.

Endophenotypes in Obsessive-Compulsive Disorder

Endophenotypes (intermediate phenotypes) represent indicators of the underlying disease process. They are considered to be more stable and reliable than clinical phenotypic markers (illness symptoms), which can be state dependent and vary considerably across patient subsets. Candidate endophenotypes have been identified in OCD and include abnormal responses on laboratory-based cognitive tests and brain-imaging changes using structural/functional magnetic resonance imaging and positron emission tomography [9, 10]. The application of novel machine-learning techniques in psychiatry provides a method for transforming group-based brain imaging data to the level of the individual patient [11]. It may reasonably be expected that within a short time frame, endophenotypes that are found to differentiate subsets of patients at the level of the group, e.g. those who do or do not respond to a certain treatment, may be transformed by such techniques into reliable biomarkers that might identify the chances of response or non-response at the individual level, in order to inform personalised treatment. In order to achieve this goal, biomarker research needs to be effectively coupled with rational clinical treatment trial methodology.

Tools and Techniques for Measuring Clinical Response

Rating Scales

Studies that investigate the determinants of the treatment response require robust and valid criteria to define degrees of clinical response. In the absence of objective biomarkers, the definition of a clinically meaningful clinical response in OCD relies upon the magnitude of clinical change as measured by rating questionnaires. Over the past three decades, the Yale-Brown Obsessive Compulsive Scale (Y-BOCS) [12, 13] has emerged as the pivotal rating scale for OCD and has been used to endorse efficacy for most of the evidence-based pharmacological treatments. The Y-BOCS is a 10-item observer-rated instrument that can be adapted as a self-rated tool. It measures the overall severity of obsessions and compulsions separately and in combination and has been shown to be sensitive to change. Items include duration, interference, distress, ability to resist and control. Post-randomisation changes in the Y-BOCS (and its variants) are usually used as the primary outcome measure in treatment trials. The scale has been adapted for use in children with OCD aged as young as 4 years of age (CY-BOCS) [14] and has also been modified for other OC spectrum disorders including body-dysmorphic disorder (BDD; BDD Y-BOCS) [15] and pathological gambling (PG-YBOCS) [16]. Application of these 'standardised' instruments facilitates the comparison of obsessive-compulsive symptom severity and changes in symptom severity across different age groups and also across related diagnoses. They may therefore be particularly apt for 'transdiagnostic' research projects, such as those proposed by the US National Institute of Mental Health in its RDoC programme [17]. Complementary scales that are also sensitive to change in OCD populations, and that may be used as secondary outcome measures, include the National Institute for Mental Health Global Obsessive-Compulsive Scale [18], the Clinical Global Impression Severity (CGI-S) and Improvement (CGI-I) scales [19], Sheehan Disability Scale (SDS) [20] and the Short-Form-36 (SF-36) [21] that, respectively, measure global OCD severity, global illness severity and improvement, psychosocial impairment and health-related disability and quality of life.

One of the main disadvantages of the Y-BOCS is the sub-division into obsession and compulsion subscales. Many patients are unable to differentiate obsessions and compulsions easily. In addition, core concepts such as avoidance [22] are largely disregarded. New scales such as the promising Dutch Dimensional Obsessive Compulsive Scale, a 10-item observer-rated scale which measures the severity of obsessive-compulsive symptoms according to time, distribution, fixation, feeling of obligation, control, fear, distress, dysfunction, avoidance and ego-dystonicity, are in the process of being validated [Denys, unpubl. data]. The Y-BOCS may also be criticised for failing to take account of the cognitive and executive impairments known to be associated with OCD [23]. The Cognitive Assessment Instrument of Obsessions and Compulsions (CAIOC) [24] is a novel 13-item tool. Its clinician and self-rated versions appear to be valid and reliable measures of the severity of functional impairment associated with OCD. Further validation, including research into the relationship of the CAIOC-13 with laboratory measures of cognitive impairment and evaluation of its sensitivity to change with treatment, is indicated.

Other OCD instruments may fulfil additional roles, e.g. the Obsessive Compulsive Inventory (OCI) [25] captures the richness of the complexity of OCD phenomenology, and the shortened version (OCI-R) [26] shows sensitivity to treatment-related change and may be suitable for naturalistic outcome studies; the Padua Inventory [27] distinguishes between worries and obsessions and may be useful in differentiating anxiety from OCD, and together with the Maudsley Obsessive-Compulsive Inventory [28] (which is not sensitive in detecting treatment effects) may be useful for registering the presence of specific obsessions and compulsions in non-clinical samples.

Criteria for Response, Remission, Relapse and Resistance

Clinical improvement, amounting to a reduction by 25% of the baseline total Y-BOCS score, has been shown to discriminate 'responders' from 'non-responders' using complementary rating scales of functional disability including the SDS and SF-36 [2], and is therefore thought to represent a clinically relevant threshold marking treatment response. However, a 25% decrease in Y-BOCS score alone does not appear large enough to signify a clinically meaningful response. For example, large-scale placebo-controlled studies such as that of Stein et al. [29] noted that a majority of patients in all treatment arms, including placebo, showed this degree of improvement, yet only about one third were 'much' or 'very much' improved on the CGI. The CGI-I captures the 'global' clinical picture and also shows convincing evidence of sensitivity to change in OCD. Combining the Y-BOCS with the CGI-I may optimise discriminatory power [30]. Therefore, a more rigorous criterion to denote a full treatment response, amounting to at least a 35% improvement on the Y-BOCS and/or a score of 2 or less (i.e. 'much' or 'very much' improved) on the CGI-I, has been proposed [31]. Consequently, 25–35% reduction in Y-BOCS score has been suggested to denote only a partial response. Remission is a higher hurdle than response. One definition requires a total Y-BOCS score of less than 16/40 [31]. However, at this level of severity, patients could still be eligible to enter some treatment trials. Stein et al. [29] therefore proposed a more stringent remission criterion, needing the total Y-BOCS score to be reduced to 10 or less and in the field of CBT, Sookman and Steketee [32] defined remission as no longer meeting OCD DSM criteria: YBOCS ≤7. In contrast, relapse has been defined as a worsening by 25% of the remission Y-BOCS score (or a CGI-I score of 6). Other plausible relapse criteria include a worsening of post-baseline Y-BOCS of ≥50%, a 5-point worsening of Y-BOCS, total Y-BOCS score ≥19, CGI-I scores of 'much' or 'very much' worse [33].

The definition of treatment resistance, representing an inadequate response following an adequate trial of treatment with good adherence, should usually be made in relation to a specific treatment, or series of treatments. Pallanti et al. [31] proposed the introduction of operational criteria for assessment of stages of response, and suggested that it should be seen as a continuum from remission to refractoriness. Treatment resistance may be defined as <25% improvement in baseline Y-BOCS [31]. Though the terms 'resistance' and 'refractory' are sometimes used interchangeably, treatment resistance may be defined as non-response following an adequate trial of one serotonin reuptake inhibitor (SRI), whilst treatment refractoriness refers to a lack of response to several trials of evidence-based treatment; according to Pallanti et al. [34], these should include three SRI agents, augmentation trials with two antipsychotics and at least 20–30 h of CBT.

Evidence-Based Treatments for Obsessive-Compulsive Disorder: Current Knowledge and Practice

Detailed discussion of the evidence base determining treatment efficacy and tolerability in OCD is beyond the scope of this chapter. Readers may refer to recent papers published by some of the authors that comprehensively review the data derived from randomised controlled trials on selected groups of individuals that provide rational or empirically derived treatment tactics for the clinical management of OCD, from treatment naïve to intractable cases [1, 35].

Guidelines for the treatment of OCD, such as the American Psychiatric Association Practice Guidelines [36] or the British Association for Psychopharmacology guidelines [37], are based upon a systematic review of outcome data from randomised controlled trials in highly selected groups of individuals, sometimes little resembling the chronic complexity of the patients seen in the naturalistic clinical setting. Therefore, while a guideline may offer a rational heuristic, it can be hard to directly translate the recommendations in the guideline to the clinical setting. It must be remembered that clinicians treat individual patients, with their own idiosyncratic profile of comorbidity, treatment history and preferences, as opposed to populations or averages. How clinicians decide which treatment to use and when, remains largely obscure (though we suspect that it may have lot more to do with intuition, heuristics and 'expertise' than it is currently fashionable to admit). Below, we summarise some of the key treatment decisions facing the clinician in everyday practice that remain difficult to resolve on an individual basis and that we believe may be enlightened by new knowledge derived from translational investigation. The decision usually involves the selection of the next stage of treatment for a patient who has responded poorly to the previous one. We include the analysis of treatment for children and adolescents with OCD because the disorder is recognised to have its origins in childhood, and therefore biomarker research may best be targeted at young people in the prodrome or early stages of illness.

Cognitive Behaviour Therapy or Serotonin Reuptake Inhibitor?

The effect sizes derived from the meta-analyses of CBT with ERP and drug trials of SSRI and clomipramine suggest equivalent efficacy for these modalities in OCD [38]. Therefore, in most guidelines, CBT or SSRI-pharmacotherapy usually constitutes the first-line recommended treatment. There are no known indicators to predict a preferential response to CBT or pharmacotherapy. For treatment-naïve adults with OCD, the choice of modality is largely left to individual preference and local availability. In the case of children and adolescents, concern about the adverse effects associated with SSRI, including the possibility of an increase in suicidal thinking or behaviour, resulted in a recommendation that CBT should be used first line in children with OCD [38]. However, compared to SSRI, CBT is less cost-effective according to at least one health-economic analysis [38]. A secondary analysis of a large randomised placebo-controlled treatment trial demonstrated that hoarding and symmetry symptoms predicted a poorer overall outcome on SSRI [39]. However, hoarding also responds poorly to CBT [39] and may indicate a particularly refractory form of illness. A priori prediction of those unlikely to respond may avoid unnecessary use of ineffective treatments.

Monotherapy or Combination Treatment?

According to current guidelines, the evidence supporting the additional benefit of combining CBT with medication is not sufficiently strong; therefore, CBT or pharmacotherapy should initially be provided as a monotherapy [37, 38]. As OCD typically responds slowly to treatment, at least 12 weeks of medication at optimised dosage and 16 h of CBT with ERP are required to test efficacy [38]. Combination strategies (e.g. CBT + SSRI) are recommended in severe illness or cases failing to respond to monotherapy [1, 35, 38]. Such strategies are costly to provide, and it would therefore be particularly helpful to determine markers that could predict, a priori, who might respond better either to monotherapy or to combination treatment.

Which Compound?

Overall, the evidence is not strong enough to support the superior efficacy or tolerability of any one SSRI in OCD [4]. In the face of equivalent efficacy of the SSRIs and clomipramine, as determined by large-scale head-to-head studies [reviewed in 1, 35, 38], deciding between SSRIs or clomipramine currently depends largely on secondary factors, including treatment tolerability and safety as well as the existence of comorbid illness and the potential for drug interactions. According to these criteria, SSRIs are usually preferred as the first choice, with clomipramine reserved for those who fail to respond to SSRIs or cannot tolerate them [38]. Guidelines [36, 40] recommended switching the SSRI if the clinical effect is incomplete after 8–12 weeks on the maximum dose, and proposed switching to clomipramine after 2 or 3 failed SSRI trials. The chance of responding to a second SRI was estimated at 40%, and to a third SRI at even less [40].

Which Dose?

SSRIs show evidence of efficacy compared to placebo across the full range of licensed doses. However, evidence from a limited number of fixed dose studies suggests that higher doses of some SSRIs (escitalopram, fluoxetine, paroxetine) are more efficacious than lower doses. Yet, higher doses are associated with a greater adverse effect burden, and it would be helpful to know in advance whether or not dose escalation is required for an individual patient. There have been no dose-finding studies of clomipramine. Daily doses ranging from 75 mg clomipramine [41] to 300 mg [42] have been found to be effective, though doses exceeding 250 mg should only be used with caution [1, 4].

Maintenance Treatment?

Whilst relapse prevention trials suggest that for those who have responded to SSRI, continuation of the treatment for at least 1 year is usually advisable to protect against relapse: however 25% of a subgroup of 'SSRI responders' in a treatment trial were nevertheless shown to relapse over a 6-month follow-up period despite being randomised to receive maintenance SSRI. In contrast, roughly 50% of the patients randomised to discontinue medication did not relapse over a similar period [33]. Knowing whether or not medication can be safely discontinued at the level of the individual patient would represent a major breakthrough in treatment planning.

High-Dose SSRI or Adjunctive Antipsychotic in SSRI-Resistant Cases?

For SSRI-resistant patients, augmentation with antipsychotic is efficacious in approximately 30% of cases [43]. One meta-analysis suggests that the presence of comorbid tic disorder may predict a favourable outcome with adjunctive antipsychotic [44]. In this meta-analysis, risperidone showed a small advantage over other antipsychotics, but the result may have been confounded by uncontrolled factors, e.g. between study differences in the response characteristics of the patients under test. Antipsychotics were generally well tolerated in the studies reviewed, with similar dropout rates in the antipsychotic and placebo groups. The only pronounced side effect was sedation in the quetiapine augmentation studies. Increased appetite and weight gain were reported in some placebo-controlled studies of second-generation antipsychotics such as olanzapine, and extrapyramidal symptoms were reported in studies of haloperidol and quetiapine. However, due to incomplete adverse event reporting in some of the studies and the brevity of the follow-up period, the meta-analysis was unable to reach a conclusion as to comparative tolerability of antipsychotics in OCD [44]. In another small, non-placebo, head-to-head study in SSRI-resistant OCD, risperidone and olanzapine showed equivalent efficacy, but risperidone was associated with more sexual dysfunction, whereas olanzapine was associated with metabolic effects and weight gain [45].

An alternative strategy to antipsychotics in SSRI-resistant OCD, which has been less rigorously investigated, but which appears relatively well tolerated, is the use of high (supra-formulary) doses of SSRI [46]. While the strength of trial evidence favours adjunctive antipsychotic, increasing the SSRI dose may be a more tolerable alternative, and can be pragmatically offered in advance of augmentation therapy. Predictors of differential treatment response and treatment tolerability at this stage of the decision-making algorithm would be particularly helpful.

Novel Compounds?

A range of pharmacological compounds are under investigation for SSRI-resistant OCD. Glutamatergic drugs, such as memantine and riluzole, anti-epileptic mood stabilisers such as lamotrigine, topiramate and pregabalin, serotonin receptor antagonists such as ondansetron, agomelatine and mirtazapine, stimulants such as D-amphetamine, and benzodiazepines such as clonazepam may all have a role, though the evidence from randomised controlled trials is not yet strong enough to unequivocally support their use [1, 4, 35]. Hypotheses deriving from pre-clinical studies that the identification of specific endophenotypic markers measurable on laboratory tests may predict a positive response to some of these compounds, e.g. OCD patients with neurocognitive changes representing motor impulsivity may respond to stimulants, reward dependant individuals may respond to mood stabilisers, are amenable to testing using translational techniques.

In-Patient Intensive Cognitive Behaviour Therapy or Somatic Therapies?

In the case of severe, enduring, refractory OCD, patients may benefit from 6 months of intensive inpatient CBT [3]. Alternatively, or in tandem, somatic treatments such as ablative neurosurgery (cingulotomy, capsulotomy) or deep brain stimulation of nodes within the corticostriatal circuitry that is thought to be implicated in OCD, may be considered [4]. These are costly, highly burdensome and potentially irreversible treatments for which a priori outcome prediction would be particularly apt.

Determining a Research-Focussed Treatment Algorithm

Placebo-controlled studies remain the ideal method to test the efficacy of a treatment and allow the determination of the specific treatment-related response [47]. They are, however, difficult to recruit to and expensive to run. In the face of established evidence-based treatments, the exposure of treatment-seeking patients to placebo simply to determine biomarkers of response may pose challenging ethical problems. Moreover, unlike a pure efficacy study, the purpose of the treatment arm in biomarker research is to anticipate a broad distribution of response rates, ranging from non-response to full response, from which biomedical correlations can be derived. It is, therefore, reasonable to omit the use of placebo and instead select standardised clinically relevant treatment strategies that resemble real-life treatment. Inclusion of a clinically representative population would be preferable to a highly selected sample as, we would argue, OCD is conspicuously heterogeneous. Again, unlike efficacy studies where the inclusion of relatively low-scoring cases may be problematic, as the treatment effect size is a function of the baseline severity and a low baseline score may obscure true differences between treatments, in biomarkers research a wide range of

Table 1. Evidence-based treatment algorithm for translational OCD studies

Stage 1	SSRI (fluvoxamine, fluoxetine, sertraline, paroxetine, citalopram and escitalopram) at optimal dose (12 weeks), or CBT (16 individual sessions), incorporating ERP[1]
Stage 2	SSRI + CBT (12 weeks)
Stage 3	SSRI + antipsychotic [risperidone (0.5–2 mg), quetiapine (≤300 mg), olanzapine (≤15 mg), aripiprazole (≤20 mg), amisulpride (200–400 mg), haloperidol (0.5–2 mg)], listed in decreasing preference; reserved for patients with documented failure to respond to a therapeutic trial of at least one SSRI and at least moderate impairment (12 weeks), or high-dose SSRI (12 weeks)
Stage 4	As per stage 3 or clinician's choice (including clomipramine, novel compounds)

Response criteria	
Full response	>35% improvement in baseline Y-BOCS scores
Partial response	≥25% improvement in baseline Y-BOCS scores
Non-response	<25% improvement in baseline Y-BOCS scores

In case of full response, the patient maintains the SSRI or SSRI + antipsychotic at the effective dose for at least one year, or CBT follow-up for one year; in case of partial or non-response, the patient moves to the next treatment stage.

[1] For adolescents, CBT is usually used first line.

inclusionary severity scores may be advantageous in determining a more representative population with a broad distribution of response criteria.

Whichever strategy one might choose, in terms of sequential treatment tactics, the result is a prescriptive or standardised algorithm, in one or other shape or form. The problem of over-generalisation therefore needs always to be kept in mind: just because a certain tactic has been shown to be efficacious in a selected sample of patients, it does not follow that it applies equally as a strategy to an entire population of patients. Based upon the current evidence-based national and international guidelines for adults and children and adolescents with OCD (e.g. UK National Institute of Clinical Excellence NICE [38], American Psychiatric Association [36], American Academy of Child and Adolescent Psychiatry [48]), we tentatively propose the following treatment algorithm as a rational, flexible and pragmatic stepped approach to detect biomarkers of treatment-response in OCD across the lifespan (table 1). We have focused this algorithm on the stages of treatment that are most relevant for the general psychiatrist; in order to investigate the most highly refractory cases, at stages of treatment beyond stage four, for whom somatic treatments in specialised centres may be considered, we would recommend a rigorous definition of treatment non-response that involves documented failure to respond to all available evidence-based treatments as the inclusion criterion.

For simplicity, the algorithm incorporates the standard measures of clinical response using the Y-BOCS, as described above [34]. Clinical changes are measured at

12-week intervals using the Y-BOCS. Sequential treatments (CBT and/or pharmaco-therapy) are provided based on whether or not the patient responds. Evaluation of additional clinically relevant response variables, such as measures of clinical global severity and improvement (CGI), depression (Montgomery Asberg Depression Rating Scale) [49], psychosocial disability (SDS), severity of functional impairment (CAOIC-13), and QOL (SF-36), as well as measures of adverse effects and treatment tolerability, would allow a more fine-grained outcome analysis.

According to the algorithm, after baseline assessment, patients are followed up prospectively under staged treatment. We suggest five treatment modalities: CBT, SSRI, CBT + SSRI, SSRI + antipsychotic, and high-dose SSRI. The order of treatment is standardised to reduce variance. However, patients may enter the algorithm at different stages according to their past treatment history if that history is well known. Some stages offer more than one modality, e.g. CBT or SSRI. In order to improve adherence, treatment at each stage should be agreed collaboratively with the patient and clinical non-attendance robustly followed up. Each treatment modality lasts for a minimum of 12 weeks. Consistent with the published guidelines (reviewed above), SSRI or CBT is the first-line treatment for adults. For adolescents, CBT is usually used first line. The SSRIs fluvoxamine, fluoxetine, sertraline and paroxetine have RCT evidence supporting efficacy in adolescents and may be preferred for this age group. Caution and frequent clinical monitoring are recommended for adolescents treated with SSRIs including, where appropriate, the Columbia-Suicide Severity Rating Scale [50]. Combined CBT and SSRI are recommended for monotherapy non-responders. Medication augmentation strategies are reserved for treatment-resistant cases in which moderate impairment in function persists despite adequate monotherapy.

Calculating the Sample Size for Treatment Cells

In the absence of prior studies, it is difficult to calculate with certainty the numbers needed in each treatment cell to detect biomarker differences that correlate with response status. Sample sizes amounting to n ≥40/subgroup are compatible with previous imaging samples and according to convention [51, 52] may indicate sufficient power to determine outcome markers for these groups. Randomised treatment trials usually report attrition rates around 25%. By engaging in collaborative care planning, dropout rates are likely to be reduced, and it would be reasonable to expect at least 60% patients to complete 12-month algorithm-based treatment under these conditions. Over this period, patients would enter at least 1 of 4 treatment modalities. Taking into account guideline recommendations for adolescents and patient preferences [53], we would predict the proportion of patients initially allocated to SSRI or CBT monotherapy may differ, and this should be factored into the power calculation to ensure no one cell is underpowered. Assimilation analysis may be used to predict the numbers moving along the stages of the algorithm, from monotherapy to CBT + SSRI and then to SSRI + AP. Based on a (1) broad recruitment profile and (2) stringent (35%) responder criterion, around 60% of participants could be expected to show a partial response/non-response to the first stages of treatment with CBT or SSRI and ≥60% a partial response/non-response to subsequent treatment.

Conclusion

OCD is typically a disabling lifespan disorder. Pharmacotherapy and psychological treatments are available but are associated with limited success for many individuals. Somatic treatments are reserved for treatment-refractory cases. Clinicians often struggle with treatment decisions in view of the lack of availability of clinical predictors of treatment response. Early exposure to treatment with a high chance of success is likely to improve the clinical outcome and reduce the health burden associated with chronic OCD. Translational research could make a significant contribution by establishing biomarkers to objectively predict treatment response (and non-response) at various stages of treatment. Such research requires collaboration between clinicians, who have the expertise in empirical treatment heuristics, and neuroscientists. Standardised treatment paradigms and methodologies provide a key component of such trials.

Acknowledgement

We wish to acknowledge our colleagues in the European College of Neuropsychopharmacology Networks Initiative and the International College of Obsessive Compulsive Spectrum Disorders for their support and guidance.

References

1 Fineberg NA, Brown A, Reghunandanan S, Pampaloni I: Evidence-based pharmacotherapy of obsessive-compulsive disorder. Int J Neuropsychopharmacol 2012;15:1173–1191.

2 Hollander E, Stein D, Fineberg NA, Marteau F, Legault M: Quality of life outcomes in patients with obsessive-compulsive disorder: relationship to treatment response and symptom relapse. J Clin Psychiatry 2010;71:784–792.

3 Boschen MJ, Drummond LM, Pillay A: Treatment of severe, treatment-refractory obsessive-compulsive disorder: a study of inpatient and community treatment. CNS Spectr 2008;13:1056–1065.

4 Fineberg N, Reghunandanan S, Simpson HB, Phillips K, Richter P, Matthews K, Stein DS, Sareen J, Brown A, Sookman D: Obsessive compulsive disorder (OCD): practical strategies for pharmacological and somatic treatment in adults, submitted.

5 Hollander E, Wong C: Psychosocial function and economic costs of obsessive compulsive disorder. CNS Spectr 1998;3:48–58.

6 Insel TS, Voon V, Nye JS, Brown VJ, Altevogt BM, Bullmore ET, Goodwin GM, Howard RJ, Kupfer DJ, Malloch G, Marston HM, Nutt DJ, Robbins TW, Stahl SM, Tricklebank MD, Williams JH, Sahakian BJ: Innovative solutions to novel drug development in mental health. Neurosci Biobehav Rev, in press.

7 Dell'Osso B, Buoli M, Hollander E, Altamura AC: Duration of untreated illness as a predictor of treatment response and remission in obsessive-compulsive disorder. World J Biol Psychiatry 2010;11:59–65.

8 Fineberg NA, Baldwin DS, Menchon JM, Denys D, Grünblatt E, Pallanti S, Stein DJ, Zohar J: Manifesto for a European research network into obsessive-compulsive and related disorders. Eur Neuropsychopharmacol 2013;23:561–568.

9 Fineberg NA, Potenza MN, Chamberlain SR, Berlin HA, Menzies L, Bechara A, Sahakian BJ, Robbins TW, Bullmore ET, Hollander E: Probing compulsive and impulsive behaviors, from animal models to endophenotypes: a narrative review. Neuropsychopharmacology 2010;35:591–604.

10 Chamberlain SR, Menzies L: Neurocognitive angle: the search for endophenotypes; in Zohar J (eds): Obsessive Compulsive Disorder: Current Science and Clinical Practice. Chichester, Wiley-Blackwell, 2012, pp 300–330.

11 Johnston BA, Mwangi B, Matthews K: Predictive classification of individual magnetic resonance imaging scans from children and adolescents. Eur Child Adolesc Psychiatry, E-pub ahead of print.

12 Goodman WK, Price LH, Rasmussen SA, Mazure C, Fleischmann RL, Hill CL, Heninger GR, Charney DS: The Yale-Brown Obsessive-Compulsive Scale. 2. Validity. Arch Gen Psychiatry 1989;46:1012–1016.

13 Goodman WK, Price LH, Rasmussen SA, Mazure C, Delgado P, Heninger GR, Charney DS: The Yale-Brown Obsessive-Compulsive Scale. 1. Development, use, and reliability. Arch Gen Psychiatry 1989; 46:1006–1011.

14 Storch EA, Murphy TK, Geffken GR, Soto O, Sajid M, Allen P, Roberti JW, Killiany EM, Goodman WK: Psychometric evaluation of the children's Yale-Brown Obsessive-Compulsive scale. Psychiatry Res 2004;129:91–98.

15 Phillips KA, Hollander E, Rasmussen SA, Aronowitz BR, DeCaria C, Goodman WK: A severity rating scale for body dysmorphic disorder: development, reliability, and validity of a modified version of the Yale-Brown Obsessive Compulsive Scale. Psychopharmacol Bull 1997;33:17–22.

16 Black DW, McNeilly DP, Burke WJ, Shaw MC, Allen J: An open-label trial of acamprosate in the treatment of pathological gambling. Ann Clin Psychiatry 2011;23:250–256.

17 NIMH Research Domain Criteria (RDoC). www.nimh.nih.gov/research/rdoc/rdoc%20wm%20proceedings.pdf (accessed 20th April 2013).

18 Insel TR, Murphy DL, Cohen RM, Alterman I, Kilts C, Linnoila M: Obsessive-compulsive disorder: a double-blind trial of clomipramine and clorgyline. Arch Gen Psychiatry 1983;46:5–12.

19 Guy W: ECDEU Assessment Manual for Psychopharmacology, revised. Rockville, US Department of Health, Education, and Welfare, Public Health Service, Alcohol, Drug Abuse, and Mental Health Administration, National Institute of Mental Health, Psychopharmacology Research Branch, Division of Extramural Research Programs, 1976, pp 76–338.

20 Sheehan DV, Harnett-Sheehan K, Raj BA: The measurement of disability. Int Clin Psychopharmacol 1996;11:89–95.

21 Ware JE, Sherbourne CD: The MOS 36-item short-form health survey (SF-36). 1 Conceptual framework and item selection. Med Care 1992;30:473–483.

22 Starcevic V, Berle D, Brakoulias V, Sammut P, Moses K, Milicevic D, Hannan A: The nature and correlates of avoidance in obsessive-compulsive disorder. Aust N Z J Psychiatry 2011;45:871–879.

23 Chamberlain SR, Blackwell AD, Fineberg NA, Robbins TW, Sahakian BJ: The neuropsychology of obsessive compulsive disorder: the importance of failures in cognitive and behavioral inhibition as candidate and endophenotypic markers. Neurosci Biobehav Rev 2005;29:399–419.

24 Dittrich WH, Johansen T, Fineberg NA: Cognitive Assessment Instrument of Obsessions and Compulsions (CAIOC-13) – a new 13-item scale for evaluating functional impairment associated with OCD. Psychiatry Res 2011;187:283–290.

25 Mataix-Cols D, Rosario-Campos MC, Leckman JF: A multi-dimensional model of obsessive-compulsive disorder. Am J Psychiatry 2005;162:228–238.

26 Abramowitz JS, Tolin DF, Diefenbach GJ: Measuring change in OCD: Sensitivity of the obsessive-compulsive inventory-revised. J Psychopathol Behav Assess 2005;27:317–324.

27 Burns GL, Keortge SG, Formea GM, Sternberger LG: Revision of the Padua Inventory of obsessive compulsive disorder symptoms: distinctions between worry, obsessions and compulsions. Behav Res Ther 1996;34:163–173.

28 Sternberger LG, Burns GL: Maudsley Obsessive Compulsive Inventory: obsessive-compulsive symptoms in a non-clinical sample. Behav Res Ther 1990; 28:337–340.

29 Stein DJ, Andersen EW, Tonnoir B, Fineberg N: Escitalopram in obsessive-compulsive disorder: a randomised, placebo-controlled, paroxetine referenced, fixed-dose, 24-week study. Curr Med Res Opin 2007; 23:701–711.

30 Hollander E, Koran LM, Goodman WK, Greist JH, Ninan PT, Yang H, Li D, Barbato LM: A double-blind, placebo-controlled study of the efficacy and safety of controlled-release fluvoxamine in patients with obsessive-compulsive disorder. J Clin Psychiatry 2003;64:640–647.

31 Pallanti S, Hollander E, Bienstock C, Koran L, Leckman J, Marazziti D, Pato M, Stein D, Zohar J: Treatment non-response in OCD: methodological issues and operational definitions. Int J Neuropsychopharmacol 2002;5:181–191.

32 Sookman D, Steketee G: Specialized cognitive behavior therapy for treatment resistant obsessive compulsive disorder; in Sookman D, Leahy R (eds): Treatment Resistant Anxiety Disorders: Resolving Impasses to Symptom Remission. New York, Routledge, 2010, pp 31–74.

33 Fineberg NA, Tonnoir B, Lemming O, Stein DJ: Escitalopram prevents relapse of obsessive compulsive disorder. Eur Neuropsychopharmacol 2007;17:430–439.

34 Pallanti S, Grassi G, Cantisani A: Approaches to treatment resistance; in Zohar J (eds): Obsessive Compulsive Disorder: Current Science and Practice. Chichester, Wiley-Blackwell, 2012, pp 99–131.

35 Fineberg NA, Reghunandanan S, Brown A, Pampaloni I: Pharmacotherapy of obsessive-compulsive disorder: evidence-based treatment and beyond. Aust N Z J Psychiatry 2013;47:121–141.

36 Koran LM, Hanna GL, Hollander E, et al: Practice guideline for the treatment of patients with obsessive-compulsive disorder. Arlington, American Psychiatric Association, 2007. http//www.psych.org/psych_pract/treatg/pg/prac_guide.cfm (accessed 15th January 2013).

37 Baldwin DS, Anderson IM, Nutt DJ, Bandelow B, Bond A, Davidson JR, den Boer JA, Fineberg NA, Knapp M, Scott J, Wittchen HU: Evidence-based guidelines for the pharmacological treatment of anxiety disorders: recommendations from the British Association for Psychopharmacology. J Psychopharmacol 2005;19:567–596.

38 National Institute of Clinical Excellence (NICE): Obsessive-compulsive disorder: core interventions in the treatment of obsessive-compulsive disorder and body dysmorphic disorder. 2006. http://www.nice.org.uk/nicemedia/pdf/cg031fullguideline.pdf (accessed 19th November 2011).

39 Stein DJ, Carey PD, Lochner C, Seedat S, Fineberg N, Andersen EW: Escitalopram in obsessive-compulsive disorder: response of symptom dimensions to pharmacotherapy. CNS Spectr 2008;13:492–498.

40 March JS, Frances A, Kahn DA, Carpenter D: The Expert Consensus Guideline series. Treatment of obsessive-compulsive disorder. J Clin Psychiatry 1997; 58:1–72.

41 Montgomery SA: Clomipramine in obsessional neurosis: a placebo-controlled trial. Pharmacol Med 1980;1:189–192.

42 De Veaugh-Geiss J, Landau P, Katz R: Treatment of obsessive compulsive disorder with clomipramine. Psychiatry Ann 1989;19:97–101.

43 Fineberg NA, Stein DJ, Premkumar P, Carey P, Sivakumaran T, Vythilingum B, Seedat S, Westenberg H, Denys D: Adjunctive quetiapine for serotonin reuptake inhibitor-resistant obsessive-compulsive disorder: a meta-analysis of randomized controlled treatment trials. Int Clin Psychopharmacol 2006;21:337–343.

44 Bloch MH, Weisenberger AL, Kelmendi B, Coric V, Bracken MB, Leckman JF: A systematic review: antipsychotic augmentation with treatment refractory obsessive-compulsive disorder. Mol Psychiatry 2006;11:622–632.

45 Maina G, Pessina E, Albert U, Bogetto F: 8-week, single-blind, randomized trial comparing risperidone versus olanzapine augmentation of serotonin reuptake inhibitors in treatment-resistant obsessive-compulsive disorder. Eur Neuropsychopharmacol 2008;18:364–372.

46 Pampaloni I, Sivakumaran T, Hawley CJ, Al Allaq A, Farrow J, Nelson S, Fineberg NA: High-dose selective serotonin reuptake inhibitors in OCD: a systematic retrospective case notes survey. J Psychopharmacol 2010;24:1439–1445.

47 Fineberg NA, Hawley C, Gale T: Are placebo-controlled trials still important for obsessive compulsive disorder? Prog Neuropsychopharmacol Biol Psychiatry 2006;30:413–422.

48 Geller DA, March J, AACAP Committee on Quality Issues: Practice parameter for the assessment and treatment of children and adolescents with obsessive-compulsive disorder. J Am Acad Child Adolesc Psychiatry 2012;51:98–113.

49 Montgomery SA, Asberg M: A new depression scale designed to be sensitive to change. Br J Psychiatry 1979;134:382–389.

50 Posner K, Brown GK, Stanley B, Brent DA, Yershova KV, Oquendo MA, Melvin GA, Greenhill L, Shen S, Mann J: The Columbia-Suicide Severity Rating Scale: initial validity and internal consistency findings from three multisite studies with adolescents and adults. Am J Psychiatry 2011;168:1266–1277.

51 Thirion B, Pinel P, Meriaux S, Roche A, Dehaene S, Poline JB: Analysis of a large fMRI cohort: statistical and methodological issues for group analyses. Neuroimage 2007;35:105–120.

52 Seghier ML, Lee HL, Schofield T, Ellis CL, Price CJ: Inter-subject variability in the use of two different neuronal networks for reading aloud familiar words. Neuroimage 2008;42:1226–1236.

53 Patel SR, Simpson HB: Patient preferences for obsessive-compulsive disorder treatment. J Clin Psychiatry 2010;71:1434–1439.

Prof. N.A. Fineberg
National Obsessive Compulsive Disorders Specialist Service, Hertfordshire Partnership NHS
University Foundation Trust, Queen Elizabeth II Hospital
Howlands, Welwyn Garden City AL7 4HQ (UK)
E-Mail naomi.fineberg@hertspartsft.nhs.uk

Author Index

Subject Index